Published by Foster Academics,
61 Van Reypen Street,
Jersey City, NJ 07306, USA
www.fosteracademics.com

Diagnosis and Prevention of Human Papillomavirus and Diseases
Edited by Joe Becker

© 2015 Foster Academics

International Standard Book Number: 978-1-63242-111-1 (Hardback)

Diagnosis and Prevention of Human Papillomavirus and Diseases

Edited by **Joe Becker**

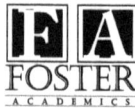

FOSTER
ACADEMICS

New Jersey

Diagnosis and Prevention of Human Papillomavirus and Diseases

Contents

Preface

This book consists of updated information regarding the diagnosis and prevention of human papillomavirus and diseases. Cervical cancer is the second most common cancer amongst women globally, and the infection with Human Papilloma Virus (HPV) has been determined as the root cause for this condition. The natural history of cervical cancer is identified by slow disease progression, making it a preventable and even curable condition when diagnosed in early stages. Pap smear and the newly introduced prophylactic vaccines are the leading prevention options. However, regardless of the availability of these primary and secondary screening techniques, the worldwide burden of this disease is unfortunately still very high. This book lays emphasis on the clinical and diagnostic conditions of HPV and related disease, featuring the current advancements in this field.

After months of intensive research and writing, this book is the end result of all who devoted their time and efforts in the initiation and progress of this book. It will surely be a source of reference in enhancing the required knowledge of the new developments in the area. During the course of developing this book, certain measures such as accuracy, authenticity and research focused analytical studies were given preference in order to produce a comprehensive book in the area of study.

This book would not have been possible without the efforts of the authors and the publisher. I extend my sincere thanks to them. Secondly, I express my gratitude to my family and well-wishers. And most importantly, I thank my students for constantly expressing their willingness and curiosity in enhancing their knowledge in the field, which encourages me to take up further research projects for the advancement of the area.

Editor

Diagnostic and Preventive Aspects of HPV-Related Diseases

Molecular Tools for Detecting Human Papillomavirus

Angela Adamski da Silva Reis,
Daniela de Melo e Silva, Cláudio Carlos da Silva and
Aparecido Divino da Cruz

Additional information is available at the end of the chapter

1. Introduction

The Human Papillomavirus (HPV) has been shown to play a causative role in anal, head and neck, oral, oropharyngeal, penile, vaginal, vulvar and cervical cancers. The last one is the second most common cancer among women worldwide [1-3]. Some types of HPV have been established as the central cause of cervical carcinoma [4-7]

Acquisition of HPV is very common, particularly among sexually active young adults, and incidence of infection with oncogenic HPV types appears to be higher than the incidence of infection with non-oncogenic types [8]. Oncogenic HPV types 16 and 18 and history of other concurrent sexually transmitted diseases were found to be significantly associated with progression to cervical cancer [1-13].

More than 100 HPV types have been identified and about 40 types can infect the genital tract. Worldwide, HPV 16 is the most common high-risk type, present in 50%, followed by HPV 18, present in 14% of cervical cancers [9]. Same types of HPV were more frequent in malignant than in benign lesions, and infection with high-risk types of HPV is now considered the major risk factor for the development of cancer of the uterine cervix [1].

Thus, the HPV infection is necessary for the development of the cervical cancer. The development of this cancer is considered to be a multistep process, where HPV is necessary but in itself an insufficient cause. Disease can only develop when there is persistent HPV infection of the cervical epithelium [3,9].

Cervical cancer is considerate a rare complication of infection with high risk HPV (HR-HPV), but every abnormal or dysplastic lesion of the cervix is potentially malignant and may develop into cervical cancer over time. The incidence is highest in developing countries, largely as a result of lack of screening programs and poor access to medical care [1]. The prevalence of HPV and the distribution of its types probably plays an important role as well. On the other hand, the relationship between others cancer types and HPV-associated is just emerging [10].

The variability in HPV-attributable proportions for non cervical cancers, in part, arises from differences in HPV detection methods across studies as well as from true geographic differences in HPV-attributable proportions [11]. Despite this variability, 90%–93% of anal cancers, 12%–63% of oropharyngeal cancers, 36%–46.9% of penile cancers, 40%–64% of vaginal cancers, and 40%–51% of vulvar cancers are potentially attributable to HPV infection [11-15].

Abnormal cervical epithelial cells can be detected microscopically following Papanicolaou (Pap) staining of conventional cervical smears or of the more homogeneous cell suspension from liquid cytology medium. This forms the basis of cervical screening programmes for detection of women at risk of disease progression, and also for incident infections [9,16]. Molecular detection of HPV provides a different approach to screening and patient management. In this chapter was described the diagnosis of HPV infection to screening cervical cancer and molecular tools to detect HPV-DNA/RNA.

2. The diagnosis of HPV infection to screening cervical cancer

Carcinoma of the uterine cervix is the second most common cancer among women worldwide, with very high mortality rates in developing countries. It was observed more than 20 years ago that some types of HPV were more frequent in malignant than in benign lesions, and infection with high-risk types of HPV is now considered the major risk factor for the development of cancer of the uterine cervix [1]. Oncogenic HPV types 16 and 18 and history of other concurrent sexually transmitted diseases were found to be significantly associated with progression to cervical cancer [5].

Studies have demonstrated a strong association between lifetime number of sexual partners and genital HPV acquisition. The acquisition of new sexual partners continues throughout all age groups. In addition, studies have shown consistently that the risk of cervical cancer can be predicted as much by a woman's own sexual behaviour as by the sexual behaviour of her husband/partner. The presence of HPV DNA in the penis and urethra of her sexual partner(s) is directly related to her HPV carrier status and therefore her risk of developing cervical cancer [13-15].

Of the genital HPVs, which are sexually transmitted, 15 are categorized as high risk and are considered the causative agents of most cervical cancers, with over 99% of cervical lesions containing viral sequences [1]. The remaining viral types are rarely found in malignancies. High-risk HPVs (HR-HPV) are also associated with many vulvar, anal and penile carcinomas and contribute to oral cancers [17], 2006). Additionally, these cancers, in contrast to cervical cancer, appear to be preferentially associated with HPV16 [11,14]. For instance, in the subset of penile cancer attributed to HPV infection, HPV 16 was found in 60,23% of cases [18]. A vaccine has recently been introduced that can prevent the initial infection by two of these high-risk types, HPV 16 and 18, which are responsible for about 70% of cervical cancers [19].

The process by which HPV facilitates tumour initiation and fosters tumour progression is an exceptional model to understand the development of many other human cancers and also allows identification of additional signalling pathways targeted in malignant progression [19]. The association between HPV and human cancer was first proposed more than three decades ago by Harald zur Hausen, and he was honored with one of two 2008 Nobel Prizes in Medicine for his isolation and characterization of HPV 16 in 1983 and later HPV 18 in cervical cancer [20]. The award recognized not only the importance of his discovery in the eventual documentation of the etiology of HPV in cervical and a number of other cancers, but also the importance of the application of his discovery to the clinical use of HPV testing and in implementation of the HPV vaccine.

Additional, many studies have demonstrated the direct role of HPV infection in the development of several human cancers [12-15,21]. HPV 16 and HPV 18 are the most frequently found HPV types in cervical cancers worldwide, being detected in approximately 50 and 20% of the cases, respectively [2-22]. For this reason, the majority of the biological studies were focused on these two HPV types.

The viral genomes are replicated in synchrony with cellular DNA replication. After cell division, one daughter cell migrates away from the basal layer and undergoes differentiation. Differentiation of HPV-positive cells induces the productive phase of the viral life cycle, which requires cellular DNA synthesis machinery. The expression of E6 and E7 deregulates cell cycle control, pushing differentiating cells into S phase, allowing viral genome amplification in cells that normally would have exited the cell cycle. The late-phase L1 and L2 proteins encapsidate newly synthesized viral genomes and virions are shed from the uppermost layers of the epithelium [19].

The induction of hyperproliferation by the E7 oncoprotein triggers apoptosis, which is blocked by the actions of the E6 oncoprotein. The cooperative actions of E6 and E7 efficiently immortalize cells and this process is augmented by the actions of the E5 protein. The ability of E6 and E7 to target crucial regulators of proliferation, apoptosis, immortalization and genomic stability collectively promotes the emergence of a clonal population of cells with a growth advantage and an increased propensity for transformation and malignant progression [19].

The best-characterized HPV 16 E6 activity is its ability to induce degradation of the tumor suppressor protein p53 via the ubiquitin pathway. This cellular protein is a transcription factor that can trigger cell cycle arrest or apoptosis in response to a large variety of cellular stresses, such as hypoxia or DNA damages. Overall, the role of p53 is to ensure the integrity of the cellular genome, preventing cell division after DNA damage or delaying it until the damage has been repaired. The induction of p53 degradation appears to be an exclusive feature of E6 proteins from the HR-HPV types [23].

Codon 72 polymorphism on the 4th exon of TP53 is involved in multiple steps of carcinogenesis and may also account for genetic differences in susceptibility to cancer [24-26]. This most common polymorphism results in a non-conservative change at codon 72 of an arginine to a proline within a proline - rich region of p53 which is known to be important for the growth suppression and apoptotic functions [25]. It has been demonstrated that the TP53 polymorphism varies according to ethnic and geographical distribution, like most human genetic polymorphisms [24].

A meta-analysis of such studies revealed that the arginine homozygous genotype is associated with an increased risk of invasive cervical cancers, but not with squamous intraepithelial lesions supporting the hypothesis that the p53 codon 72 polymorphism may have a principal role in progression to HPV-related cancer, rather than in initiation of the neoplasia [27].

For prevention and early detection of cervical cancer, it is important to detect not only cervical intraepithelial changes, but also to identify the presence of HR-HPV and its type as well. If the results of HR-HPV test are positive, the possibility of cervical intraepithelial neoplasia (CIN) can be prognosticated even if there are no cytologic changes in the cervix. The possibility for regression of CIN 2 cervical changes caused by HPV type 16 is lower compared with cervical changes caused by other HR-HPV types. The risk of mild cervical changes leading to severe cervical changes (CIN 3) is higher when detecting HR-HPV types, especially HPV type 16, compared with lower-risk HPV types. HR-HPV-positive women, even without cytologic changes, have a 210-fold higher risk of developing CIN 3 in 6 years as compared with HR-HPV-negative women [28].

Starting in the late 1960s significant advances were made in understanding the cellular changes leading to invasive cervical cancer, but it was not until 1976 that Meisels and Fortin first established HPV as the etiologic agent in an abnormal cervical cytologic finding (koilocytotic atypia) [20]. The advent of screening to identify and treat cervical cancer precursor lesions, CIN, has led to a substantial reduction in the incidence of cervical cancer in those countries where routine screening is in place. Conversely, most cervical cancer-related mortality occurs in countries where there is no routine cervical screening, although Pap's smear is a cost effective screening method in low resource settings [10].

Cervical screening is considered to have been the most effective cancer-screening test ever introduced and in developed countries with organized programmes. A successful screening programme however is dependent on understanding and acceptance of the need for a particular test, the need for further investigation of abnormalities and particularly, the need for quality assurance of all parts of the system [29].

In the evaluation by IARC in 2005 was concluded that there is sufficient evidence that screening women ages 35 to 64 for cervical cancer precursors by conventional cytology every 3 to 5 years within high-quality programs reduces incidence of invasive cervical cancer by at least 80% among those screened [6]. Despite the large amount of data available on the value of HPV-DNA testing for the detection of cervical cancer precursors, both in the primary cervical screening and in the management of 'borderline' or Atypical Squamous Cells of Undetermined Significance (ASCUS) cytology, HPV-DNA tests have not always and correctly been translated into clinical practice by clinicians and within national cervical screening programs [30-31].

Although Pap's smears have reduced the incidence of cervical cancer by over 80% in the United States, cervical cancer is the second leading cause of cancer deaths in women worldwide, and effective implementation of the HPV vaccine and continued screening should dramatically reduce the incidence of these cancers [19]. Cervical cytologic testing or colposcopy is an acceptable method for managing women over the age of 20 years with ASCUS, but HPV-DNA testing is the preferred approach. Several population-based studies have established that tests for HR-HPV DNA have higher clinical sensitivity than cytology in detecting cervical intrae-pithelial neoplasia (CIN) of grades 2 and above (CIN2+), and that combined HPV and cytology testing shows the highest negative predictive values (NPV) for CIN2+ [31-69]. Thus, the HPV DNA test should be used in conjunction with Pap's smear test wherever feasible and affordable or potentially as a stand-alone test [32], because both combined has been shown to greatly improve the ability to detect pre-cancerous states [33].

In general, the prevalence of HPV is higher in young women compared to women over 30 years [34-35]. Most HPV infections are transient [9,36] and natural history studies have shown that HPV DNA is detectable in cells from the cervix for less than a year in most infected women. Therefore, the presence or absence of HPV DNA at a single time point is a poor indicator of lifetime exposure. To mitigate this problem, serological tools to detect HPV antibodies have been developed.

However, the serological assays have only limited accuracy and HPV cannot be grown in conventional cell cultures. As infection with HPV is followed by a humoral immune response against the major capsid protein [37], with antibodies remaining detectable for many years, serology is not suitable for distinguishing present and past infections. Consequently, accurate diagnosis of HPV infection relies on the detection of viral nucleic acid [9,38].

The Hybrid Capture Assay I (HC1) was first introduced by Digene in 1995 [39]. HC1 was a relatively fast, liquid hybridization assay designed to detect 14 HPV types divided into high-risk types (HPV 16, 18, 31, 33, 35, 45, 51, 52 and 56) and low-risk types (HPV 6, 11, 42, 43, and 44). Initially, this was to be used to augment the sensitivity of conventional Pap testing and to provide a meaningful negative predictive value for assessing cervical dysplasia [20].

The second generation of Hybrid Capture Asssay, the hybrid capture-II (HC2) DNA test - Digene (Now Qiagen, Valencia, Calif Gaithersburg, MD, USA), which uses a micro titer plate instead of tubes and has been approved by the US Food and Drug Administration (FDA) for DNA- HPV identification [40], as an adjunct to cervical screening in the US women in aged 30 years and over. HC2 is a semiquantitative measure of viral load relative to 1pg/ml and uses RNA-labeled probes for targeting DNA sequences from 13 high-risk HPV (16, 18, 31, 33, 35, 39, 45, 51, 52, 56, 58, 59, and 68) 5 low-risk types (6, 11, 42, 43 and 44) [7,40-41].

Although its use has become the standard in many countries, it has several limitations including the inability to identify specific types and the lack of internal control for the amount of input DNA 7,40-42]. In addition, the reliance on sample volume as a proxy for cellularity may give rise to false negatives in samples with few infected cells. The lack of a negative control within the test also prevents detection of false negatives due to procedural or reagent problems. Another source of concern is the fact that the HR-HPV probe set is not all-inclusive. Women with unusual types may have a true-negative HC2 test yet still harbor a virus capable of causing cancer [43].

Studies comparing HC2 and Polymarese Chain Reaction (PCR) results have also shown that the hybrid capture probes are not entirely type specific [43]. The detection limit of approximately 5000 genome is the power of HC2 and it makes it less sensitive than PCR and cross-reactivity of the two probe cocktails can reduce the clinical relevance of a positive result [20,40].

Despite the HC2 present some limitations [33], this assay has shown high sensitivity for the detection of CIN of grade 2 and worse (CIN2+) and it was recently recommended to be used as a benchmark for performance assessment of new candidate HPV tests for primary cervical cancer screening in women of 30 years and older. The emergence of competing platforms like the Linear Array (Roche) and INNO-LiPA HPV (Innogenetics) has led to the development of some new elements by Qiagen that are designed to counteract perceived advantages of alternative tests [43]. This others platforms are commonly used in the HPV typing assays and follow up of persistent infections to monitor the presence of specific HPV genotypes [44].

Has been demonstrated that HC2 has proven its effectiveness in large clinical trials and everyday practice, but the search continues for markers with superior specificity for high-grade disease without excessive corresponding loss of sensitivity. A number of new assays have been developed for molecular and immunostaining platforms with the intention of meeting this need [43].

As a screening test, cervical cytology for CIN has reduced the incidence of mortality worldwide [45], however this methodology has a limited sensitivity. So, as described by [46] a shift from conventional cytology to a molecular approach integrated into cervical cancer screening is the most likely solution to the goals of improved screening in both the developed and developing world. Therefore, molecular tests have become available for clinical and research purposes in response to the need for identifying infection during earlier stages and improving patient follow-up [9,40].

A modified, experimental Hybrid Capture assay named Hybrid Capture 3 uses RNA probes, as in Hybrid Capture 2, but in combination with biotinylated capture oligonucleotides that are directed to unique sequence regions within the desired target to increase test specificity [47]. The assay has been developed further to reduce cross-reactivity while maintaining sensitivity and for use either on DNA or RNA as targets. A recent comparison study concluded that, at the optimal cut-off points, Hybrid Capture 2 and 3 had similar screening performance characteristics for high-grade lesions diagnosed at the enrolment visit [48].

Hybrid Capture 3 (HC3) is being evaluated as the next generation of hybrid capture clinical assays that target 13 oncogenic HPV types for the detection of cervical precancerous cervical intraepithelial neoplasia grade 3 (CIN3). A primary technical distinction between HC3 and HC2 is that HC3 employs a biotinylated DNA oligonucleotide specific for selected HPV DNA sequences for the capture of the DNA-RNA complexes on streptavidin-coated wells, whereas HC2 uses wells coated with polyclonal antibody against DNA-RNA complexes for hybrid capture. The use of capture oligonucleotide instead of an immobilized antibody also diminishes the possibility of nonspecific RNA-DNA hybrids, present as the result of improperly alkali-denatured specimens, from binding to the microplate well and consequently may reduce false positivity for HC3 compared to HC2 [48].

This ratio assay may reflect the natural pattern of HPV mRNA expression that occurs during the progression of disease in cervical epithelium. After initial infection, polycistronic, pre-mRNA is transcribed from HPV DNA that exists either as circular, extrachromosomal episomes or as DNA that is integrated into the chromosome. As pre-malignant lesions progress, the abundance of mRNAs that encode the oncogenes, such as E6 and E7 (E6–7), may increase and the mRNAs encoding non-oncogenic HPV proteins, such as E2 and L1, may decrease [49]. The incidence of HPV integration may reduce further transcripts encoding E2 and other downstream genes, such as L1, because integration usually occurs at the E2 loci [50]. The E2 gene product is an important down-regulator of oncogenic E6–7 expression [19]. Thus, lower E2 levels may correlate with disease progression. Therefore, it may be useful to measure the ratio of E6–7 over E2 transcripts in cervical specimens and compare this ratio with the severity of disease [51].

In the study [48] was compared the performance of a prototype version of the Hybrid Capture 3 (HC3) human papillomavirus (HPV) DNA assay to the current generation Hybrid Capture 2 (HC2) assay, both of which target 13 oncogenic HPV types, for the detection of cervical intraepithelial neoplasia grade 3 and cancer (CIN3+) with cervicovaginal lavage specimens collected at enrollment into a 10-year cohort study at Kaiser Permanente. The authors suggest that HC3 may be a slightly more sensitive, equally specific test for the detection of CIN3+ over the duration of typical screening intervals compared to its predecessor, HC2. The increased sensitivity of HC3 compared to HC2 appears to be the result of increased detection of CIN3+ in women who were 30 years of age or older and were cytologically negative. They emphasize that further validation studies of HC3 are needed with more clinically relevant cervical specimens.

Diagnosis of HPV infection relies on the detection of the viral DNA in clinical samples; thus accurate detection and genotyping of HPV are of critical importance for determining the prevalence of HPVs in a given population and for determining the risks associated with infections of a particular type [52]. The first evaluation of the use of HPV testing in a potential clinical application was published in 1989 by Tidy et al. on the detection of HPV 16 by PCR both in normal and in dyskaryotic smears from 21 women. The results was sufficiently compelling to predict that HPV testing might eventually supplement cytologic analysis of cervical samples in screening [20].

PCR is a highly sensitive technique and allows testing on samples with less tissue or fewer cells [7,46]. Multiplex HPV genotyping methods based on hybridization to fluorescently labeled beads have also been reported [53]. These methods are capable of detecting very small copy numbers of virus, and extremely high sensitivities have been reported. However, because HC2 has been established as the criterion standard for clinical treatment algorithms, such high positive rates are actually a drawback rather than an advantage for clinical use. The relative complexity of PCR-based methods, concerns about contamination of the laboratory by PCR products, and patent protection on some aspects of the technology have further hindered widespread adoption of this approach [43].

The sensitivity and specificity of PCR based methods vary, depending mainly on the primer set, the size of the PCR product, the reaction conditions and efficacy of the DNA polymerase used in the reaction, the spectrum of HPV types amplified, the ability to detect multiple types and the availability of a type-specific assay. PCR can theoretically produce 109 copies from a single double stranded DNA molecule after 30 cycles of amplification. Therefore, care must be taken to avoid false-positive results derived from cross-contaminated specimens or reagents. Several procedures are available to avoid the potential problems of using PCR protocols for HPV DNA detection [30].

The limitations associated with PCR-based HPV-DNA detection are related to primer selection and optimal protocol standardization [46,54]. The PCR assay most likely to be amendable to broad screening and/or surveillance applications are based on consensus primer amplification of a broad spectrum of genotypes which are subsequently differentiated by type-specific oligonucleotide probe hybridization. The most commonly used consensus PCR target is the highly conserved L1 open reading frame (ORF), of genital HPV genomes [52]. Among these are the single pair of consensus primers GP5/6 [55] and its extended version GP5+/6+ [35,56] and the MY09/11 degenerate primers [57] and its modified version, PGMY09/11 [30,58] and SPF 10 [59]. In addition, none of these assays can be automated or deployed on a high-throughput platform, features that are essential for an assay intended for use with a large volume of patients [60].

The viral nucleic acid must be preserved to avoid false-negative results caused by degradation by endogenous endonucleases. This is especially important when analyzing HPV-RNA transcripts. To assess the integrity of genomic DNA in the specimen and its suitability for molecular analysis, adequate controls, such as β-globin gene amplification or spiking of the sample with known positive material, are crucial. Several commercially available sampling kits, originally intended for cytology (e.g. PreservCyt, CytycCorp.) adequately preserve nucleic acids for molecular diagnosis even after prolonged storage at ambient temperatures [61].

The commercial HPV assays are based on L1 or E1 PCR for high-risk HPV DNA detection and genotyping are now available from different companies: AmplicorR and Linear Array (Roche Molecular Systems, CA, USA), INNO-LiPAR (Inngenetics, Ghent, Belgium), PapiloCheck (Greiner Bio-One GmbH, Germany), Multiplex HPV Genotyping Kit (Multimetrix GmmbH, Heildelberg, Germany) [Table 01]. After amplifying parts of the L1 region, such assays hybridize the resulting PCR product to a detection and visualization unit (microarray or a reverse line blot) [62].

HPV-DNA assays can be performed using the same specimen as used for cytological examination, which is an important logistic aspect of routine clinical testing. However, a cervical scrape is only a small sample of the cervical epithelium and sampling errors may influence cytology grading. Only a portion of the cervical cell suspension is used for DNA isolation with only a fraction of the isolated DNA being used for specific DNA detection. Therefore, if a specimen only contains a limited number of HPV-DNA copies, sampling errors may produce inconsistencies even in a sensitive assay. Furthermore, the outcome of a HPV-DNA assay can vary depending on the menstrual cycle [9].

Luminex (xMAP) suspension array technology is based on polystyrene beads that are internally dyed with various ratios of two spectrally distinct fluorophores. Different molecules such as individual oligonucleotide probes can be coupled to different bead sets with specific absorption spectra. These sets are combined to a suspension array and allow up to 100 different probes to be measured simultaneously in a single reaction (multiplexing) [62].

This technology can potentially be fully automated, dramatically decreasing the personal cost component of the assay; this assay has been used for the genotyping of 45 HPV types with

PGMY09/11 PCR, 22 HPV types with GP5+/6+ PCR 15 HPV types with YBT L1/GP-1 PCR, and 18 HPV types with GP5+/6+ PCR. These multiplex HPV genotyping (MPG) methods have been compared with other well established HPV detection methods such as HC2, restriction fragment length polymorphism (RFLP) and DNA chip technology for the evaluation of their performance. However, none of these well established assays are perfect and suitable for the "gold standard". Sequencing gives the most conclusive genotype information, although it is the most labor intensive. However, sequencing is the most desirable way to validate HPV genotyping methods [62].

Assay name	HPV genotypes detected	Detection technology	DNA and HPV gene detected	Producer
Hybrid captureHigh-risk 2 (HC2)	16,18,31,33,35,39,45,51,52,56,58,59,6 8 Low –risk 6, 11, 42, 43, 44	Sandwich capture molecular	DNA, *L1*	Qiagen (MD, USA)
Cervista	16, 18 and bulk (31, 33, 35, 39, 45, 51, 52, 56, 58, 59, 66, 68)	Invader chemistry	DNA, *L1, E6, E7*	Hologic (WI, USA)
Cobas HPV test	16, 18 and bulk (31, 33, 35, 39, 45, 51, 52, 56, 58, 59, 66, 68)	Real-time PCR	DNA, *L1*	Roche (Rotkreuz, Switzerland)
Abbott´s Real Time High Risk HPV	16, 18 and bulk (31, 33, 35, 39, 45, 51, 52, 56, 58, 59, 66, 68)	Real-time PCR	DNA, *L1*	Abbott (IL, USA)
Clinical Array	6, 11, 16, 18, 26, 31, 33, 35, 39, 40, 42, 43, 44, 45, 51, 52, 53, 54, 56, 58, 59, 61, 62, 66, 68, 70, 71, 72, 73, 81, 82, 83, 84, 85, 89.	PCR/microarray	DNA, *L1*	Genomica (Madrid, Spain)
Linear Array	6, 11, 16, 18, 26, 31, 33, 35, 39, 40, 42, 45, 51, 52, 53, 54, 55, 56, 58, 59, 61, 62, 64, 66, 67, 68, 69, 71, 71, 72, 73, 81, 82, 83, 84.	PCR/reverse hybdridization line blot	DNA, *L1*	Innogenetics (Gent, Belgium)
INNO-LiPA Genotyping Extra	6, 11, 16, 18, 26, 31, 33, 35, 39, 40, 43, 44, 45, 51, 52, 53, 54, 56, 58, 59, 66, 68, 69, 70, 71, 73, 74, 82.	PCR/reverse hybdridization line blot	DNA, *L1*	Innogenetics (Gent, Belgium)
PapilloCheck	6,11, 16, 18, 31, 33, 35, 39, 40, 42, 43, 44/55, 45, 51, 52, 53, 56, 58, 59, 66, 68, 70, 73, 82	PCR/microarray	DNA, *L1*	Greiner BioOne (Frickenhaunsen, Germany)

* Modified from [62]

Table 1. Commercial HPV-DNA assays

3. HPV nucleic acid detection

Detection of HPV E6/E7 messenger RNA (mRNA) is an indicator of HPV oncogenic activity and may be used as a clinically predictive marker to identify women at risk of developing high-grade cervical dysplastic lesions and cervical carcinoma [63]. This method has been proposed as a more specific marker for cervical dysplasia and cancer than HPV DNA [64]. Several assays have been designed to detect mRNA of the E6 and E7 transforming genes of HPV. The level of E6 and E7 gene expression is increased in high-grade lesions compared with low-grade lesions. These tests have high specificity for detecting disease and could potentially serve as functional discriminators between high-risk and low-risk infections [19].

Initial studies comparing HPV DNA and RNA detection (using consensus PCR and PreTect HPV-Proofer) in women with ASCUS and mild dysplasia on cervical cytology showed that twice as many women were positive for HPV DNA compared with those with HPV RNA positivity. They also demonstrated that while both tests were highly sensitive for detection of CIN2+ (85.7%), HPV RNA detection was far more specific for detection of high-grade lesions (84.9% vs 50%) [65].

The PreTect HPV-Proofer (NorChip AS, Klokkarstua, Norway) is a commercially available real-time multiplex nucleic acid sequence-based amplification (NASBA) assay, also called NucliSENS EasyQ (bioMérieux, Marcy l'Etoile, France). This assay is based HPV detection using HPV DNA plasmids and detects E6/E7 mRNA of the five most common HPV types, HPV16, 18, 31, 33, and 45 [64,66]. These five types have been shown to account for about 82% of cervical cancer worldwide, but their prevalence varies between different geographical regions [67].

In comparison to HPV DNA tests, NASBA-based HPV detection showed better results in terms of specificity for high-grade cervical lesions, while its sensitivity is lower. Currently, it is difficult to know whether the differences in diagnostic accuracy are a result of the larger type detection range and high analytical sensitivity of the HPV DNA tests. To elucidate this issue, experimental confirmation that RNA is the sole target of HPV NASBA is required [64].

NASBA-positive women are 69.8 times more likely to be diagnosed with CIN2+ within 2 years of testing than NASBA negative women. Thus, the addition of HPV mRNA triage to cervical screening programmers may decrease the incidence of false-negative results while also allowing the time interval between screening events to be increased for those women who are HPV DNA and RNA negative [63]. Several studies on the relative performance of NASBA have been conducted in Europe with an indication that this test is more specific than other tests, including the APTIMA and HC2 assays to identify CIN 2+ [65,68-70]. This indicates that the NASBA assay can be used reliably to obtain simultaneous type-specific information for the five genotypes targeted by the test. This is an appealing feature given the indication for the identification of types 16 and 18 in risk stratification and better clinical management of women with a positive HPV test [71].

On the other hand, there have been reports that the NASBA technique can detect DNA, causing false-positive results [64,72]. However, NASBA can serve as a better triage test than HPV DNA to reduce colposcopy referral in both ASCUS and low grade squamous intraepithelial lesion (LSIL). It is also more efficient than cytology for the triage of HPV DNA-positive women. Nevertheless, its low sensitivity demands a strict follow-up of HPV DNA positive-mRNA negative cases [73].

APTIMA (Gen-Probe, San Diego, CA) is a commercially available mRNA test for HPV, which detects mRNA of HR-HPV types (HPV 16, 18, 31, 33, 35, 39, 45, 51, 52, 56, 58, 59, 66, and 68), based on transcription-mediated amplification [66,74]. There is indication that the APTIMA test has clinical sensitivity similar to that of HC2 [74], but with higher specificity for detection of dysplasia and improved clinical specificity over that of HC2, which is designed to detect DNA of the same HPV types, except for type 66 [66]. The germany study concluded that APTIMA had a sensitivity similar to but a specificity significantly higher (P < 0.0001) than the HC2 test for the detection of CIN2+. that he AHPV assay was significantly more sensitive and significantly more specific than cytology for the detection of disease [75]. The assay is sensitive and very specific for detection of high-risk HPV, which may improve patient management and reduce the cost of care. However, APTIMA does not specify the individual HPV types detected [76].

In study carried out as part of a multicenter study in Canada which was assessed the clinical usefulness of testing for E6/E7 mRNA and other molecular biomarkers in cervical cancer screening in comparison with HPV DNA testing and cytology. A point worth noting is that 61 (15.9%) of 384 CIN 2+ cases were found in women with normal cytology at the time of enrollment, and 70.5% and 86.9% of these were positive by NASBA and HC2, respectively. This reinforces the importance of incorporating HPV testing or repeat cytology in cervical cancer screening. Also, a separate analysis of unsatisfactory cytology indicated an enriched population of CIN 2+ [71].

This reflects the inherent limitation of cytology-based evaluation. Regardless, the positivity with NASBA or HC2 was dependent on the number of genotypes covered by the respective tests and their prevalence in different grades of cytologic and histologic lesions. Furthermore, the lesion progression is more strongly associated with types 16 and 18, and there are indications that an HPV test that distinguishes types 16 and 18 from other oncogenic types may be more useful as it could identify women at greater risk of cervical cancer [71].

Microfluidic approaches in diagnostics achieve significant reagent volume reduction and thus cost-drive innovation, potentially achieving widespread penetration in non-hospital, non-specialized environments. However, microfluidic approaches are not without their challenges. The field of "lab-on-a-chip" (LOC) diagnostics has grown rapidly from this basic need, and it is fast accelerating towards a "sample-in answer-out" platform for molecular diagnostics. NASBA technology with real-time fluorescence measurement was adapted to detect HPV mRNA in cervical specimens and cervical cell lines. The isothermal nature of NASBA greatly simplifies amplification strategies for nucleic acid detection on chip. This platform has huge potential within "point-of-care"(POC) diagnostics as up to 16 different targets can be detected simultaneously for each clinical sample analyzed [77].

In recent study from Norway, the prototype NASBA platform presented amplification efficiency of has been compared to an industry gold standard for HPV detection with encouraging results. By this, we have demonstrated the subcomponents of a complete integrated in vitro diagnostic system: from clinical sample input to sample preparation to amplification to detection, thus advancing towards a "sample-in, answer-out" diagnostic platform. The prototype NASBA platform combined extraction and amplification in a microfluidic device consisting of extraction and NASBA chips. In addition, the adopted NASBA method offers the unique characteristics of isothermal amplification, greatly simplifying the thermocycling requirements for the system: effectively allowing a "blackbox" technology to be developed encompassing amplification and detection simultaneously in a real-time format. The Authors described this technology platform is not limited to diagnostics of cervical precancer and cancer, but it has enormous potential in the monitoring and diagnosis of gene activity in areas such as infectious disease, oncology, immune response to allergens, immunotherapies, and chemotherapies [77].

The mRNA assays with real-time PCR may be a useful tool in investigation of as well as in primary screening for cervical neoplasias, and it might be worthwhile to consider which genotypes to include in further investigations to optimize sensitivity and specificity, especially in a post vaccine era, when it may be necessary to reconsider HPV testing strategies [66].

3.1. MicroRNA analysis in Human Papillomavirus (HPV)

MicroRNAs (miRNAs) are noncoding regulatory RNAs 18-25 nucleotides in size that are derived from RNA polymerase II (pol II) transcripts of coding or noncoding genes. MiRNAs most often function by binding to the 3′ UTRs of target messenger RNAs, whereby they induce mRNA degradation or translational repression [78]. Many miRNAs are tissue- or differentiation-specific, and their temporal or short-lived expression modulates gene expression at the posttranscriptional level by base-pairing with complementary nucleotide sequences of target mRNAs [79-80]. The functions of miRNAs are still largely unknown, but it seems that they are important in the regulation of cellular gene expression and behavior [81,82].

As of August 2012, the miRBase database (http://www.mirbase.org/) [112] had collected 21,264 entries representing hairpin precursor pre-miRNAs. Human genome contains ~ 416 miRNA genes encoding 1048 distinct mature miRNAs from every chromosome except Y. Approximately 113 miRNA genes encode a cluster of miRNAs and produce ~ 390 miRNA sequences. Bioinformatics prediction shows that each miRNA targets ~ 200 RNA transcripts directly or indirectly, and up to one-third of the total number of human mRNAs are targets of more than one miRNA [81]. So, the actions of miRNAs exert profound effects on gene expression at the posttranscriptional level in almost every biological process. However, miRNA expression itself, similar to any other transcription mediated by pol II, is regulated both at the transcriptional and posttranscriptional levels.

Many cellular transcription factors, including c-Myc, p53, and E2F, have been described to regulate miRNA transcription. Oncogenic HPV E6 induces degradation of p53 and E7 mediates degradation of pRB to release E2F from the pRB–E2F complex, it is conceivable that oncogenic HPV infection causes aberrant expression of cellular miRNAs [81]. Other factors involved in miRNA maturation and processing after transcription are Drosha (an RNase-II endonuclease that produces pre-miRNA from pri-miRNA), DGCR8 (DiGeorge syndrome critical region gene 8, a double-stranded RNA-binding protein needed for Drosha activity), exportin 5 (for pre-miRNA export), Dicer (an RNase-III enzyme that produces mature miRNA from pre-miRNA), TRBP (a Dicer partner), and Ago2 (a major component for RISC) [81,83-84].

In the study [81] was profiled 455 miRNAs via miRNA microarray in 4 cervical cancer tissues and 4 normal cervical cancer tissues and they found significant overexpression of 18 miRNAs and underexpression of 15 miRNAs cervical cancer tissues compared to normal cervical cancer tissues [85]. In the analysis from157 cellular miRNAs via the TaqMan MicroRNA Human Early Panel Kit (Applied Biosystems) in 10 early stage squamous cell carcinomas and 10 normal cervical samples. The authors found overpression of 68 miRNAs and underexpression of two in the cervical carcinomas versus normal cervical samples [86].

A recent review published [81] presented that cervical cancer represents a unique tumor model for understanding how viral E6 and E7 oncoproteins deregulate the expression of the miR-15/16 cluster, miR-17-92 family, miR-21, miR-23b, miR-34a, and miR-10b/93/25 cluster via the E6-p53 and E7-pRb pathways. miRNAs may influence the expression of papillomavirus gene in a differentiation-dependent manner by targeting viral RNA transcripts. Genome-wide profiling of miRNA signatures has indicated that aberrant, increased or decreased, miRNA expression is common in most human tumors [83,86]. The table 2 [81] presented a summary of miRNA expression profiling studies in cervical cancer, as illustrated below, in three distinct studies.

In the study conducted in 2011 was found significant overexpression of 18 miRNAs and underexpression of 2 miRNAs in cervical cancer tissues compared to normal cervical tissues via TaqMan MicroRNA arrays. Those authors demonstrated, via individual qRT-PCR assays, significant overexpression of miR-16, miR-21, miR-106b, miR135b, miR-141, miR-223, miR-301b and miR-449a, and underexpression of miR-218 and miR-433 in cervical cancer and dysplasia from normal cervical compared to normal cervical tissue. Their results showed that miR-21, miR-135b, miR-223 and miR-301b were overexpressed in the cervical cancer tissue compared to both normal and cervical dysplasia tissue. So, those authors concluded that such miRNAs are good candidates for markers of progression from normal to dysplasia to cancer [85].

Another recent study published in 2011 was analyzed six paired normal and cervical cancer tissues by using the same miRNA array plataform and showed an increased expression of 12 miRNAs and decreased expression of 11 miRNAs, as presented in table 2 [87]. The study presented by [88] found increased expression of miR-21 in cervical cancer and a decreased expression of both miR-143 and miR-145. Those data together indicated that cervical cancer expresses no or very little of the miR-143/145 cluster. A PCR-based miRNA assay was used to analyze 102 cervical cancer samples [89] and the authors identified miR-200a and miR-9 as two molecular markers that could be used to predict cervical cancer survival.

In the analysis [90] was investigated 802 unknown and 122 predicted human miRNAs via CaptialBio mammalian miRNA arrays V 3.0 in 13 HPV-16 and HPV-18 positive cervical cancers and their adjacent normal tissues. The authors found that miR-141 is overexpressed and miR-218 is underexpressed in cervical cancer compared to normal cervical tissue. In the study [111] analyzed miRNA expression via microarray in 5 cervical squamous cell carcinomas that appeared to be HPV-negative and 5 normal cervical tissues and they found that miR-21 to be overexpressed in the cervical cancer samples.

MiR-21 is the most highly overexpressed miRNA in numerous cancers and it down regulates the tumor suppressor PTEN in non-small cell lung cancer and in hepatocellular cancer, in which PTEN regulation leads to overexpression of matrix metalloproteinases MMP2 and MMP9 [85]. These proteins promote cellular migration and invasion. MiR-21 also targets the tumor suppressor genes tropomyosin I (TPM1), programmed cell death 4 (PDCD4) and maspin, and the latter two have been implicated in tumor invasion and metastasis [91]. Increased miR-21 expression in cervical cancer may be attributable to both E6 and E7. Such viral oncoproteins play important roles in regulating cellular miRNA expression and their function can be reduced due to epigenetic modification of miRNA genes. Identification of a panel of miRNAs that can be used as early biomarkers in cervical cancer is potentially useful to determine disease behavior and prognosis. They may also provide new targets for anticancer therapy [85].

Until now, there are evidence indicating that HPV regulation of cellular miRNA expression most likely occurs through viral E6 and E7 [81], although oncogenic HPVs do not produce viral miRNAs, they are responsible for the aberrant expression of oncogenic or tumor suppressive miRNAs. High-risk E6 and E7 interact separately with several dozens or even hundreds of cellular factors and these interactions could lead to increased or decreased expression cellular miRNAs. Some of the altered miRNA expression could be a result from both E6 and E7. It is known that the main function of oncogenic HPV E6 is to target p53 for degradation [81-93]. As a transcription factor, p53 plays an important role in the transcription of numerous coding and noncoding genes [92-94] and it seems that oncogenic HPV is capable of regulating the expression of many cellular miRNAs via p53 [81], and its downstream targets are miR-34a and miR-23b, increasing cell growth and migration in cervical tissues.

miRNA	Chromosome location	Wang et al [108]	Li et al [109]	Witten et al [110]
miR-15[a]	13q14.2	Up		
miR-15b	3q25.33	Up	Up	
miR-16	13q14.2	Up	Up	
miR-17-5p	13q31.3	Up	Up	
miR-20a	13q31.3	Up	Up	
miR-20b	Xq26.2	Up	Up	
miR-21	17q23.1	Up	Up	Up
miR-93	7q22.1	Up	Up	
miR-106a	Xq26.2	Up	Up	
miR-146a	5q34	Up		
miR-148a	7p15.2	Up		
miR-155	21q21.3	Up		Up
miR-181c	19p13.13	Up		
miR-182	7q32.2	Up	Up	Up

miRNA	Chromosome location	Wang et al [108]	Li et al [109]	Witten et al [110]
miR-183	7q32.2	Up		
miR-185	22q11.21	Up	Up	
miR-223	Xq12	Up		
miR-224	Xq28	Up	Up	
miR-324-5p	17p13.1	Up		
miR-10b	2q31.1		Down	Down
miR-29a	7q32.3	Down	Down	
miR-30b	8q24.22	Down		
miR-34a	1p36.22	Down	Down	
miR-125a	19q13.41	Down		Down
miR-125b	11q24.1		Down	Down
miR-126	9q34.3	Down	Down	
miR-127	14q32.2	Down	Down	
miR-133a	18q11.2	Down		
miR-133b	6p12.2	Down		Down
miR-143	5q32	Down	Down	Down
miR-145	5q32	Down		
miR-191	3p21.31	Down		
miR-218	4p15.31;5q34	Down	Down	
miR-378 (422b)	5q32	Down		
miR-422a	15q22.31	Down		
miR-424	Xq26.3	Down	Down	Down
miR-450	Xq26.3	Down	Down	Down
miR-455	9q32	Down	Down	
miR-574	4p14	Down		

Up: upregulated in cervical cancer; down, downregulated in cervical cancer.[81].

Table 2. Summary of miRNA signatures in cervical cancer.

4. Clinical utility of molecular HPV diagnosis

The incidence of cervical cancer in the decades to come might in fact increase in developing countries due to the aging of the population and the persistent absence of adequate screening programs [95]. In countries with screening, the target of preventive efforts has shifted from cervical cancer detection to the diagnosis and treatment of cancer precursor lesions. However, the morphologic basis of the screening test cannot be substantially improved, inherently diminishing the accuracy for precursor lesion diagnosis. In these countries, a false negative Pap test occurs in 30% of all cervical cancers diagnosed and another 10% is attributable to errors in following up abnormal cytology reports [95,96].

Despite this limitation, a significant reduction in cervical cancer has been achieved with cytology-based technology and screening strategies [95]. HR-HPV DNA testing is currently recommended for triage of cytological diagnoses of ASCUS, as a cotest with the Pap smear in the general screening of women ≥30 years of age, and for follow-up of women after colonoscopy and treatment [97].

Histological examination of colposcopy-guided biopsies is still considered the "gold standard" in the assessment of cervical lesions; however, the histologic assessment of these lesions is limited to the interpretation of the morphology, with little to no information regarding the risk of persistence, progression, or regression. In addition, histologic assessment of cervical lesions is complicated by interobserver variability. The main interpretive categories include distinguishing normal from dysplasia (CIN) of any grade and low-grade (CIN1) lesions from high-grade (CIN2/3) lesions. Errors in histologic diagnosis lead to either overtreatment of patients who will not benefit from intervention or, conversely, undertreatment of patients with clinically significant high-grade lesions that received false negative diagnoses [98].

Contemporaneous cervical cancer screening guidelines from the American Cancer Society (ACS) and the American College of Obstetricians and Gynecologists (ACOG) in effect acknowledged the extremely high sensitivity of FDA-approved Pap and HPV co-testing by specifically accepting lengthened screening intervals for women who test negative on both cytology and HPV tests [103]. There is ample evidence that the detection of HPV DNA in cervical samples has a higher sensitivity for cervical cancer and precancerous lesions than the Pap test and high-quality HPV tests are routinely used in prevention programs in some developed countries [99].

Although the recent introduction of a highly effective prophylactic HPV vaccine has great promise for the prevention of persistent infections and precancerous lesions, cervical cancer screening will still be required because the current vaccines do not protect against all carcinogenic HPV types and do not treat preexisting HPV infections and related disease [97]. Since persistent infection with HR-HPV is a risk factor for progression to cervical cancer and with the advent of HPV vaccines, it is increasingly relevant to perform HPV genotyping to identify oncogenic HPV vaccine types. HPV genotyping is of clinical interest, since the risk of developing a precancerous lesion is between 10%, and 15% with HPV types 16 and 18, and below 3% for all other high-risk types combined. Genotyping information could provide more information regarding risk-stratification as well as persistence of infection [98].

While current guidelines and recommendations consistently advise on vaccinating young girls before their sexual debut, natural history studies indicate that all sexually active women are at risk of new oncogenic HPV infections and of development of cervical lesions and cancer throughout their lives. The reviewed data suggest that most sexually active women have the potential to benefit from HPV vaccination, with the exception of those with current infections with both oncogenic HPV vaccine types. Women of all ages should be able to make a well-informed decision when considering HPV vaccination [99].

Screening protocols are likely to be modified taking advantage of the higher validity of HPV tests as compared to the conventional Pap smear. Many clinical trials have compared HPV DNA testing and cytology in screening scenarios and concluded that HPV test offers a greater sensitivity (in the range of 30%) and a reduced specificity (in the range of 8%) as compared to cytology. Moreover HPV tests are less demanding in terms of manpower and quality control and automated equipments are available for high throughput performance [100]. Other biomarkers are under evaluation to increase the specificity of screening programs and for the triage of HPV positive women with normal cytology. These include HPV typing, p16 INK immunostaining and others [101].

p16INK4a has been successfully deployed for the classification of HPV-related disease for several reasons: the expression of p16INK4a is directly linked to the HPV oncogenic action, since continuous expression of E7 is necessary to maintain the malignant phenotype, the expression of p16INK4a is independent of the HPV type, and therefore, genotyping does not need to be performed, and the expression of p16INK4a by cycling cells is a specific marker of HPV-E7 overexpression or other events that inactivate Rb by immunochemistry. Additionally, improving diagnostic accuracy and reproducibility, the use of p16INK4a immunohistochemistry may help in identifying CIN1 lesions that are associated with HR-HPV types; these lesions are at an increased risk for progression to high-grade dysplasia or carcinoma [98]. Thus, the clinical assessment of HPV infection uses a combination of diagnostic cytologies, such as the Pap test in association with complementary DNA test and hostp16INK4a [101].

The new guideline regarding screening for the early detection of cervical precancerous lesions and cancer was published by the ACS and American Society for Colposcopy and Cervical Pathology (ASCC) in American Journal of Clinical Pathology [102]. The new guideline includes a review of molecular screening tests and strategies, it suggest that perhaps the largest immediate gain in reducing the burden of cervical cancer incidence and mortality could be attained by increasing access to screening (regardless of the test used) among women who are currently unscreened or screened infrequently. Incorporation of HPV testing may offer advantages over what is already a successful screening strategy if utilized (ie, cytology) [103]. Incorporation of HPV testing into cervical cancer screening strategies has the potential to allow both increased disease detection and increased length of screening intervals. The recommendations are described in the Table 3.

Population	Screening Method*	Management of Screen	Results Comments
Aged <21 years (y)	No screening		HPV testing should not be used for screening or management of ASC-US in this age group
Aged 21-29 years (y)	Cytology alone every 3 y	HPV-positive ASC-US† or cytology of LSIL or more severe: Refer to ASCCP guidelines2.	HPV testing should not be used for screening in this age group

Population	Screening Method*	Management of Screen	Results Comments
		Cytology negative or HPV negative ASC-US†: Rescreen with cytology in 3 y	
Aged 30-65 years (y)	HPV and cytology "cotesting" every 5 y (preferred)	HPV-positive ASC-US or cytology of LSIL or more severe: Refer to ASCCP guidelines2 HPV positive, cytology negative: Option 1: 12-mo follow-up with contesting Option 2: Test for HPV16 or HPV16/18 genotypes • If HPV16 or HPV16/18 positive: refer to colposcopy • If HPV16 or HPV16/18 negative: 12-mo follow-up with cotesting Cotest negative or HPV-negative ASC-US: Rescreen with cotesting in 5 y	Screening by HPV testing alone is not recommended for most clinical settingst.
	Cytology alone every	HPV-positive ASC-US† or cytology of LSIL or more severe: Refer to ASCCP guidelines2 Cytology negative or HPV-negative ASC-US†: Rescreen with cytology in 3 y	
Aged "/>65 years (y)	No screening following adequate negative prior screening		Women with a history of CIN2 or a more severe diagnosis should continue routine screening for at least 20 y
After hysterectomy	No screening		Applies to women without a cervix and without a history of CIN2 or a more severe diagnosis in the past 20 y or cervical cancer ever
HPV vaccinated	Follow age-specific recommendations (same as unvaccinated women)		

ASCCP, American Society for Colposcopy and Cervical Pathology; ASC-US, atypical squamous cells of undetermined significance; CIN2, cervical intraepithelial neoplasia grade 2; HPV, human papillomavirus; LSIL, low-grade squamous intraepithelial lesion.

* Women should not be screened annually at any age by any method.

† ASC-US cytology with secondary HPV testing for management decisions. * Modified from [102].

Table 3. Summary of Recommendations of The American Society for Colposcopy and Cervical Pathology

On the other hand, educative action to prevent cervical and non cervical cancers, which are part of basic health actions, should be considered a professional commitment to the population's quality of life and a care quality commitment, emphasizing patients' autonomy in self-care. In the study in Brazil aimed to evaluate the applicability of an educational booklet that contained information for the general population about promotion and prevention of infections and neoplasic process caused by the HPV. The authors enphatized it is necessary to promote and improve campaigns to the population about the HPV and its relations with the neoplasic process to preventive strategies [104].

Proper condom use as a primary prevention measure should remain a top priority for health officials. Campaigns with a primary aim to increase sexually transmitted infection (STI) knowledge and awareness with the intention of influencing risk perceptions amongst those sexually active, may not effectively translate into an increase in prevention behaviors. To reach the public health goal of reducing STI prevalence, barriers to engaging in STI prevention need to be addressed, including preventive strategies [105].

Education should not only be considered an extra activity, but an action that redirects practices at health promotion as a whole. Suggests that preventive knowledge about the natural history of cervical and non cervical cancer and, such as use of HPV vaccination in both sex will decrease the incidence of HPV associated cancers and has the potential to be of great significance to high-risk female and male populations, the largest group to suffer from HPV-associated cancers within this greater population [105].

In addition, molecular tools are a relatively new division of laboratory medicine that detects, characterizes, and/or quantifies nucleic acids to assist in the diagnosis of human disease. Molecular assays augment classical areas of laboratory medicine by providing additional diagnostic data either in a more expeditious manner or by providing results that would not be obtainable using standard methodologies. These methods are used for detecting infectious agents have several advantages when compared to classical approaches, because these methods generally do not require growth in culture media, like HPV, which cannot be grown in conventional cell cultures [106].

In this context, researchers benefit from having a variety of molecular diagnostic tests at their fingertips; however, the clinical laboratories in the United States have a more limited selection of FDA-approved tests for HPV. Many of the HPV diagnostic kits available in regions such as Europe and Canada have not been approved for clinical use in the United States. Meanwhile, laboratories may choose to use non-approved tests as analyte specific reagents (ASRs) or home brews, although more extensive validation is required in these cases [59].

Regardless of the technical method used, careful consideration is necessary in the evaluation of diagnostic techniques for HPV screening. Most infectious disease tests strive for the highest possible analytical sensitivity, and PCR is typically the optimal method to achieve that standard. However, the more important standard for HPV screening is not analytical sensitivity but clinical sensitivity and specificity. Clinical utility of HPV screening is based on the prediction of cervical cancer, not simply the presence of the virus. Especially in young adult populations, detecting the HPV virus has little clinical use because the vast majority of these cases will self-resolve and never develop into cancer. The high sensitivity of PCR is thus a detriment in HPV screening, because PCR can detect even miniscule amounts of virus that may have no clinical significance [59].

There are many advantages to the PCR technology for such screening applications, including automation capabilities, turnaround time, multiplexing, sensitivity/specificity, multiple specimen types, and small-specimen volume. The major concern with the in vitro amplification technologies is the potential for contamination [107]. PCR require that laboratories determine a threshold of detection representing a clinically significant result. Likewise, the detection of non cancer-causing, low-risk strains of HPV has virtually no clinical utility. Knowing that a low-risk HPV strain is present does not have an impact on the clinical management of a patient with cutaneous or mucosal warts. In order to prevent superfluous laboratory testing, clinicians should also heed the ASCCP guidelines for the management of women with or without cytological abnormalities [59].

The clinical laboratory must evaluate many factors in the adoption of an appropriate HPV test, including consideration of the population being served. In underprivileged areas, for example, HPV screening tests with less than optimal clinical sensitivities and specificities may still far surpass current cervical cancer screening methods. As new data emerge from recently established HPV screening methods, researchers and clinicians will continue to strive toward the goal of early and accurate detection of cervical cancer [59].

5. Conclusion

Molecular biology techniques with different sensitivity and specificity have facilitated the characterization of the entire HPV genome, where different functional regions are identified, as a profile of their gene expression. Additionally, molecular tools have been recognized as the most appropriate method to identify and type HPV genomes because of its higher sensitivity and specificity. Although the cervical cytology for CIN has been used to reduce the incidence of mortality worldwide, molecular technologies continue to evolve for many molecular diagnostic applications. Novel strategies for detection and genotyping are important to complement the screening programmes for HPV detection in women at risk of cervical cancer.

It is also important to mention the WHO Global HPV LabNet as a WHO initiative established to support the world-wide implementation of HPV vaccines through improved laboratory standardization and quality assurance of HPV testing and typing methods to promote international comparability of results. The major methods for achieving progress towards this goal are developing international biological standards as well as preparing and validating proficiency panels to qualify methods. And finally, the incorporation of HPV testing into cervical cancer screening strategies has the potential to allow both increased disease detection and increased length of screening intervals. The recommendations are described above (Table 3) and follows the so-called "Meyer-criteria" that present scientific evidence for minimal criteria for an HPV test.

Acknowledgements

This chapter was written by the researchers of the HPV Study Group in Goiânia-GO, Brazil. The authors thank S. Quail for English support.

Author details

Angela Adamski da Silva Reis[1], Daniela de Melo e Silva[2], Cláudio Carlos da Silva[3] and Aparecido Divino da Cruz[3]

1 Federal University of Goiás - Biological Sciences Institute - Department of Biochemistry and Molecular Biology, Brazil

2 Federal University of Goiás - Biological Sciences Institute - Department of General Biology, Brazil

3 Pontifical Catholic University of Goiás.- Department of Medicine and Biology, Brazil

References

[1] Villa LL. Biology of genital human papillomavirus. International Journal of Gynecology and Obstetrics 2006; 94 (1) S3-S7.

[2] Bosch FX, Lorincz A, Munoz N, Meijer CJ, Shah KV. The causal relation between human papillomavirus and cervical cancer. Journal of Clinical Pathology 2002;55(4) 244-65.

[3] Steenbergen RD, de Wilde J, Wilting SM, Brink AA, Snijders PJ, Meijer CJ. HPV-mediated transformation of the anogenital tract. Journal of Clinical Virology 2005;32 (S1) S25-33

[4] Walboomers JM, Jacobs MV, Manos MM, Bosch FX, Kummer JA, Shah KV. Human papillomavirus is a necessary cause of invasive cervical cancer worldwide. The Journal of Pathology 1999;189(1)12-9.

[5] Muñoz N, Castellsagué X, de González AB, Gissmann L. Chapter 1: HPV in the etiology of human cancer. Vaccine 2006; 24 (3) S3/1-10.

[6] International Agency for Research on Cancer: Monographs on the Evaluation of Carcinogenic Risks to Humans-Human papillomaviruses. Lyon: IARC Press (90) 16-36, 2007.

[7] Lie AK, Kristensen G. Human papillomavirus E6/E7 mRNA testing as a predictive marker for cervical carcinoma. Expert Review of Molecular Diagnostics's. 2008; 8(4) 405-15.

[8] Baseman JG, Koutsky LA. The epidemiology of human papillomavirus infections. Journal of Clinical Virology 2005; 32(1) S16-24

[9] Molijn A, Kleter B, Quint W, van Doorn L-J. Molecular diagnosis of human papillomavirus (HPV) infections. Journal of Clinical Virology 2005; (32S) S43–S51.

[10] Palefsky JM. Human Papillomavirus-Related Disease in Men: Not Just a Women's Issue. Journal of Adolescent Health 2010; 46(2) S12-S19.

[11] Chaturvedi, A.K. (2010)Beyond Cervical Cancer: Burden of Other HPV-Related Cancers Among Men and Women. Journal o f Adolescent Health 2010; (46) S20–S26.

[12] Giuliano AR, G A, & Nyitray AG. Epidemiology and pathology of HPV disease in males. Gynecologic Oncology 2010; 117(2)1 S15-S19.

[13] Giuliano AR, Tortolero-Luna G, Ferrer E, Burchell AN, de Sanjosé S, Kjaer SK, Muñoz N, Schiffman M. & Bosch FX. Epidemiology of Human Papillomavirus Infection in Men, Cancers other than Cervical and Benign Conditions. Vaccine 2008; 26(10) K17-K28.

[14] Gillison ML. Human Papillomavirus-Related Diseases: Oropharynx Cancers and Potential Implications for Adolescent HPV Vaccination. Journal of Adolescent Health 2008; 43(4) S52-S60.

[15] Castellsague X, Bosch FX, Munoz N, Meijer CJ, Shah KV, de Sanjose S. Male circumcision, penile human papillomavirus infection, and cervical cancer in female partners. The New England Journal of Medicine 2002;346(15)1105–12.

[16] Cuschieri KS, Cubie HA. The role of human papillomavirus testing in cervical screening. Journal of Clinical Virology 2005; 32(1) S34-42.

[17] Parkin DM, Bray F. Chapter 2: The burden of HPV-related cancers. Vaccine 2006; 24 (3) S3/11-25.

[18] Miralles-Guri C, Bruni L, Cubilla AL, Castellsagué X, Bosch FX, Sanjosé S. Human papillomavirus prevalence and type distribution in penile carcinoma. Journal of Clinical Pathology 2009; 62 (10) 870–878.

[19] Moody, C.A. & Laimins, L.A. Human papillomavirus oncoproteins: pathways to transformation. Nature Reviews - Cancer 2010; 10(8) 550-560.

[20] Cox JT. History of the use of HPV testing in cervical screening and in the management of abnormal cervical screening results. Journal of Clinical Virology 2009; S1 (45) S3 S12.

[21] Bosch FX, Burchell AN, Schiffman M, Giuliano AR, de Sanjose S, Bruni L, Tortolero-Luna G, Kjaer SK, Muñoz N. Epidemiology and Natural History of Human Papillo-

mavirus Infections and Type-Specific Implications in Cervical Neoplasia. In: ICO Monograph Series on HPV and Cervical Cancer: General Overview. Vaccine 2008; 26(10) K1-K16.

[22] Muñoz N, Bosch FX, de Sanjose S, Herrero R, Castellsague X, Shah KV. Epidemiologic classification of human papillomavirus types associated with cervical cancer. The New England Journal of Medicine 2003; 348(6) 518–27.

[23] Ghittoni R, Accardi R, Hasan U, Gheit T, Sylla B, Tommasino M. The biological properties of E6 and E7 oncoproteins from human papillomaviruses. Virus Genes 2010; 40(1) 1-13.

[24] Reis AAS, Silva DM, Curado MP & da Cruz AD. Involvement of CYP1A1, GST, 72TP53 polymorphisms in the pathogenesis of thyroid nodules. Genetics and Molecular Research 2010; 9(4) 2222-2229.

[25] Tornesello ML, Duraturo ML, Guida V, Losito S, Botti G, Pilotti S, Stefanon B, De Palo G, Buonaguro L, Buonaguro FM. Analysis of TP53 codon 72 polymorphism in HPV-positive and HPV-negative penile carcinoma. Cancer Letters 2008; 269 (1) 159–164

[26] Almeida PS, Manoel WJ, Reis AAS, Silva ER. & Saddi VA. TP53 codon 72 polymorphism in adult soft tissue sarcomas. Genetics and Molecular Research 2008; 7(4) 1344-1352.

[27] Koushik A, Platt RW & Franco EL. p53 codon 72 polymorphism and cervical neoplasia: a meta-analysis review. Cancer Epidemiology Biomarkers & Prevention 2004; 13(1) 11–22.

[28] Jariene K, Vaitkiene D, Bartusevičius A, Tvarijonavičienė E, Minkauskiene M, Nadišauskiene R, Kruminis V, Kliučinskas M. Prevalence of Human Papillomavirus Types 16, 18, and 45 in Women With Cervical Intraepithelial Changes: Associations With Colposcopic and Histological Findings. Medicina (Kaunas) 2012;48(1) 22-30.

[29] Miller AB. Quality assurance in screening strategies: reviews. Virus Research 2002; 89:295-9.

[30] International Agency for Research on Cancer: IARC Handbooks of Cancer Prevention Vol.10. Cervix Cancer Screening. Lyon: IARC Press; 2005.

[31] Origoni M, Cristoforoni P, Costa S, Mariani L, Scirpa P, Lorincz A, Sideri M. HPV-DNA testing for cervical cancer precursors: from evidence to clinical practice. E cancer medical science 2012; (6) 258-273.

[32] Katyal S, Mehrotra R. Complementary Procedures in Cervical Cancer Screening in Low Resource Settings. Journal of Obstetrics & Gynaecology of India 2011;61(4) 436-438.

[33] Baleriola C, Millar D, Melki J, Coulston N, Altman P, Rismanto N, Rawlinson W. Comparison of a novel HPV test with the Hybrid Capture II (hcII) and a reference

PCR method shows high specificity and positive predictive value for 13 high-risk human papillomavirus infections. Journal of Clinical Virology 2008; (42) 22–26.

[34] Evander M, Edlund K, Gustafsson A, Jonsson M, Karlsson R, Rylander E, Wadell G.Human papillomavirus infection is transient in young women: a population-based cohort study. The Journal of Infection Disease 1995;171(4)1026-30.

[35] de Roda Husman A-M, Walboomers JMM, van den Brule AJC, Meijer CJLM, Snijders PJF. The use of general primers GP5 and GP6 elongated at their 3_ ends with adjacent highly conserved sequences improves human papillomavirus detection by PCR. Journal of General Virology 1995;(76)1057–62.

[36] Moscicki AB. Genital infections with human papillomavirus (HPV). The Pediatric Infection Disease Journal. 1998;17(7) 651-2.

[37] Dillner J. The serological response to papillomaviruses. Cancer Biology 1999; (9) 423-430.

[38] Koliopoulos G, Valasoulis G, ZilakouE. An update review on HPV testing methods for cervical neoplasia. Expert Opinion on Medical Diagnostics 2009; (3) 123–131.

[39] Clavel C, Masure M, Bory JP, Putaud I, Mangeonjean C, Lorenzato M. Hybrid Capture II-based human papillomavirus detection, a sensitive test to detect in routine high-grade cervical lesions: a preliminary study on 1518 women. British Journal of Cancer 1999; 80(9) 1306-1311.

[40] Munoz M, Camargo M, Soto-De Leon SC, Rojas-Villarraga A, Sanchez R, Jaimes C, Perez-Prados A, Patarroyo ME, Patarroyo MA. The diagnostic performance of classical molecular tests used for detecting human papillomavirus. The Journal Virological Methods 2012;185(1)32-8.

[41] Vernick JP, Steigman CK. The HPV DNA virus hybrid capture assay: what is it--and where do we go from here? Medical Laboratory Observer 2003; 35(3) 8-10.

[42] Poljak M, Kovanda A, Kocjan BJ, Seme K, Janˇcar N, Vrtaˇcnik-Bokal E. The Abbott RealTime High Risk HPV test: comparative evaluation of analytical specificity and clinical sensitivity for cervical carcinoma and CIN3 lesions with the Hybrid Capture 2 HPV DNA test. Acta Dermatoven APA 2009;(18)94–103.

[43] Thrall MJ, Mody DR. Clinical Human Papillomavirus Testing Modalities: Established Techniques and New Directions. Pathology Case Reviews 2011; 16(2) 55-61.

[44] Venturoli S, Leo E, Nocera M, Barbieri D, Criccaa M, Costa C, Santini D, Zerbini ML. Comparison of Abbott RealTime High Risk HPV and Hybrid Capture 2 for the detection of high-risk HPV DNA in a referral population setting. Journal of Clinical Virology 2012; (53) 121-124.

[45] Keegan H, Mc Inerney J, Pilkington L, Grønn P, Silva I, Karlsen F, Bolger N, Logan C, Furuberg L, O'Leary J, Martin C. Comparison of HPV detection technologies: Hybrid capture 2, PreTect HPV-Proofer and analysis ofHPV DNA viral load in HPV16,

HPV18 and HPV33 E6/E7 mRNA positive specimens. Journal of Virology Methods 2009;155(1) 61-6.

[46] Gravitt PE, Coutlée F, Iftner T, Sellors JW, Quint WG, Wheeler CM. New technologies in cervical cancer screening. Vaccine 2008; 26 (S10) K42-52.

[47] Lorincz A, Anthony J. Advances in HPV detection by hybrid capture. Papillomavirus Rep 2001;12 145-54.

[48] Castle PE, Lorincz AT, Scott DR, Sherman ME, Glass AG,Rush BB, Wacholder S, Burk RD, Manos M M, Schussler JE, Macomber P, Schiffman M. Comparison between Prototype Hybrid Capture 3 and Hybrid Capture 2 Human Papillomavirus DNA Assays for Detection of High-Grade Cervical Intraepithelial Neoplasia and Cancer. Journal of Clinical Microbiology 2003; 41(9) 4022–4030.

[49] Doorbar J. Papillomavirus life cycle organization and biomarker selection. Disease Markers 2007; 23(4)297-313.

[50] Vinokurova S, Wentzensen N, Kraus I, Klaes R, Driesch C, Melsheimer P, Kisseljov F, Dürst M, Schneider A, von Knebel Doeberitz M. Type-dependent integration frequency of human papillomavirus genomes in cervical lesions. Cancer Res. 2008;68(1) 307-13.

[51] Lowe B, Fulbright A, Nazarenko I. A hybrid-capture assay to detect HPV mRNA ratios in cervical specimens. Journal of Virology Methods 2012 ;179(1) 142-147.

[52] Roberts CC, Swoyer R, Bryan JT, Taddeo FJ. Comparison of real-time multiplex human papillomavirus (HPV) PCR assays with the linear array HPVgenotyping PCR assay and influence of DNA extraction method on HPV detection. Journal of Clinical Microbiology 2011; 49(5) 1899-906.

[53] Pagliusi SR, Dillner J, Pawlita M, Quint WG, Wheeler CM, Ferguson M. Chapter 23: International Standard reagents for harmonization of HPV serology and DNA assays--an update. Vaccine 2006; 24(S3) 193-200.

[54] Iftner T, Villa LL. Chapter 12: Human papillomavirus technologies. J Natl Cancer Inst Monogr. 2003;(31) 80-8.

[55] van den Brule AJ, Snijders PJ, Gordijn RL, Bleker OP, Meijer CJ, Walboomers JM.General primer-mediated polymerase chain reaction permits the detection of sequenced and still unsequenced human papillomavirus genotypes in cervical scrapes and carcinomas. International Journal of Cancer 1990; 45(4) 644-9.

[56] Jacobs MV, Snijders PJ, van den Brule AJ, Helmerhorst TJ, Meijer CJ, Walboomers JM. A general primer GP5+/GP6(+)-mediated PCR enzymeimmunoassay method for rapid detection of 14 high-risk and 6 low-risk human papillomavirus genotypes in cervical scrapings. Journal of Clinical Microbiology 1997;(35)791-5.

[57] Manos MM, Kinney WK, Hurley LB. Identifying women with cervical neoplasia: us-
      ing human papillomavirus testing for equivocal Papanicolaou results. Journal of
      American Medicine Association 1999;(281)1605-1610.

[58] Gravitt PE, Peyton CL, Apple RJ. Genotyping of 27 human papillomavirus types by
      using L1 consensus PCR products by a single hybridization, reverse line blot detec-
      tion. Journal of Clinical Microbiology 1998;(36)3020–3027.

[59] Arney A, Bennett KM. Molecular Diagnostics of Human Papillomavirus. LabMedi-
      cine 2010; (41) 523-530.

[60] Chung MY, Kim Y-W, Bae SM, Kwon EH, Chaturvedi PK, Battogtokh G, Ahn WS.
      Development of a Bead-Based Multiplex Genotyping Method for Diagnostic Charac-
      terization of HPV Infection. PLoS ONE 2009; 7 (2) e32259. doi:10.1371

[61] Sherman ME, Schiffman MH, Lorincz AT, Herrero R, Hutchinson ML, Bratti C. Cer-
      vical specimens collected in liquid buffer are suitable for both cytologic screening
      and ancillary human papillomavirus testing. Cancer 1997; (81) 89-97.

[62] Rebolj M, Pribac I, Lynge E. False-positive Human Papillomavirus DNA tests in cer-
      vical screening: it is all in a definition. European Journal of Cancer 2011;47(2) 255-61.

[63] Astbury K, Martin CM, Ring M, Pilkington L, Bolger N, Sheils OM, O'Leary JJ. Fu-
      ture molecular aspects of cervical cytology. Current Diagnostic Pathology 2006; (12)
      104-113.

[64] Boulet GA, Micalessi IM, Horvath CA, Benoy IH, Depuydt CE, Bogers JJ. Nucleic
      acid sequence-based amplification assay for human papillomavirus mRNA detection
      and typing: evidence for DNA amplification. Journal of Clinical Microbiology 2010;
      48(7) 2524-2529.

[65] Molden T, Kraus I, Karlsen F, Skomedal H, Nygård JF, Hagmar B. Comparison of hu-
      man papillomavirus messenger RNA and DNA detection: a cross-sectional study of
      4,136 women >30 years of age with a 2-year follow-up of high-grade squamous intra-
      epithelial lesion. Cancer Epidemiology, Biomarkers & Prevention 2005;14(2) 367-372.

[66] Andersson E, Karrberg C, Thomas R, Blomqvist L, Zetterqvist B-M, Ryd W, Lindh
      Magnus, Horal Peter. Type-Specific Human Papillomavirus E6/E7 mRNA Detection
      by Real-Time PCR Improves Identification of Cervical Neoplasia. Journal of Clinical
      Microbiology 2011; 49(11) 3794–3799.

[67] Clifford G M, Smith JS, Aguado T, Franceschi S. Comparison of HPV type distribu-
      tion in high-grade cervical lesions and cervical cancer: a meta-analysis British Journal
      of Cancer 2003; 89(1) 101-105.

[68] Cushieri KS, Cubie HA, Whitley MW, Seagar AL, Arends MJ, Moore C. Multiple
      high-risk HPV infections are common in cervical neoplasia and young women in a
      cervical screening population. Journal of Clinical Pathology 2004;(57) 68-72.

[69] Molden T, Nygard JF, Kraus I, Karlsen F, Nygard M, Skare GB, Skomedal H, Thoresen SO, Hagmar B. Predicting CIN2+ when detecting HPV mRNA and DNA by PreTect HPV-proofer and consensus PCR: A 2-year follow-up of women with ASCUS or LSIL Pap smear. Internacional Journal of Cancer 2005;114(6) 973-976.

[70] Szarewski A, Ambroisine L, Cadman L, Austin J, Ho L, Terry G. Comparison of predictors for high-grade cervical intraepithelial neoplasia in women with abnormal smears. Cancer Epidemiology, Biomarkers & Prevention 2008; (17) 3033-3042

[71] Ratnam Samuel, Coutlee F, Fontaine D, Bentley J, Escott N,Ghatage P, Gadag V, Holloway G, Bartellas E, Kum Nick, Giede C, Lear A Clinical Performance of the PreTect HPV-Proofer E6/E7 mRNA Assay in Comparison with That of the Hybrid Capture 2 Test for Identification of Women at Risk of Cervical Cancer. Journal of Clinical Microbiology 2010; 48(8) 2779–2785.

[72] Rodriguez-Lazaro D, Lloyd J, Ikonomopoulos J, Pla M, Cook N. Unexpected detection of DNA by nucleic acid sequence-based amplification technique. Molecular and Cellular Probes 2004; 18:251-253.

[73] Benevolo M, Vocaturo A, Caraceni D, French D, Rosini S, Zappacosta R, Terrenato I, Ciccocioppo L, Frega A, Rossi PG. Sensitivity, Specificity, and Clinical Value of Human Papillomavirus(HPV) E6/E7 mRNA Assay as a Triage Test for Cervical Cytology and HPV DNA Test. journal of Clinical Microbiology 2011; 49(7) 2643-2650.

[74] Ratnam Samuel, Coutlee Francois, Fontaine Dan, Bentley James, Escott Nicholas, Ghatage P, Gadag V, Holloway G, Bartellas E,Kum N, Giede C, Lear A. Aptima HPV E6/E7 mRNA Test Is as Sensitive as Hybrid Capture 2 Assay but More Specific at Detecting Cervical Precancer and Cancer. Journal of Clinical Microbiology 2011; 49(2) 557-564.

[75] Clad A, Reuschenbach M, Weinschenk J, Grote R, Rahmsdorf J, Freudenberg N. Performance of the Aptima High-Risk Human Papillomavirus mRNA Assay in a Referral Population in Comparison with Hybrid Capture 2 and Cytology. Journal of Clinical Microbiology 2011; 49(3) 1071-1076.

[76] Dockter J, Schroder A, Hill C, Guzenski L, Monsonego J, Giachetti C. Clinical performance of the APTIMA® HPV Assay for the detection of high-risk HPV and high-grade cervical lesions. Journal of Clinical Virology 2009; 45(S1) S55-61.

[77] Gulliksen A, Keegan H, Martin C, O'Leary J, Solli LA, Falang IM, Grønn P, Karlgard A, Mielnik MM, Johansen IR, Tofteberg TR, Baier T, Gransee R, Drese K, Hansen-Hagge T, Riegger L, Koltay P, Zengerle R, Karlsen F, Ausen D, Furuberg L.Towards a "Sample-In, Answer-Out" Point-of-Care Platform for Nucleic Acid Extraction and Amplification: Using an HPV E6/E7 mRNA Model System. Journal of Oncology 2012; 905024. doi: 10.1155/2012/905024

[78] Farh KK, Grimson A, Jan C, Lewis BP, Johnston WK, Lim LP, Burge CB, Bartel DF. The widespread impact of mammalian MicroRNAs on mRNA repression and evolution. Science 2005; (310) 1817-1821.

[79] Lewis BP, Burge CB, Bartel DP. Conserved seed pairing, often flanked by adenosines, indicates that thousands of human genes are microRNA targets. Cell 2005; (120)15-20.

[80] Grimson A, Farh KK, Johnston WK, Garrett-Engele P, Lim LP, Bartel DP. MicroRNA targeting specificity in mammals: determinants beyond seed pairing. Molecular Cell 2007; 91-105.

[81] Zheng ZM, Wang X. Regulation of cellular miRNA expression by human papillomaviruses. Biochimica et Biophysica Acta 2011; (1809) 668-677

[82] Deftereos G, Corrie SR, Feng Q, Morihara J, Stern J, Hawes SE, Kiviat NB. Expression of MIr-21 and MIr-143 in Cervical Specimens Ranging from Histologically Normal through to Invasive Cervical Cancer. Plos One 2011; 6(12) 1-8.

[83] Farazi TA, Spitzer JI, Morozov P, Tusch T. mRNAs in human cancer. Journal of Pathology 2011; (223) 102-115.

[84] Cullen BR. Viruses and microRNAs. Nature Genetics 2006; (38) S25-S30.

[85] McBee WC, Gardiner AS, Edwards RP, Lesnock JL, Bhargava R, Austin RM, Guido RS, Khan, S.A. MicroRNA Analysis in Human Papillomavirus (HPV)-Associated Cervical Neoplasia and Cancer. Carcinogenesis and Mutagenesis 2011; 2 (1) 2-9.

[86] Lee JW, Choi CH, Choi JJ, Park YA, Kim SJ, H SY, Kim T-J,Lee J-H, Kim B-G, Bae DS. Altered MicroRNA Expression in Cervical Carcinomas. Clinical Cancer Research 2008; 14 2535-2542.

[87] Li Y, Wang F, Xu J, Ye F, Shen Y, Zhou J, Lu W, Wan X, Ma D, Xie X. Progressive miRNA expression profiles in cervical carcinogenesis and identification of HPV related target genes for mir-29. Journal of Pathology 2011; (224) 484-495.

[88] Lui WO, Pourmand N, Patterson BK, Fire A. Patterns of Known and novel small RNAs in human cervical cancer. Cancer Research 2007; 6031-6043.

[89] Hu X, Schwartz JK, Lewis-Jr JS, Huettner PC, Rader JS, Deasy JO, Grigsby PW, Wang X. A microRNA expression signature for cervical cancer prognosis. Cancer Research 2010; (70) 1441-1448.

[90] Rao Q, Shen Q, Zhou H, Peng Y, Li J, Lin Z. Aberrant microRNA expression in human cervical carcinomas. Medicine Oncology 2012; 29(2) 1242-1248.

[91] Zhu S, Wu H, Wu F, Nie D, Sheng S, Mo YY. MicroRNA-21 targets tumor suppressor genes in invasion and metastasis. Cell Research 2008; (18)350-359

[92] Suzuki HI, Yamagata K, Sugimoto K, Iwamoto S, Kato S, Miyazono K. Modulation of microRNA processing by p53. Nature 2009; (460) 529-533.

[93] Green DR, Kroemer G. Cytoplasmatic functions of the tumour suppressor p53. Nature 2009; (458) 1127-1130

[94] Riley T, Sontag E, Chen P, Levine A. Trasnscriptional control of human p53.-related genes. Nature Review Molecular Cellular Biology 2008; (9) 402-412.

[95] Bosch X & Harper D. Prevention strategies of cervical cancer in the HPV vaccine era. Gynecologic Oncology, 2006; 103 (1) 21-24.

[96] Nirchio V, Lipsi R, Fusilli S, Ciccone E, Murino L, Santangelo A, Romano F, Di Taranto AM, Pedà D, Castriota M, Antonetti R, Bondi A. HPV infection: comparison between morphological studies and molecular biology. Pathologica 2008;100(3) 149-55

[97] Marks A, Castle PE, Schiffman M, Gravitt PE. Evaluation of Any or Type-Specific Persistence of High-Risk Human Papillomavirus for Detecting Cervical Precancer. Journal of Clinical Microbiology 2012; 50(2) 300. DOI:10.1128/JCM.05979-11.

[98] Hwang SJ, Shroyer KR. Biomarkers of Cervical Dysplasia and Carcinoma. Journal of Oncology 2012;9 doi:10.1155/2012/507286

[99] Moy LM, Zhao FH, Li LY. Human papillomavirus testing and cervical cytology in primary screening for cervical cancer among women in rural China: comparison of sensitivity,specificity, and frequency of referral. International Journal of Cancer 2010; (127) 646–56.

[100] Castellsagué X, Schneider A, Kaufmann AM, Bosch FX. HPV vaccination against cervical cancer in women above 25 years of age:key considerations and current perspectives. Gynecologic Oncology 2009; (115) S15-S23.

[101] Satra M, Vamvakopoulou DN, Sioutopoulou DO, Kollia P, Kiritsaka A, Sotiriou S, Antonakopoulos G, Alexandris E, Costantoulakis P, Vamvakopoulos NC. Sequence-based genotyping HPV L1 DNA and RNA transcripts in clinical specimens. Pathology – Research and Practice 2009; (205) 863–869.

[102] Saslow D, Solomon D, Lawson HW, Killackey Maureen, Kulasingam SL, Cain J, Garcia FAR, Moriarty AT, Waxman AG, Wilbur DC, Wentzensen N, DownsJr LS, Spitzer M, Moscicki AB, Franco EL, Stoler MH, Schiffman M, Castle PE, Myers ER. American Cancer Society, American Society for Colposcopy and Cervical Pathology, and American Society for Clinical Pathology Screening Guidelines for the Prevention and Early Detection of Cervical Cancer. American Journal of Clinical Pathology 2012; (137) 516-542.

[103] Katki HA, Kinney WK, Fetterman B, Lorey T, Poitras NE, Cheung L, Demuth F, Schiffman M, Wacholder S, Castle PE. Cervical cancer risk for women undergoing concurrent testing for human papillomavirus and cervical cytology: a population-based study in routine clinical practice. Lancet Oncology 2011; 12(7) 663-72.

[104] Reis AAS, Monteiro CD, de Paula LB, da Silva RS, da Cruz AD. Human papillomavirus and public health: cervical cancer prevention. Ciência e Saúde Coletiva 2010; 15(1) 1060-2010.

[105] Reis AAS,da Cruz AD, The impact of Human Papillomavirus on Cancer Risk in Penile Cancer. In: Broeck DV. (ed.) Human Papillomavirus and Related Disease -From Bench to Bedside - A clinical Perspective. Rijeka: In Tech; 2011. p.319-348.

[106] Ferreira-Gonzalez A, Garrett C. Laboratory-Developed Tests in Molecular Diagnostics. In: Coleman WB and Tsongalis GJ. (2ªed.) Molecular Diagnostics for the Clinical Laboratorian. New Jersey: Human Press Inc; 2006. p247-256.

[107] Voytek TM.,Tsongalis GJ, Human Papillomavirus. In: Coleman WB and Tsongalis GJ. (2ªed.) Molecular Diagnostics for the Clinical Laboratorian. New Jersey: Human Press Inc; 2006. p447-451.

[108] Wang X, Tang S, Le SY, Lu R, Rader JS, Meyers C, Zheng ZM. Aberrant expression of oncogenic and tumor suppressive microRNAs in cervical cancer is required for cancer cell growth. Plos One 2008; 3(7) e2557.

[109] Li Y, Wang F, Xu J, Ye F, Shen Y, Zhou J, Lu W, Wan X, Ma D, Xie X. Progressive miRNA expression profiles in cervical carcinogenesis and identification of HPV related target genes for mir-29. Journal of Pathology 2011; 224 484-495

[110] Witten D, Tibshirani R, Gu SG, Fire A, Lui WO. Ultra-high throughput sequencing-based small RNA discovery and discrete statistical biomarkers analysis in a collection of cervical tumors and matched controls. BMC Biology 2010; 8 58.

[111] Zhang Y, Dai Y, Huang Y, Ma L, Yin Y, Tang M, Hu C. Microarray profile of micro-ribonucleic acid in tumor tissue from cervical squamous cell carcinoma without human papillomavirus Journal of Obstetrics and Gynaecology Research 2009; 35(5) 842-849

[112] miRBase: the microRNA database. http:// www.mirbase.org/ (accessed 19 August 2012).

Chapter 2

Molecular Diagnosis of Human Papillomavirus Infections

Santiago Melón, Marta Alvarez-Argüelles and
María de Oña

Additional information is available at the end of the chapter

1. Introduction

Human Papillomavirus (HPV) is arguably the most common sexually transmitted agent worldwide, either in its clinical (genital warts) or subclinical presentation in men and women. The main interest in HPV relates to its recognized as a causal and necessary factor for cervical cancer one of the most common cancers in women (80% of cases in most developing countries, with an annual incidence of almost half a millon and a mortality rate of approximately 50%) [1-5], and other types of cancer, such as penis, anal or oral cancer [6].

The overall prevalence of HPV in cervix in women in the general population is 10%. This prevalence is higher in the less developed world than in more developed regions [7, 8]. A review of studies has also shown prevalence of HPV in men as usually 20% or greater, depending on population tested and the type and number of anatomic sites evaluated [9].

HPV infection is most common in sexually active young women 25 years of age or younger but cervical cancer is common in older woman, suggesting infection at younger age and slow progression to cancer [10].

The most significant predictor for adquiring HPV infection in men or women appears to be the life time number of sexual parteners [11,12,13]. For women, the sexual activity of their partner(s) is also important, with increased risk of adquiring HPV if their partner had, or currently has, other partners [12].

Not all women infected with high-risk HPV develop cervical cancer, other factors are necessary: genotype, persistent infection, viral variants, viral load, integration, coinfection, age of 30 years old, inmunosupresión, smoking, condom use, coinfections, long-term use of oral contraceptives, parity and circumcision. [10, 12, 14-24]

About 189 HPV genotypes have been sequence and classified according to their biological niche, oncogenic potential and phylogenetic position [25]. From them, about 40 can infect the genital tract [26]. HPV types are classified based on their association with cervical cancer and precursor lesion into low-risk types (**LR-HPV)**, which are found mainly in genital warts, high-risk types (**HR-HPV)**, which are frequently associated with invasive cervical cancer and undetermined risk types (table 1) [27, 28, 29].

Risk category	HPV types
High-risk	16,18,31,33,35,39,45,51,52,56,58,59,68,73,82
Low-risk	6,11,40,42,43,44,54, 61,70,72, 81, 83, 89
Undetermined risk	26,53,66

Table 1. HPV types classification according their oncogenic potential

Worldwide, HPV-16 is the most common HPV type across the spectrum of HPV related cervical lesions. In women with ICC (invasive cervical cancer), the most common HPV types are HPV-16,18,33,45,31 and 58 [30, 31], but among these genotypes, certain variants have linked to different clinical outcomes. It is now generally accepted that HPV has co-existed with its human host over a very long period of time and has evolved into multiple evolutionary lineages [25, 32]. Intratypic variants of HPV16 have been identified from different geographic locations and are classified according to their host ethnic groups as European (including prototypes and Asian types), Asian American, African and North American [33]. Through epidemiological and in-vitro experimental studies, natural variants of HPV16 have shown substantial differences in pathogenicity, immunogenicity and tumorigenicity. IARC Study [34] and IARC Meta-analysis [31] are very robust in identifying that HPV-16 and 18 contibute approximately 70% of all ICC. HPV-16,18 and 45 are the three most relevant types in cervical adenocarcinoma [30]. The geographical variation in type distribution is of minor significance variation.

Among men and women, cancers of the ano-genital tract and their precursor lesions have been strongly linked to infection with sexually transmited human papillomavirus. In men, HPV infection has been strongly associated with anal cancer and is associated with approximately 85% of the anal squamous cell cancers that accur annually worldwide. Likewise, approximately 50% of cancers of penis have been associtated to HPV infection [35]. Genital warts are a common sexually transmitted condition with an estimated prevalence of 1-2% of young adults [36]. Although having genital warts is not associated with mortality, represent a significant public health problem (clinical symptoms and psychosocial problems) and healthcare costs for society [37-39]. More than 90% of genital warts are related to HPV-6 and 11 (low risk genotypes) in general these types are not associated with malignant lesions, however 20-50% of these also contained coinfection with oncogenic HPV types [39-41].

On the other hand, between 33-72% of oropharyngeal cancers, and 10% of cancer of the larynx may be attributed to HPV infection [42-44].

2. Etiopathogenesis of HPV

The HPV virion has a double-stranded, circular DNA genome of approximately 7900bp, with eight overlapping open reading frames, comprising early (E), and late (L) genes and an untranslated long control region, within an icosahedral capsid. The L1 and L2 genes encode the mayor and minor capsid proteins. The capsid contains 72 pentamers of L1, and a pproximately 12 molecules of L2. The early genes regulate viral replication and some have transformation potential. Late genes L6 and L7 code for structural capsid proteins which encapsidate the viral genome. (Figure 1).

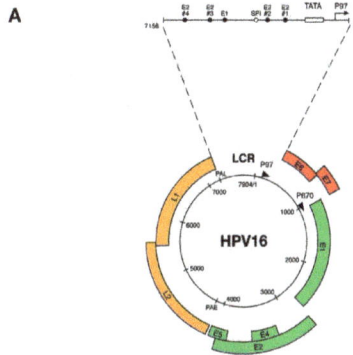

Figure 1. Organization of the HPV genome. Adapted from Doorbar J. [45]

Infection by papillomaviruses requires that virus particles gain access to the epithelial basal layer and enter the dividing basal cells. Having entered the epithelial tissues, the HPV virus enters the nucleus of a basal epithelial cell, where early genes E1 and E2 are expressed, replicating the viral genome and transcribing messenger RNA needed for viral replication; in addition to its role in replication and genome segregation, E2 can also act as a transcription factor and can regulate the viral early promoter and control expression of the viral oncogenes (E6 and E7). At low levels, E2 acts as a transcriptional activator, whereas at high levels E2 represses oncogene expression [45]. As the host cells differentiate, genes E4 and E5 assist in the production of the viral genome by controlling epidermal growth factor. E6 and E7 are viral oncogenes which now become important. E6 causes degradation of the tumour suppressor gene p53, while E7 completes for retinoblastoma protein (pRb), allowing the transcription factor E2F to drive cell proliferation processes. The p16 protein, encoded by the suppressor gene CDKN2A (MTS1, INK4A) at chromosome 9p21, is an inhibitor of cyclin dependent kinases (cdk)which slows cell cycle by inactivating the function of the complex-cdk4 and cdk6-cyclin D. These complexes regulate the control point of the G1 phase of the cell cycle with subsequent phosphorylation and inactivation of retinoblastoma (pRb), which E2F released and which allows cells to enter S phase. It has been demonstrated existence of a correlation between pRb and p16 reciprocal, which is why there a strong overexpression of p16 both in carcinomas as in lesions premalignant cervix. In cervical cancer, pRb is functionally inactivated from the initial stages of cervical carcinogenesis as a consequence of expression of HPV E7 gene. Genes E6 and E7 therefore act to remove two principle mechanisms of cell defence, and drive the cell replication machinery towards production of new virus particles. E6 and E7 are also known to promote oncogenesis. [45]

On the other hand, integration of HPV-DNA into the host DNA is a well known topic in cervical cancer. Integration of HPV 16 DNA correlates with dysfunction of HPV E1 or E2 ORF, which are active during HPV replication. E2 loss of function allows up-regulation of E6 and E7 oncoproteins, because E2 is a repressor of E6 and E7. (Figure 2).

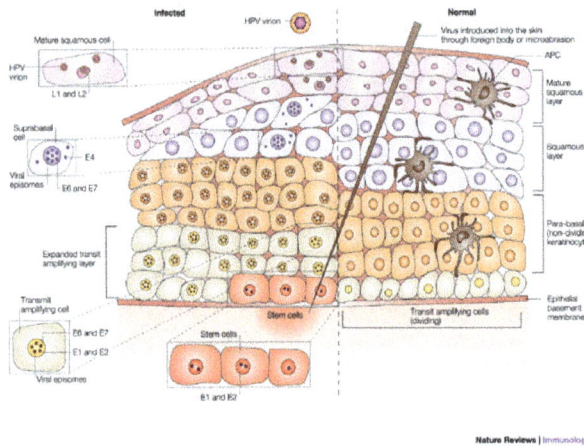

Figure 2. The location in squamous epithelium of the main stages of the papillomavirus life cycle. [46]

3. Diagnosis of HPV infections

Despite the promising outcomes, vaccination does not exempt from performing periodic control visits, because the effects of the vaccine at 15-20 years and the role other genotypes with oncogenic capacity not included in the vaccine may play are still unknown. Furthermore, there is still a large population of women which has had no access to it. Then, secondary prevention by screening and treatment will continue to be crucially important in cervical cancer prevention programs. Moreover, the fact that infection by HPV provokes long-term symptomatology demands a close follow-up (screening) of those individuals susceptible to infection in order to avoid related problems.

Currently, cervical cancer screening is acknowledged as the most effective approach for cervical cancer control. The primary screening and diagnostic methods have been cytology and histology, but two limitations of the Pap smear exist: low specificity leading to the need for repeat screening at relatively short intervals and cervical cancer screening, based on Pap smear, remains beyond the economic resources of nation in developing world. This economic disparity has meant that cervical cancer incidence and mortality rates in the developing world have remained high, with large reductions in these rates being limited primarily to the industrialized world. Thus, the reduction of cervical cancer in developing nations remains an unmet need of high priority. Since the link between HPV and cervical cancer is known and numerous large scale studies have been done, molecular methods to detect HPV DNA in clinical specimens (vaginal, urethral, paraurethral, anal or pharyngeal exudates, biopsies, and, especially, endocervical exudates) have been introduced into screening algorithms.

Increased sensitivity has important clinical outcomes because reduce mortality and an elongation of screening, and implies better compliance with screening and lower cost [47]. An Italian study showed that HPV-based screening is more effective than cytology in preventing invasive cervical cancer, by detecting persistent high-grade lesions earlier and providing longer low-risk period [48].

HPV serves as paradigm for the use of NAATs for its diagnosis and typification due to how difficult it is to obtain the virus via cell cultures or to develop indirect diagnosis techniques [49].

The first protocols for detect HPV were described about 20 years ago, using L1 consensus primers PCR systems, particularly MY09/11 and GP5+/6+ [50-52]. These primer systems have been widely used to study the natural history of HPV and their rule in the development of genital cancer [53-55]. Nowadays, several kits are commercially available which allow for the detection of the virus or the detection and typification of the most relevant HPVs: Amplicor HPV test and Linear array HPV Genotyping test (Roche Diagnostics, Switzerland), Innolipa HPV Genotyping Extra (Innogenetics, Belgium), Biopat kit (Biotools, Spain) or Clart Papillomavirus 2 (Genómica, Spain). The latter uses microarray technology to increase the number of hybridizations in a reduced space. Besides genome amplification, direct hybridization protocols on the sample (hybrid capture) approved by the FDA for diagnosing HPV in women (Hybrid Capture II, Digene, USA) is also used. These protocols identify high and low-risk genotypes without specifying the infecting genotype.

The sensitivity of such methods has left out cytological methods (Papanicolau), which are less sensitive and specific. This high degree of sensitivity allows to extending the period between control visits of women to 5 or 6 years [56, 57].

3.1. Signal amplification systems

The Hybrid Capture II system (HCII, Digene, USA) is a non radioactive signal amplification method based on the hybridization of the target HPV-DNA to labeled RNA probes in solution. The resulting RNA-DNA hybrids are captured onto microtiter wells and are detected by specific monoclonal antibody and chemiluminiscence substrate, providing a semi-quantitative measurement of HPV-DNA. Two different probe cocktails are used, one containing probes for five low-risk gentypes: HPV 6, 11, 42,43 and 44 and the other containing probes for 13 high-risk genotypes: HPV 16,18,31,33,35,39,45,51,52,56,58,59 and 68.

However, HCII has some limitations. It distinguishes between the high-risk and low-risk groups but does not permit identification of specific HPV genotypes. Hybrid Capture II (HCII) has been shown to have similar analytic sensitivity to some PCR methods for HPV DNA detection [58], but present cross-reactivity of the two probe cocktails can reduce the clinical relevance of a positive result [59, 60].

The Hybrid Capture III (HCIII, Digene, USA) is being evaluated as the next generation of hybrid capture clinical assays. A primary technical distinction between HCIII and HCII is that HCIII employs a biotinylated DNA oligonucleotide specific for selected HPV DNA sequences (HPV16 and HPV18) for the capture of the DNA-RNA complexes on streptavidin-coated wells, to reduce false positivity [59].

3.2. Target amplification systems (PCR)

Type specific primers designed to amplify exclusively a single HPV genotype can be use but multiple type-specific PCR reactions must be performed separately to detect the presence of HPV in a sample. This method is labor-intensive, a little bit expensive and the type –specificity of each PCR primer set should be validated. Alternatively, consensus or general PCR primers can be used to amplify a broad-spectrum of HPV types: genome amplification protocols (PCR) with degenerate primers targeted towards the L1 gene fragment (MY09/MY11) allow for the detection of a wide range of viral subtypes, which are then identified with specific probes [50, 61]. Other consensual primers (PGMY, GP5+/GP6+ or SF10) used on the same target enhance diagnostic sensitivity [52, 62, 63]. Thanks to these protocols, the low and high cancer progression risk genotypes were identified [25].

Amplification protocols have also experimented great advancements with the application of real-time PCR, which reduces reaction times (e.g. HPV RealTime test, Abbot, USA; GenoID, Hungary). In fact, it is now possible to automate the whole process (Cobas® 4800 HPV Test with 16/18 Genotyping, Roche Diagnostics, Switzerland).

Type-specific PCR primers can be combined with fluorescent probes to real-time detection [64-66] although multiplexing several type specific primers within one reaction can be technically difficult. Broad-spectrum PCR primers have also been used in real-time PCR [67, 68].

The HCII method and consensus PCR assays are currently the most frecuently applied. In last years, RT-PCR is being introduced in clinical microbiology laboratories.

3.3. Full spectrum genotyping

About 40 different HPV types (involved in human genital infections) have been identified based on DNA sequence analysis so far, with a subset of these being classified as high risk. DNA of these types is found in almost all cervical cancers, however, regional variation in the distribution of certain HPV types should be taken into account in the composition of screening "cocktails" for high-risk HPV types from different populations [29]. The diversity of virus types and the incidence of multiple infections have made it necessary to develop reliable methods to identify the different genotypes, for epidemiological studies as well as for the patient follow up [69]. Over the last few years, virus genotyping has become an important way to approach cervical cancer. Then HPV genotype detection could increase specificity in a routine screening program or in post –treatment follow-up (i.e. test of cure) by differentiating transient and sequential infection from persistent infection [70-72].

Population-based genotyping characterizations pre- and post-vaccination will be important to determinate vaccine effectiveness and potential unmasking of niche replacements by non-vaccines HPV types in cytologically normal women and women with low and high grade lesions.

Genotyping assays have been developed, like GP5+/6+ reverse line blot, or MY90/11 dot-blot. Based in these technologies, specific kits have been comercializated: PGMY09/11 linear array (Linear Array® HPV genotyping test; Roche Molecular Systems, Switzeland) and SPF10 LiPA 25 (Inno-LiPA® HPV test, Innogenetics, Belgium). The assays are based on consensus broad spectrum PCR which are subsequently differentiated by type-specific oligonucleotide probe hybrydizacion. These assays have the ability to identify multiple several viruses in cases of multiple infections. In the last years, others assays for HPV genotyping has been commercial-ised and introduced in clinical and research laboratories with full or partial automation (PapilloCheck HPV-Screening Test, Greiner Bio-One; Clart HPV2, Genomica, Infiniti HPV Genotyping assay, Autogenomics; Cobas 4800 HPV Test, Roche diagnostics; Real Time High Risk HPV test, Abbott Molecular) [73]

As already reported and in spite of its limitations, sequencing could be considered the gold standard for HPV genotyping, due to the possibility of identifying virtually all virus types without mistaken classifications through cross-reactions among similar types, which can occur using tests based on hybriditation [74, 75]. Nevertheless, it was disadvantaged at identifying genotypes in samples with multiple infections, in which viral sequences overlap and it is not possible to distinguish the various types [74, 76].

In any case, genotyping is a technology that has to be incorporated in the HPV surveillance. Waiting for massive sequencing, now the most promising field is automated methods, because simplifies the testing procedure, increases the sample processing capability, minimizes the human errors, facilitates the quality assurance, reduces the cost and can be developed in multiples laboratories.

4. Screening and progression prognostic biomarkers technologies

Because molecular testing for HR-HPV DNA may detect infection too early in the process, with only a small subset of women developing disease that progresses to cancer, there is interest in defining secondary markers that have potential application in identification of women who need to be followed more closely because they are at higher risk of developing high-grade lesions [77]; especially, when the positive predictive value of current screening strategies will be diminished in a vaccinated population [78]. Then, the impetus for new screenig or progre-sion technologies in the developed world is thus predominately driven by the need to increase positive predictive value and reduce over-manegement of low-grade and often transient abnormalities.

In these situations, several surrogate markers are in research.

4.1. HPV viral load

Several studies have suggested that a high HPV-DNA viral load may be a candidate marker that could help identify women at greater risk of CIN progression [64, 65, 79, 80]. It has been reproted that average HPV DNA copy number increases significantly with the grade of CIN mainly for HPV 16, but not for other HR-HPV types [81-83]. Some studies have pointed out that high viral load in cytological normal epithelium could also be a risk factor for neoplasic progression but other studies suggested an important limitation to the utility in screening algorithms for the sustancial overlap oh HPV load values between women without and with CIN and the common presence of more than one carcinogenic HPV type [64, 84].

Real- time PCR techniques have been developed to quantify HPV in clinical samples. Moreover, the HCII provides semiquantitative measurement of HPV–DNA, and some studies have demonstrated that the estimated HCII load correlated well with the precise load generated by RT-PCR [85-86]. However, real-time PCR assays more accurately measure HPV 16 viral load by adjusting the signal obtained for HPV 16 DNA with the amount of cellular DNA calculated for amplification of a human gene, therefore providing a more accurate viral load [64, 65, 87, 88]. However, due to low multiplicity for different HR-HPV types, real-time PCR methods are not suitable as a high-throughput screening tool.

4.2. HPV mRNA

Although HR-HPV genotypes are associated with any grade of dysplasia, these types can be detected in a significant proportion of women with normal cytology. It is konwn that HPV E6 and E7 genes are overexpressed throughout the thickness of epithelial cells in high-grade lesions and cancer. Then, mRNA could be more efficient than cytology for the triage of HPV DNA-positive women, and provides high speficity for high grade cervical intraepithelial neoplasia identification [69, 89-93].

Some authors have developed a real time reverse transcriptase amplificatios (RT–PCR) for HPV detection strategies and suggested that it may be more specific for the detection of symtomatic infections and quantitative increased coordinately with severity of the lesion [94, 95].

These assays incorporates NASBA amplification of E6/7 mRNA transcripts prior to type specific detection via molecular beacons for HPVs 16,18,31,33,and 45. Initial data, on the pronsotic value and specificity for underlying disease, is promising, but the value of this method compared with DNA based assays remains to be determined in large-scale prospective studies [96,97].

Detection of human papillomavirus (HPV) E6/E7 oncogene expression may be more predictive of cervical cancer risk than test HPV-DNA.Commercial test targeting HPV mRNA has been developed: NucliSENS-EasyQ® HPV E6/E7 mRNA assay (Biomerieux, USA) and Aptima HPV test (Gen-Probe, USA) both are a type-specific E6/E7 mRNA test for HR-HPV types performed in one NASBA reaction NucliSENS-EasyQ® HPV E6/E7 mRNA assay detected HPV 16,18,31,33 and 45 with detection and genotyping and Aptima HPV test detects E6/E7 mRNA of 14 oncogenic types HPV16,18,31,33,35,39,45,51,52,56,58,59,66, and 68.

4.3. HPV integration (E2/E6-7 ratio)

Most HR-HPV infections are either latent or permissive. Latent infections are not very well defined, but it is assumed that the viral genome is maintained as an episome in the basal and parabasal cells of the epithelium without inducing obvious phenotypic alterations in the host cell.

The transformation process is characterized by the deregulation of viral oncogenes E6 and E7 in cycling cells which ultimately results in chromosomal instability and the accumulation of mutations. The underlying mechanisms for deregulation are manifold. Integration of the HPV genome is a characteristic step in cervical carcinogenesis and its appearance correlates with the progression of precancerous lesions (CIN2/3) to invasive carcinoma [98-100].

However, integration is not mandatory in this process and was shown to be HPV-type dependent. Vinokurova and colleagues observed that HPV16, 18 and 45 were substantially more often present in an integrated state compared with HPV types 31 and 33 [101].

The loss of the viral E2 gene is a common consequence of HPV integration. This event may lead to an elevated expression of the oncogenes E6 and E7 due to the fact that E2 is no longer able to repress the expression of the viral oncogenes in trans [102, 103]. However, in a recent analysis of biopsy material no correlation between the expression levels of viral oncogene transcripts and the physical state of the viral genome was found [104.

Several investigators have also focussed on the impact integration may have on the host genome. Methods for detection of integrated HPV have been described [87, 105. However, they are affected by similar limitations described for HPV viral load. On the other hand, cervical epithelial cells for women with CIN may simultaneously countain episomal and integrated HPV DNA. Recent data suggest that integration frequency in CIN3 and ICC is variable by HPV genotype, further reducing the desired gains in specificity [101].

4.4. E6-T350G HPV 16 variant

A variety of HPV types have been characterized on the basis of differences greater than 10% in L1 gene sequence [25]. Isolates of the same type are referred to as "variants" when the nucleotide sequences of their coding genes differ by less than 2%, or when the non-coding region (LCR) differs by as much as 5% [106]. HPV 16 is one of the most important HPV genotypes wich cause serius cervical disorders, but amoung these genotypes, certains variants have been linked to different clinical outcomes. HPV 16 variants have been grouped into six distinct phylogenetic branches: E (European), AA (Asian-American), Af1(African 1), Af2 (African 2), NA (North American), As (Asian) with different geographic distributions. Most

HPV16 variants from European and North American samples were classified as European prototype (EP) [107]. Several studies have shown that the infection by the European L83V HPV16 variant, harbouring a nucleotide substitution at position 350 in the E6 gene (E6-T350G), is a risk factor for advanced cervical disease although some discrepant results have also been found [21, 104, 108, 109].

Detection of HPV variant has been performed mainly by Sanger sequencing, pyrosequencing or high resolution melting analysis [110, 111]. A new one-step allelic discrimination real time PCR assay to detect the E6-T350G HPV 16 variant was evaluated in clinical samples, this novel allelic discrimination assay is a fast sensitive and specific method [24].

4.5. p16 enzyme linked inmunosorbent assay

Protein p16 is a cell cycle regulation protein which accumulates in abnormal epithelial cells infected with HR-HPVs as a result of a loss of negative regulation by the retinoblastoma protein induced by E7 expresion [112]. In immunostaining studies, p16 (INK4a) has shown potential as a marker of high grade cervical intraepithelial neoplasia (CIN) and invasive cervical cancer [113, 114]. A recent literature report demonstrates different p16 accuracy according to different anatomical sub-sites. In this complex scenario the p16-IHC test alone or in association to CDKN2a promoter methylation could be used only as screening methods but need to be associated with molecular tests in order to detect HPV-DNA and to assess its integration status. Furthermore, non-dysplastic cells, particulary methaplastic, atrophic and endocervical cells, may display p16 immunoreactivity, thereby reducing specificity [115].

4.6. Methylation profile

Methylation of CpG islands within gene promoter regions can lead to silencing of gene expression. Methylation of tumor-relevant genes has been identified in many cancers: p16 methylation is the paradigm for epigenetic inactivation of a tumor suppressor gene, leading to abrogation of cell cycle control, escape from senescence, and induction of proliferation.

Methylation has been detected already at precancerous stages, suggesting that methylation markers may have value in cervical cancer screening [116]. Furthermore, methylated DNA is a stable target and allows for flexibility of assay development.The detection of methylated genes from cervical specimens is technically feasible and represents a source for detecting potential biomarkers of relevance to cervical carcinogenesis. In particular, there is the ultimate hope of finding methylation markers that, among HPV-infected women, would indicate the presence of CIN2+ and risk of cancer.

A clear role of methylation in carcinogenesis has been demonstrated only for 6 genes (DAPK1, RASSF1, CDKN2A, RARB, MLH1, and GSTP1 [117].

During the last years, several new platforms have been developed that allow for accurate high-throughput genome-wide DNA methylation profiling [118]. Markers or marker panels identified in these approaches could be translated to smaller scaled assays such as Methylight to be used in cervical cancer screening, but their use is in research.

4.7. Human telomerase RNA component (hTERC)-gain

It has been generally accepted that carcinogenesis involves the progressive accumulation of genetic abnormalities. Gain at 3q is a common feature of squamous-cell carcinoma (SCC), with an overlapping area of gain at 3q26 having been reported in SCC at different anatomic sites [119], including cervix of the uterus [120, 121].

The human telomerase RNA component (hTERC) gene, localized on chromosome 3q26, encodes the RNA component of human telomerase, and acts as a template for the addition of the repeat sequence [122]. Genetic studies have shown that amplification of *hTERC* gene might be an early event commonly involved in the progression of CIN to cervical cancer [123-127].

Amplification of hTERC gene has been identified in many tumor samples and immortalized cell lines using techniques such as fluorescence in situ hybridization (FISH) and Southern blot analysis, suggesting that transcription is upregulated during tumorigenesis [128]. Lan YL et al. confirm that measuring hTERC gene gain could be a useful biomarker to predict the progression of CIN-I or –II to CIN-III and cervical cancer [129]. The present limitation to this assay is the technical complexity and requeriment of highly trained individuals to interpret the FISH staining, however automated methods for reading TERCH FISH slides are under development.

4.8. Other proliferation/cell cycle markers

HPV contributes to neoplastic progression predominantly through the action of two viral oncoproteins (E6 and E7) and is manifested by changes in the expression of host cell cycle regulatory proteins [130]. Such differentially expressed host proteins and nucleic acids may have a role as "biomarkers" of dysplastic cells.

To date, a wide array of molecular markers has been evaluated. Three markers that have shown the greatest potential are the cyclin dependant kinase inhibitor p16^{INK4} [131, 132] and the DNA replication licensing proteins CDC6 (cell division cycle protein 6) and MCM5 (mini chromosome maintenance 5) [133]. Some authors found that three markers showed a linear correlation between their presence or absence and the grade of dysplasia [132].

5. Summary

In summary, the relevance of HPV infections requires a close monitoring, especially in certain groups o individuals (e. i. Women older than 30 years old). The accuracy of methos using NAATs has emerged as election in the control of HPV infection. But the search is ongoing for safer: more precise markers which may allow for a better control of the infection [134]. These markers include genome quantification via real-time PCR, viral integration into the human genome via E2-E1/E6-E7 genes ratio or the search of viral variants by sequencing, pyrose-quencing or allelic discrimination techniques [24, 109, 135].

Addition of new technologies into existing, highly efective screening programs are considered according to the ability to increase the efficiency of the program (high sensitivity with reduction in unnecessary follow-up of minor, transient infection) [136].

The table 2 presents a summary of the technologies relative to their intended or perceived benefit and limitations compared to existing screening and progression prognostic biomarkers methods [136].

Technology	Benefits	Limitations
HCII	Non radioactive signal amplification method	Not identification of specific HPV genotypes
	Distinguishes between the high-risk and low-risk HPV	Cross-reactivity between high-risk and low-risk HPV
	Similar analytic sensitivity to some PCR methods for HPV DNA detection	
PCR	Non radioactive signal amplification method	Contamination
	Low cost	
	Amenable to use with many-samples	
HPV genotyping	Discrimination of HPV-18/18 from other high-risk types may have greater positive predictive value.	Moderate to high complexity even with standardized commercial reagents.
	May differentiate sequential infection with different types from persistent infection with the same type.	Very difficult to establish consensus primer-based genotyping de novo with adequate quality control
	Useful for test of cure.	Algorithms may be too complicated to be readily translated into clinical practice.
	Amenable to use with self-sampling.	High cost
	Compatible with many collection buffers.	
	Objective output.	
HPV mRNA	Potential to increase specificity	Moderate to high complexity
	Objective output.	RNA less stable, not compatible with some common collection buffers
		Compatibility with self-sampling unknown
		High cost
HPV viral load	Potential to increase specificity	High complexity
	Objective and quantitative output.	Not pronostic (except for HPV 16)
		Requires type-specific quantitation
		High cost

Technology	Benefits	Limitations
HPV integration	Potential to increase specificity	Moderate complexity for DNA methods
	Objective output.	Very high complexity to detect integrated transcripts
		Integrated DNA may not be transcriptionally active
		Requires type-specific assay
		Common occurrence of mixed episomal and integrated HPV in cervical intraepithelial neoplasia
		High cost
p16 enzyme liked inmunobsorbent assay	Single analyte (p16protein) to detect infection with any high-risk HPV	Moderate complexity
	May increase specificity by detecting active infection	Compatibility with self-sampling unknown
	Subjective output	Not compatible with all collection buffers
	Cost may be lower than DNA/RNA test	Order of sampling may affect performance
		Low specifity
Methylacion profile	As a marker of disease and not infection, may increase specificity	High complexity
	Compatible with urine sampling	Sensitivity limited; questionable reproducibility
	Objective output.	High cost
TERC-gain	As a marker of disease and not infection, may increase specificity	Very high complexity
	Subjective output	High cost
	May be useful as a pronostic marker	
Other proliferation/ cell cycle markers	As a marker of disease and not infection, may increase specificity	High complexity
	Subjective output	Questionable reproducibility
		High cost

TERC: telomerase RNA component. Adapted from Gravitt et al [135]

Table 2. Screening and progression prognostic biomarkers technologies.

Author details

Santiago Melón, Marta Alvarez-Argüelles and María de Oña

Virology Unit (Microbiology Service), Hospital Universitario Central de Asturias (HUCA), Oviedo, Asturias, Spain

References

[1] Ferlay J, Bray F, Pisani P, Parkin DM. Globocan 2000: cancer incidence, mortality and prevalence world wide.IARC CancerBase no.5. Lyons, France: IARC press 2001.

[2] Parkin DM, Bray F, Ferlay J, Pisani P. Estimating the world cancer burden: Globocan 2000. Int J Cancer 2001; 94:153-6.

[3] Zur Hausen H. Papillomaviruses and cancer: from basic studies to clinical application. Nat Rev Cancer 2002;(2):342-50.

[4] Bosch FX, Lorincz A, Muñoz N, Meijer CJ, Shah KV. The casual relation between human papilomavirus and cervical cancer. J Clin Pathol 2002;55:244-65.

[5] Steenbergen RDM, de WildeJ, Wilting SM, Brink AATP, Snijders PJF, Meier CJLM. HPV-mediated transformation of the anogenital tract. J Clin Virol 2005; 32(suppl):43-51.

[6] Georgieva S, Iordanov V, Sergieva S. Nature of cervical cancer and other HPV-associated cancers. J Buon 2009(14): 391-8.

[7] Castellsague X, de San José S, Aguado T, Louie KS, Bruni L, Muñoz et al., editors. HPV and Cervical cancer in the world. 2007 Report. WHO/ICO Information Centre on HPV and Cervical cancer (HPV Information Centre). Vaccine 2007; 25(suppl 3).

[8] De San José S, Diaz M, Castellsague X, Clifford G, Bruni L, Muñoz N et el. Worldwide prevalence and genotype distribution of cervical human papillomavirus DNA in women with normal cytology: a meta-analysis. Lancet Infect Dis 2007;7(7):453-9.

[9] Dunne EF Nielson CM, Stone KM, Markowitz LE, Giuliano AR.Prevalence of HPV infection among men: a systemic review of the literature. J Infect Dis 2006; 194:1044-57.

[10] Molano M, van den Brule A, Plummer M, Weiderpass E, Poso H, Arslan A, por el HPV Study group. Determinants of clearance of human papillomavirus infections in Colombian womens with normal cytology: a population –based, 5 years follow-up study. Am J Epidemiol. 2003;158:486-94.

[11] Partridge JM, Koutsky LA. Genital human papillomavirus infection in men. Lancet Infect Dis 2006; 6:21-31.

[12] Vaccarella S, Franceschi S, Herrero R, Muñoz N, Snijders PJ, Clifford GM, et al. Sexual behaviour, condom use, and human papillomavirus: pooled analysis of the IARC

human papilomavirus prevalence surveys. Cancer Epidemiol Biomarkers Prevention 2006;15: 326-33.

[13] Wiley D, Masongsong E. Human Papillomavirus: the burden of infection. Obstet Gynecol Surv.2006:61(suppl)3-14.

[14] Smith JS, Herrero R, Bosetti C, Muñoz N, Bosch FX, Eluf-Neto J, Castellsagué X, Meijer C, van den Brule A, Franceschi S, Ashley R, por el International Agency for Research on Cancer (IARC) Multicentric Cervical Cancer Study Group. Herpes simplex virus-2 as a human papillomavirus cofactor in the etiology of invasive cervical cancer. J Nat Cancer Inst. 2002;94:1604-13.

[15] Castellsagué X, Muñoz N. Cofactors in human papillomavirus carcinogenesis-role of parity, oral contraceptives, and tobacco smoking. J Natl Cancer Inst Monogr. 2003;31.20-28.

[16] Palefsky JM, Holly EA. Inmunosuppression and co-infection with HIV. J Natl Cancer Inst Monogr. 2003;31:41-6.

[17] Hopman AH, Kamps MA, Smedts F, Speed EJ, Herrington CS, Ramaekers FC. HPV in situ hybridization: impact of different protocols on the detection of integrated HPV. Int J Cancer.2005;115:419-28.

[18] Khan M, Castle P, Lorincz A, Wacholder S, Sherman M, Scott D, et al. The elevated 10-year risk of cervical precancer and cancer in women with human papillomavirus (HPV) type 16 or 18 and the possible utility of type-specific HPV testing in clinical practice. J Natl Cancer Inst. 2005;97:1072-9.

[19] Trimble C, Genkinger J, Burke A, Hoffman S, Helzlisouer K, Diener-West M, et al. Active and passive cigarette smoking and the risk of cervical neoplasia. Obstet Gynecol. 2005;105:174-81.

[20] Tseng HF, Morgenstern H, Mark T, Peters RK. Risk factors for penile cancer: results of a population-based case-control study in Los Angeles Country (United States). Cancer Causes Control 2005;2:298.

[21] Grodzki M, Besson G, Clavel C, Arslan A, Franceschi S, Birembaut P,et al. Increased risk for cervical disease progression of French women infected with the human papillomavirus type 16 E6-350G variant. Cancer Epidemiol Blomarkers Prev. 2006;15:820-2.

[22] Peter M, Rosty C, Couturier C, Radvanyi F, Teshima H, Sastre-Garau X. MYC activation associated with the integration of HPV DNA at the MYC locus in genital tumors. Oncogene. 2006;25:5985-93.

[23] Winer R, Hughes J, Feng Q, O'Reilly S, Kiviat N, Colmes K, et al. Condom use and the risk of genital human papillomavirus infection in young woman. N Engl J Med . 2006; 354:2645-54.

[24] Perez S, Cid A, Araujo A, Lamas MJ, Saran MT, Alvarez MJ, et al. A novel real-time genotyping assay for detection of the E6-350G HPV 16 variant. J Virol Methods 2011; 173(2)357-63.

[25] Bernard HU, Burk RD, Chen Z, van Doorslaer K, Hausen Hz, de Villiers EM. Classification of papilllomaviruses (PVs) based on 189 PV types and proposal of taxonomic amendments. Virology 2010; 401(1):70-79.

[26] De Villiers EM. Taxonomic classification of papillomaviruses. Papillomavirus Rep 2001;12:57-63.

[27] Davies P, Kornegay J, Iftner T. Current methos of testing for human papilomavirus. Best Pract Res Clin Obstet Gyneacol 2001; 15:677-700.

[28] Van der Brule AJ, Pol R, Fransen-Daalmeijer N, Schouls LM, Meijer CJLM, Snijders PJ. GP5+/6+ PCR followed by reverse line blot analysis enables rapid and high-throughput identification of human papilomavirus genotypes. J Clin Microbiol 2002; 40:779-87.

[29] Muñoz N, Bosch FX, de Sanjosé S, Herrero R, Castellsagué X, Shah KV, et al. Epidemiological classification of human papillomavirus types associated with cervical cancer. N. Engl.J.Med. 2003:348;518-27.

[30] Castellsague X, Diaz M, de San José S, Muñoz N, Herrero H, Franceschi S. et al. Worldwide human papillomavirus etiology of cervical adenocarcinoma and its factors: implications for screnning and prevention. J Nat Cancer Inst 2006; 985:303-15.

[31] Smith JS, Lindsay L, Hoots B, Keys J, Franceschi S, Winer R, et al. Human papilomavirus type distribution in invasive cervical cancer and high-grade cervical lesions: a meta-analysis update. Int J Cancer 2007; 121(3):621-32.

[32] Bernard HU, Calleja-Macias IE, Dunn ST. Genome variation of human papillomavirus types: phylogenetic and medical implications. Int J Cancer. 2006;118:1071-6.

[33] Picconi MA, Alonio LV, Sichero L, Mbayed V, Villa LL, Gronda J, et al. Human papillomavirus type-16 variants in Quechua aboriginals from Argentina. J Med Virol. 2003;69:546-52.

[34] Muñoz N, Bosch FX, Castellsague X, Diaz M, de San José S, Hammouda D et al. Against which human papilomavirus types shall we vaccinate and screen? The international perspective. Int J Cancer 2004; 111(2):278-85.

[35] Lont AP, Kroon BK, Horenblas S, Gallee MP, Berkhof J, Meijer CJ et al . Presence of high-risk human papillomavirus DNA in penile carcinoma predicts favorable outcome in survival. Int J Cancer 2006; 119(5):21078-81.

[36] Fairley CK, Donovan B. What can surveillance of genital warts tell us? Sex Health. 2010;7(3):325-7.

[37] Insigna RP, Dasbach EJ, Elbasha EH. Assessing the annual economic burden of preventing and treating anogenital human papilomavirus related disease in the US:

analytic framework and review of the literature. Pharmacoeconomics 2005; 23(11): 1107-22.

[38] Brown RE, Breugelmans JG, Theodoratou D, Bernard S. Cost of detection and treatment of cervical cancer, cervical dysplasia and genital warts in the UK. Curr Med Res Opin 2006;22(4):663-70.

[39] Lacey CJ, Lowndes CM, Shah KV. Chapter 4: Burden and management of non-cancerous HPV-related conditions: HPV 6/11 disease. Vaccine 2006.Aug 21;24 (suppl 3):35-41.

[40] Potocnik M, Kocjan BJ, Seme K, Poljak M. Distribution of human papilomavirus (HPV) genotypes in genital warts from males in Slovenia. Acta Dermatoven APA 2007;16(3): 91-6.

[41] Cremin S, Menton JF, Canier L, Horgan M, Fanning I.J. The prevalence and genotype of human papilomavirus on cervical samples from an Irish female population with external genital warts. Hum Vaccin Immunother 2012; 8 (7): 916-920.

[42] IARC .Cancer incidence in five continents, Vol IX. IARC Scientific Publications No. 160.Lyon:IARC, 2007.

[43] IARC. Human papilomavirus.IARC Monographs on the Evaluation of carcinomagenic risk to humans.2007, Vol.90.Lyon.

[44] D'Souza G, Kreimer AR, Viscidi R, Pawlita M, Fakhry C, Koch WM, et al. Case control study of human papilomavirus and oropharyngeal cancer. N Engl J Med 2007;356(19): 1944-56.

[45] Doorbar J. Molecular biology of human papilomavirus infection and cervical cancer. Clinical Science 2006; 110: 525–41.

[46] Frazer IH. Prevention of cervical cancer through papilomavirus vaccination. *Nature Reviews Immunology 2004;* 4:46-55

[47] Origoni M, Cristoforoni P, Costa S, Mariani L, Scirpa P, Lorincz A, et al. HPV-DNA testing for cervical cancer precursors: from evidence to clinical practice. e-cancer 2012; 6:258.

[48] Ronco G, Giorgi-Ross P, Caorzzi F et al for the NewTechnologies for Cervical Cancer screening (NTCC) Working Group. Efficacy of human papilomavirus testing for the detection of invasive cervical cancers and cervical intraepithelial neoplasia: a rando-mised controlled trial. Lancet Oncol, 2012; 11:259-57.

[49] Dillner J. The serological response to papilomavirus. Semin Cancer Biol 1999; 9:423-30.

[50] Manos MM, Ting Y, Wright DK, Lewis JA, Broker TR, Wolinsky SM. Use of polymerase chain reaction amplification for the detection of genital human papillomaviruses. Cancer Cells 1989; 7:209–14.

[51] Bauer HM, Greer CE, Mannos MM. Determination of genital human papillomavirus infection using consensus PCR. C.s. Herrington and J.O.D Mc Gee (ed.). Diagnostic

molecular pathology: a practical approach. Oxford University Press, Oxford, United Kingdom. 1992; p.132-152.

[52] Jacobs MV, Snijders PJ, van den Brule AJ, Helmerhorst TJ, Meijer CJ, Walboomers JM. A general primer GP5+/GP6+-mediated PCR-enzyme inmunnoassay method for rapid detection of 14 high-risk and 6 low-risk human papilomavirus genotypes in genital scrapings. J Clin Microb.1997;35:791-5.

[53] Schiffman M, Bauer H, Hoover R, Glass AG, Cadell DM, Rush BB, et al.Epidemiologic evidence showing the HPV infection causes most cervical intraepithelial neoplasia. J Natl Cancer Inst. 1993; 85:958–64.

[54] Kjaer SK, van den Brule AJ, Bock JE, Poll PA, Engholm G, Sherman ME, et al. Human papillomavirus—the most significant risk determinant of cervical intraepithelial neoplasia. Int J Cancer 1996; 65:601–06.

[55] Ho GY, Bierman R, Beardsley L, Chang CJ, Burk RD. Natural history of cervicovaginal papillomavirus infection in young women. N. Engl. Med. 1998; 338:423-8.

[56] Dillner J, Rebolj M, Birembaut P, Petry KU, Szarewski A, Munk C, et al. Long term predictive values of cytology and human papillomavirus testing in cervical cancer screening: joint European cohort study. BMJ 2008; 337:a1754.

[57] De Oña M, Álvarez-Argüelles ME, Torrents M, Villa L, Rodríguez-Feijoo A, Palacio A, et al. Prevalence, evolution, and features of infection with human papillomavirus: a 15-year longitudinal study of routine screening of a women population in the north of Spain. J Med Virol 2010; 82:597-604.

[58] Bozzetti M, Nonnenmacher B, Mielzinska I, Villa L, Lorincz A, Breitenbach V et al. Comparision between Hybrid Capture 2 and polymerase chain reaction results among women at low-risk for cervical cancer. Ann Epidemiol 2000; 10:466.

[59] Castle PE, Schiffman M, Burk RD, Hildesheim A, Herrero R, Bratti MC, et al. Restricted cross-reactivity of hybrid capture 2 Test with low-risk human papillomavirus types. Cancer Epidemiol. Biomark. Prev. 2002; 11:1394-9.

[60] Poljak M, Marin IJ, Seme K, Vince A. Hybrid Capture II HPV test detects at least 15 human papilomavirus genotypes not included in its current high-risk probe cocktail. J Clin Virol 2002: 25(suppl 3):89-97.

[61] Ting Y, Manos MM. Detection and typing of genital human papillomaviruses, p. 356-367. In: M. Innis, D. Gelfand, J. Sninsky, and T. White (ed.), PCR Protocols: A Guide to Methods and Applications. 1990 Academic Press, Inc., San Diego, Calif.

[62] Kleter B, van Doorn LJ, Schrauwen L, Molijn A, Sastrowijoto S, ter Schegget J, et al. Development and clinical evaluation of highly sensitive PCR-reverse hybridization line probe assay of detection and identification of anogenital human papillomavirus. J Clin Microbiol 1999; 37:2508-17.

[63] Gravitt PE, Peyton CL, Alessi TQ, Wheeler CM, Coutlée F, Hildesheim A, et al. Improved amplification of genital human papillomaviruses. J Clin Microbiol 2000; 38: 357-61.

[64] Josefsson AM, Magnusson PK, Ylitalo N, Sorensen P, Qwar-forth-Tubbin P, Andersen PK,et al. Viral load of human papilomavirus 16 as a determinant for development of cervical carcinoma in situ: a nested case-control study. Lancet, 2000.355:2189-93.

[65] Ylitalo N, Josefsson A, Melbye M, Sorensen P, Frisch M, Andersen PK et al. A prospective study showing long-term infection with human papillomavirus 16 before the development of cervical carcinoma in situ. Cancer Res 2000; 60:6027-32.

[66] Tucker RA, Unger ER, Holloway BP, Swan DC. Real-Time PCR-based fluorescent assay for quantitation of human papilomavirus types 6,11,16 and 18. Mol Diagn 2001;6:39-47.

[67] Strauss S, Desselberger U, Gray JJ. Detection of genital and cutaneus human papillomavirus types: differences in the sensitivity of generic PCRs, and consequences for clinical virological diagnosis. Br J Biomed Sci 2000; 57:221-5.

[68] Cubie HA, Seagar AL, McGoogan E, Whitehead J, Brass A, Arends MJ, et al. Rapid real-time PCR to distinguish between human papillomavirus types 16 and 18. Mol Pathol 2001;54:24-9.

[69] Sotlar K, Stubner A, Diemer D, Menton S, Menton M, Dietz K, Wallwiener D, Kandolf R, Bültmann B. Detection of high-risk human papillomavirus E6 and E7 oncogene transcripts in cervical scrapes by nested RT-polymerase chain reaction. J Med Virol. 2004;74(1):107-16.

[70] Schiffman M. Integration of human papilomavirus vaccination, cytology and human papillomavirus testing. Cancer 2007;111(3)145:53.

[71] Wright Jr TC, Massad LS, Dunton CJ, Spitzer M, Wilkinson EJ, Solomon D. 2006 consensus guidelines for the management of women with abnormal cervical screening test. J low Genit Tract Dis 2007;11(4):201-22.

[72] Rodriguez AC, Shiffman M, Herrero R, Wacholder S, Hildesheim A, Castle PE, et al. Rapid clearance of human papillomavirus and implications for clinical focus on persistent infections. J Natl Cancer Inst 2008;100(7):513-7.

[73] Torres M, Fraile L, Echevarría JM, Hernández-Novoa B, Ortiz M. Humana Papillomaviru (HPV) Genotyping: automation and application in routine laboratory testing. Open Virol J, 2012; 6:144-150.

[74] Serrano ML, Correa M, Medina O, Melgarejo D, Bravo MM. Tipificación de vírus del papiloma humano mediante secuencia directa en mujeres com citología normal. Rev Colomb Cancer. 2003;7: 18-24.

[75] Fontaine V, Mascaux C, Weyn C, Bernis A, Celio N, Lefevre P, et al. Evaluation of combined general primer-mediated PCR sequencing and type-specific PCR strategies

for determination of human papillomavirus genotypes in cervical cell specimens. J Clin Microbiol 2007;45: 928-34.

[76] Choi YD, Jung WW, Nam JH, Choi HS, Park CS. Detection of HPV genotypes in cervical lesions by the HPV DNA chip and sequencing. Ginecol Oncol 2005;98: 369-75.

[77] Schiffman M, Kjaer SK. Natural history of anogenital human papillomavirus infection and neoplasia. J Natl Cancer Inst Monogr. 2004 ;31:14-9.

[78] Clifford GM, Gallus S, Herrero R, Muñoz N, Snijders PJ, Vaccarella S, et al. Wordwide distribution of human papilomavirus types in cytologically normal womwn in the IARC HPV prevalence surveys: a pooled analysis. Lancet 2005;366(9490):991-8.

[79] Van Duin M, Snijders PJ, Schrijnemakers HF, Voorhorst FJ, Rozendaal L, Nobbebhuis MA, et al. Human papilomavirus 16 load in normal and abnormal cervical scrapes: an indicator of CIN II/III and viral clearance. Int J Cancer 2002; 98:590-5.

[80] Carcopini X, Henry M, Olive D, Boubli L, Tamalet C. Detection and quantification of human papillomavirus genital infections: virological, epidemiological, and clinical applications. Med Mal Infect 2011;41 (29):68-79.

[81] Gravitt PE, Peyton CL, Wheeler C, Apple R, Higuchi R, Shah KV. Reproducibility of HPV 16 and HPV 18 viral load quantitation using TaqMan real-time PCR assays. J Virol Methods 2003; 112: 23–33.

[82] Weissenborn SJ, Funke AM, Hellmich M, Mallmann P, Fuchs PG, Pfister HJ, et al. Oncogenic human papillomavirus DNA loads in human immunodeficiency virus-positive women with high-grade cervical lesions are strongly elevated. J Clin Microbiol 2003;41: 2763–67.

[83] Tábora N, Ferrera A, Bakkers J, Massuger L, Melchers WJG. High HPV 16 Viral Load is Associated with Increased Cervical Dysplasia in Honduran Women.Am J Trop Med Hyg 2008; 78(5):843-6.

[84] Fontaine J, Hankins C, Mayrand MH, Levre J, Money D, Gagnon S et al. High levels of HPV-16 DNA are associated with high-grade cervical lesions in women at risk or infected with HIV. AIDS 2005;19(8):785-94.

[85] Sun CA, Liu JF, Wu DM, Nieh S, Yu CP, Chu TY. Viral load of high-risk human papillomavirus in cervical squamous intraepithelial lesions. Int J Gynaecol Obstet 2002; 76: 41–7.

[86] Dalstein V, Riethmuller D, Pretet JL, Le Bail Carval K, Sautiere JL, Carbillet JP, et al. Persistence and load of high-risk HPV are predictors for development of high-grade cervical lesions: a longitudinal French cohort study. Int J Cancer 2003; 106: 396–403.

[87] Nagao S, Yoshinouchi M, Miyagi Y, Hongo A, Kodama J, Itoh S, et al. Rapid and sensitive detection of physical status of human papillomavirus type 16 DNA by quantitative real-time PCR. J Clin Microbiol 2002;40: 863–7.

[88] Peitsaro P, Johansson B, Syrjanen S. Integrated human papillomavirus type 16 is frequently found in cervical cancer precursors as demonstrated by a novel quantitative real-time PCR technique. J Clin Microbiol 2002; 40: 886–91.

[89] Castle PE, Dockter J, Giachetti C, Garcia FA, Mc Cormick MK, Mitchell Al, et al. A cross-sectional study of a prototype carcinogenic human papilomavirus E6/E7 messenger RNA assay for detection of cervical precancer and cancer. Clin Cancer Res 2007; 13(9): 2599-605.

[90] Arbyn M, Ronco G, Cuzick J, Wentzensen N, Castle PE. How to evaluate emerging technologies in cervical cancer screening? Int J Cancer. 2009;125(11):2489-96.

[91] Halfon P, Benmoura D, Agostini A, Khiri H, Martineau A, Penaranda G, et al. Relevance of HPV mRNA detection in a population of ASCUS plus women using the NucliSENS EasyQ HPV assay. J Clin Virol. 2010;47(2):177-81.

[92] Benevolo M, Vocaturo A, Caraceni D, French D, Rosini S, Zappacosta R, et al. Sensitivity, specificity, and clinical value of human papillomavirus (HPV) E6/E7 mRNA assay as a triage test for cervical cytology and HPV DNA test. J Clin Microbiol. 2011;49(7):2643-5.

[93] Perez S, Iñarrea A, Lamas MJ, Saran MT, Cid A, Alvarez MJ, et al. Human Papillomavirus (HPV) E6/E7 mRNA assay as a triage test after HPV16 and 18 DNA detection. J Med Virol, 2012; in press.

[94] Lamarcq L, Deeds J, Ginzinger D, Perry J, Padmanabha S, Smith Mc Cune K. Measurements of human papilomavirus transcripts by real time quantitative reverse transcription polymerase chain reaction in samples colledted for cervical cancer screening. J Mol Diagn 2002;4(2):97-102.

[95] Wang-Johanning F, Lu DW, Wang Y, Johnson MR, Johanning GL. Quantitation of human papillomavirus 16 E6 and E7 DNA and RNA in residual material from ThinPrep papanicolau test using realtime polymerase chain reactions analysis. Cancer 2002; 94(8):2199-210.

[96] Kraus I, Molden T, Erno LE, Skomedal H, Karlsen F, Hagmar B. Human papillomavirus oncogenic expression in dysplastic portio; an investigation of biopsies fron 190 cervical cones. Br J Cancer 2004;90:1407-13.

[97] Lie AK Risberg B, Delabie J, Begum S, Rimalla R, Hagen B. DNA versus RNA based methods for HPV testing in screening evaluation of Hybrid Capture II and pre-tect HPV proofer in Norway 2004. In: Proceedings of the 21st International Papillomavirus Conference; 2004.p.55 [abstract].

[98] Kalantari M, Calleja-Macias IE, Tewari D, Hagmar B, Lie K, Barrera-Saldana HA, et al. Conserved methylation patterns of human papillomavirus type 16 DNA in asymptomatic infection and cervical neoplasia. J.Virol. 78: 12762-2.

[99]   Wentzensen N, Vinokurova S, von Knebel Doeberitz M. Systematic review of genomic integration sites of human papillomavirus genomes in epithelial dysplasia and invasive cancer of the female lower genital tract. Cancer Res 2004;64. 3070-04.

[100] Pett M, Coleman N. Integration of high-risk human papillomavirus: a key event in cervical carcinogenesis? J Pathol 2007;212: 356–67.

[101] Vinokurova S, Wentzensen N, Kraus I, Klaes R, Driesch C, Melsheimer P, et al. Type dependent integration frecuency of human papilomavirus genomes in cervical lesions. Cancer Res 2008;68(1)307-13.

[102] Baker CC, Phelps WC, Lindgren V, Braun MJ, Gonda MA, et al. Structural and transcriptional analysis of human papillomavirus type 16 sequences in cervical carcinoma cell lines. Journal of virology 1987;61: 962–971.

[103] Romanczuk H, Howley PM. Disruption of either the E1 or the E2 regulatory gene of human papillomavirus type 16 increases viral immortalization capacity. Proceedings of the National Academy of Sciences of the United States of America 1992;89: 3159–63.

[104] Hafner N, Driesch C, Gajda M, Jansen L, Kirchmayr R, Runnebaum IB et al. Integration of the HPV16 genome does not invariably result in high levels of viral oncogene transcripts. Oncogene 2008;27: 1610–7.

[105] Luft F, Klaes R, Nees M, Duerst M, Heilmann V, Melsheimer P, et al. Detection of integrated papillomavirus sequences by ligation-mediated PCR (DIPS-PCR) and molecular characterization in cervical cancer cells. Int J Cancer 2001; 92(1):9-17.

[106] Bernard HU, Calleja-Macias IE, Dunn ST. Genome variation of human papillomavirus types: phylogenetic and medical implications. Int J Cancer. 2006; 118:1071–6.

[107] Yamada T, Mannos MM, Peto J, Greer CE, Muñoz N, Bosch FX, et al. Human papillo-mavirus type 16 sequence variation in cervical cancers: a wordwide perspective J Virol 1997;71 :2463-72.

[108] Xi LF, Kiviat NB, Hildesheim A, Galloway DA, Wheeler CM, Ho J, et al. Human papilomavirus type 16 and 18 varianst: race-related distribution and persistence. J Natl Cancer Inst 2006; 98: 1045-52.

[109] Zuna RE, Moore WE, Shanesmith RP, Dunn ST, Wang SS, Schiffman M, et al. Associ-ation of HPV16 E6 variants with diagnostic severity in cervical cytology samples of 354 women in a US population. Int J Cancer 2009;125: 2609-13.

[110] Sabol I, Cretnik M, Hadzisejdić I, Si-Mohamed A, Matovina M, Grahovac B, Levanat S, Grce M. A new approach for the evaluation of the human papillomavirus type 16 variability with high resolution melting analysis. J Virol Methods. 2009;162(1-2):142-7. Epub 2009 Aug 5.

[111] Swan DC, Limor JR, Duncan KL, Rajeevan MS, Unger ER. Human papillomavirus type 16 variant assignment by pyrosequencing. J Virol Methods. 2006;136(1-2):166-70.

[112] Klaes R, Friedrich T, Spitkovsky D, Ridder R, Rudy W, Petry U et al. Overexpression of p16 as a specific marker for dysplastic and neoplastic epithelial cells of the cervix uteri. Int J Cancer 2001;92:276–84.

[113] O'Neill CJ, McCluggage WG. p16 expression in the female genital tract and its value in diagnosis. Adv Anat Pathol. 2006;13(1):8-15.

[114] Mao C, Balasubramanian A, Yu M, Kiviat N, Ridder R, Reichert A, et al. Evaluation of a new p16(INK4A) ELISA test and a high-risk HPV DNA test for cervical cancer screening: results from proof-of-concept study. Int J Cancer. 2007 1;120(11):2435-8.

[115] Wentzensen N, Bergeron C, Cas F, Eschenbach D, Vinokurova S, von Knebel Doeberitz M. Evaluation of a nuclear score for p16INK4a-stained cervical squamous cells in liquid-based cytology samples. Cancer Cytopathology 2005; 105(6):461–7.

[116] Esteller M. Epigenetics in cancer. N Engl J Med. 2008 Mar 13;358(11):1148–59.

[117] Wentzensen N, Sherman ME, Schiffman M, Wang SS. Utility of methylation markers in cervical cancer early detection: appraisal of the state-of-the-science. Gynecol Oncol. 2009;112(2):293-9.

[118] Gargiulo G, Minucci S. Epigenomic profiling of cancer cells. Int J Biochem Cell Biol. 2009;41(1):127-35.

[119] Sugita M, Tanaka N, Davidson S, Sekiya S, Varella-Garcia M, West J, et al. Molecular definition of a small amplification domain within 3q26 in tumors of cervix, ovary, and lung. Cancer Genet Cytogenet. 2000;117:9–18.

[120] Hopman AH, Theelen W, Hommelberg PP, Kamps MA, Herrington CS, Morrison LE, et al. Genomic integration of oncogenic HPV and gain of the human telomerase gene TERC at 3q26 are strongly associated events in the progression of uterine cervical dysplasia to invasive cancer. J Pathol. 2006;210:412–9.

[121] Caraway NP, Khanna A, Dawlett M, Guo M, Guo N, Lin E,et al. Gain of the 3q26 region in cervicovaginal liquid-based pap preparations is associated with squamous intrae-pithelial lesions and squamous cell carcinoma. Gynecol Oncol. 2008;110:37–42.

[122] Meyerson M. Role of telomerase in normal and cancer cells. J Clin Oncol. 2000;18:2626–34.

[123] Ramsaroop R, Oei P, Ng D, Kumar N, Cotter PD. Cervical intraepithelialneoplasia and aneusomy of TERC: assessment of liquid-based cytological preparations. Diagn Cytopathol 2009; 37: 411-5.

[124] Sui W, Ou M, Dai Y, Chen J, Lan H, Yan Q, et al. Gain of the human telomerase RNA gene TERC at 3q26 is strongly associated with cervical intraepithelial neoplasia and carcinoma. Int J Gynecol Cancer 2009; 19: 1303-1306.

[125] Zhang Y, Wang X, Ma L, Wang Z, Hu L. Clinical significance of hTERC gene amplifi-cation detection by FISH in the screening of cervical lesions. J Huazhong Univ Sci Technolog Med Sci 2009; 29: 368-71.

[126] Jalali GR, Herzog TJ, Dziura B, Walat R, Kilpatrick MW. Amplification of the chromo-
        some 3q26 region shows high negative predictive value for nonmalignant transforma-
        tion of LSIL cytologic finding. Am J Obstet Gynecol 2010, 202. 501.e1 e5.

[127] Jiang J, Wei LH, Li YL, Wu RF, Xie X, Feng YJ, et al. Detection of TERC amplification
        in cervical epithelial cells for the diagnosis of high-grade cervical lesions and invasive
        cancer: a multicenter study in China. J Mol Diagn 2010; 12: 808-17.

[128] Guilleret I, Yan P, Guillou L, Braunschweig R, Coindre JM, Benhattar J. The human
        telomerase RNA gene (hTERC) is regulated during carcinogenesis but is not dependent
        on DNA methylation. Carcinogenesis. 2002;23:2025–2030.

[129] Lan YL, Yu L, Jia CW, Wu YM, Wang SY. Gain of human telomerase RNA gene is
        associated with progression of cervical intraepithelial neoplasia grade I or II. Chin Med
        J (Engl). 2012;125(9):1599-602.

[130] Giannoudis A, Herrington SC. Human papillomavirus variants and squamous
        neoplasia of the cervix. J Pathol 2001;193:295–302.

[131] Klaes R, Benner A, Friedrich T, Ridder R, Herrington S, Jenkins D,et al. p16INK4A
        immunohistochemistry improves interobserver agreement in the diagnosis of cervical
        intraepithelial neoplasia. Am J Surg Pathol, 2002;26:1389–99.

[132] Murphy N, Ring M, Killalea AG, Uhlmann V, O'Donovan M, Mulcahy F,et al.
        p16INK4A as a marker for cervical dyskaryosis: CIN and cGIN in cervical biopsies and
        ThinPrep™ smears. J Clin Pathol 2003;56:53–63.

[133] Bonds L, Baker P, Gup C, Shroyer KR. Immunohistochemical localization of CDC6 in
        squamous and glandular neoplasia of the uterine cervix. Arch Pathol Lab Med
        2002;126:1162–8.

[134] Grce M, Matovina M, Milutin-Gasperov N, Sabol I. Advances in cervical cancer control
        and future perspectives. Coll Antropol 2010;34:731-6.

[135] Tamalet C, Richet H, Carcopino X, Henry M, Leretraite L, Heid P, et al. Testing for
        human papillomavirus and measurement of viral load of HPV 16 and 18 in self-
        collected vaginal swabs of women who do not undergo cervical cytological screening
        in Southern France. J Med Virol 2010;82:1431-7.

[136] Gravitt PE, Coutlée F, Iftner T, Sellors JW, Quint WGV, Wheeler CM. New technologies
        in cervical cancer screening. Vaccine 2008, 26(suppl) 42-52.

Chapter 3

HPV Diagnosis in Vaccination Era

Fátima Galán-Sánchez and
Manuel Rodríguez-Iglesias

Additional information is available at the end of the chapter

1. Introduction

Diagnostic methods for the detection of HPV should increase standardization and reproducibility due to two significant events in the future: the epidemiological monitoring changes in a vaccinated population and the involvement of HPV in tumors of other anatomical sites.

It will be necessary to diagnose HPV in processes other than cervical cancer, and we refer not only to their involvement in tumors with a demonstrated relationship, as in the anal region, but also to other locations in which their participation is suggested, as in the oropharyngeal tumors. Standardization in the collection and sample processing will be crucial in order to achieve accurate results involving an aid in the diagnosis and prognosis of these processes and their possible prevention.

However, the future challenge will be presented with the changes caused by the vaccination campaigns and their influence on the prevalence of cytological abnormalities and screening programs that will need to be designed according to the new status. There are already published results showing a decrease in the incidence of HPV in young women vaccinated Australia and confirm the estimates of predictive models [1].

Vaccination impact monitoring requires a multidisciplinary collaboration with technical and information support adequate to provide significant evidence to justify changes in health measures. However, screening should remain as an important strategy in cervical cancer control in both vaccinated and unvaccinated people. The reduction in incidence in young women after mass vaccination of adolescents together with greater range in controls and improved sensitivity of HPV testing draws a picture with attractive screening programs more efficient and cost effective in disease control.

The availability of sensitive diagnostic assays for HPV, reproducible and cost effectively will be critical in the monitoring of current vaccines and the design and implementation of vaccination programs. The HPV vaccine offers a unique opportunity to fight against cancer and diseases associated with HPV infection.

2. HPV epidemiology: The changes coming

Although the risk of cervical cancer was long known to be associated with risky sexual behavior in both the woman and her partner, it was not until around 3 decades ago that HPV was identified the likely culprit by Dr. Zur Hausen, whose work in cervical cancer won him the Nobel Prize. The development of superior molecular techniques advanced the field rapidly cementing the association between HPV and cervical cancer. This finding quickly led scientists to examine HPV's association with other anogenital cancers in women including vulvar, vaginal and anal cancers and in men, penile and anal cancers [2]. Most recently, oropharyngeal cancers have joined the list of HPV-associated cancers. Although HPV was found to be associated with these other anogenital cancers, most of the work continues to focus on cervical cancers since it remains 20 times more common than any of the other HPV-associated cancers. This phenomenon is likely due to the vulnerability of the cervix to HPV. Although the mechanisms are not well understood, the transformation zone (TZ) is likely one of the most vulnerable epithelia to HPV's carcinogenic powers [3]. The TZ change of columnar epithelium to stratified epithelium Mullerian urogenital area in the ectocervix. In the puberty columnar epithelium differentiates into stratified squamous epithelium. Metaplastic tissue is more vulnerable to HPV because its thickness to the basal layer is smaller and the virus requires cells in differentiation state for their survival, which is accelerated in metaplastic tissues [4]. It is likely that this metaplastic tissue supports viral persistence which is essential for cancer development. Interestingly metaplastic tissue is also found in the anal and tonsillar tissue.

According to a recent meta-analysis that included data from more than 1 million women in 59 countries, the prevalence of genital HPV infection among those with normal cytology ranges from 1.6% to 41.9% [5]. The estimated average global prevalence of HPV in this particular study was 11.7%. This study, along with others [6], reported an interesting trend in the female age-specific distribution of HPV whereby there is a first peak at younger ages (< 25 years) in all regions; and in the Americas, Africa and Europe, a clear second peak among individuals 45 years or older. The first peak, which comes shortly after sexual debut for most women, is generally attributed to higher levels of sexual activity with multiple partners and low viral immunity. After the first peak, a consistent age-related decline in HPV prevalence has been documented in numerous epidemiological studies. Although the reason for the smaller second peak at middle age still remains unclear, possible explanations include immunosenescence, hormonal changes prior to menopause, changes in male/female sexual behavior, cohort effects, or perhaps higher rates of HPV persistence at older ages [7]. However, new sexual exposures and latent reactivation are often invoked as explanation for the second peak of HPV prevalence observed in older women, particularly in Latin America [6]. Studies in humans are unable to directly demonstrate establishment of latency and induction of reactivation from the latent state. However, animal models of papillomavirus infection have provided sufficient experimental evidence for papillomavirus latency [8]. HPV infects basal epithelial cells at sites of microtrauma, likely a normal consequence of sexual intercourse. Infected basal cells induced to differentiate to fill the wound will result in active papillomavirus infection. A few infected basal stem cells will retain HPV, but do not differentiate, and these infected cells are unlikely to be sampled using standard exfoliative techniques employed in most epidemiologic studies, which sample only the surface epithelium. Thus, HPV in a basal stem cell may remain undetectable until triggered to differentiate by undetermined stimuli such as wound repair and hormonal regulation [9]. With high cellular turnover in the cervical epithelium, one may expect relatively constant detection of HPV in this model. However, it is likely that a reactivated infection subsequent to latently infected stem cell differentiation is immediately recognized and brought under control by a functional memory immune response resulting in very short duration of active infection. This model would be consistent with the increase in new HPV DNA detection immediately following memory T cell depletion in acute HIV and in sexually abstinent women with chronic HIV infection [10, 11]. The relatively lower rates of recurrent HPV DNA detection in healthy populations suggests that the normal immune response is able to retain recurrence, but that background reactivation is common and likely associated with short duration of detectable viral DNA [12].

Among sexually active males, genital HPV infection is also very common; however, prevalence varies widely depending on geographic region, risk group, anatomical site, sampling method, and HPV testing methodology [13, 14]. In a recent systematic review, Smith et al [15] estimated HPV prevalence to be between 1% and 84% in low-risk sexually active men, and between 2% and 93% in high risk men. HPV infection declines substantially after about 30 years of age, The prevalence of HPV infection in males generally remains constant or declines only slightly with age after peak prevalence. One possible explanation for this is that men experience a higher rate of reinfection compared to women. Anal cancer is very rare in the general population, but much more common in well defined, high-risk populations, including women with a previous cervical precancer, men having sex with men (MSM), and immune-compromised individuals. Infection with carcinogenic human papillomavirus (HPV) has been increasingly recognised to cause anal cancer and Machalek et al [16] recorded a prevalence of high-risk anal HPV in HIV-positive MSM of 73.5%.

In 1995, the International Agency for Research on Cancer (IARC) first classified HPV types 16 and 18 as carcinogenic to humans, but based on more recent evidence, the list of carcinogenic HPV types has been expanded to include a total of 13 mucosotropic anogenital HPV types as being definite or probable carcinogens (grade 1 or 2a) based on their frequent association with invasive cervical cancer (ICC) and cervical intraepithelial neoplasia (CIN) [17]. The oncogenic types (mostly HPV 16) are also causally implicated in other cancers, including penile, anal, vulvar and vaginal cancers [18, 19]. The remaining genital types (e.g., HPV types 6, 11, 42, 43, 44 and some rarer types) are considered to be of low or no oncogenic risk [20]. However, these types may cause subclinical and clinically visible benign lesions known as flat and acuminate condylomata, respectively.

In descending order, the most common HPV types implicated in cervical cancer globally are: 16, 18, 58, 33, 45, 31, 52, 35, 59, 39, 51 and 56 [21]. HPV types 16 and 18 are the most dominant types implicated in cervical cancer in all continents, being responsible for ~ 70% of ICC cases globally. In many studies, estimating the fraction of cervical cancer cases attributable to the different HPV types is difficult due to the high prevalence of multiple type infections. For example, a recent meta-analysis estimated the prevalence of co-infection (≥ 2 HPV types) in tumor specimens at 15.7% [21]. Other recent meta-analyses and cross sectional studies evaluating the worldwide distribution of HPV infections consistently reveal the same HPV prevalence patterns [5, 22]. This widespread circulation of HR-HPV types strengthens the potential for a phenomenon known as type-replacement, i.e., an increase in other non-vaccine genotypes following HPV vaccination. However, based on evidence that HPVs evolve very slowly and that HPV types do not normally compete with one another during natural infection [23-25], it is still unlikely that some other HPV type(s) will evolve to fill the niche currently occupied by vaccine target types. Furthermore, phase III trials evaluating both bivalent and quadrivalent vaccines indicate partial cross-type protection (cross-immunity) against many phylogenetically related HPV types [26-28], suggesting that the benefit from vaccination may be even greater than expected.

Infection of the oral cavity with high risk HPV is also now recognized as an important cause of oral and oropharyngeal cancers [29]. However, unlike cervical cancer in which 100% of cases are attributable to infection with HPV, only 25–35% of these cancers are attributable to HPV [2, 30]; the major risk factors being alcohol and tobacco use. Among cases of oral/oropharyngeal cancer linked to HPV infection, HPV 16 is by far the most common type detected in tumor specimens [31, 32]. Based on evaluation of risk factor profiles for cancers of the head and neck, comparing HPV 16-positive and HPV 16-negative cases, some researchers have decided that these should actually be considered distinct cancers [33]. In their study, sexual behavior (but not alcohol or tobacco use) was an important predictor of head and neck cancers among HPV 16-positive subjects, meanwhile the opposite was observed for HPV 16-negative subjects.

HPV 16 is the most common in all the HPV associated anogenital and oropharyngeal cancers therefore the HPV vaccines currently on the market are likely to make a significant impact on all these cancers in women and in men. In contrast, the role of HPV in penile cancers is less understood. Trauma and inflammation appear to be important risks suggesting that tissue damage and/or repair processes play a role in cancer development [34]. The natural history of HPV in the penis is also not well described. Although there is a histologic equivalent of the precancerous CIN 3 found in men, referred to as penile intraepithelial neoplasia (PIN), nothing is known about the natural history of these lesions and whether they have the same potential as CIN 3 (~ 12%) to progress to invasive cancer. One intriguing observation is that the penile cancer has a much lower prevalence than cervical cancer and yet the prevalence of HPV is much higher in the genitals of men than what is observed in women. Across all ages, HPV is found 2–4 times more common in the genital area of men than seen in women and the decline observed with age in women is not seen in men with similar prevalence across all ages. In contrast, the natural history of HPV in anogenital area in men behaves similar to HPV in women [35] in that HPV appears to be rapidly cleared so by 6–8 months, most infections are undetected. These observations and the fact that antibodies to HPV are less common in men than in women suggest that most infections in men are relatively superficial and clearance is likely directed by local innate immune responses, but not by memory immune responses [36]. Since men do not appear to develop adequate HPV specific immune responses, they are not protected from re-infection. This is another argument for HPV vaccination in men. It may be that sexually active males would benefit from vaccination. Benefits would include prevention of penile, anal and oropharyngeal cancers and prevention of infections would, in theory, also benefit women [37].

After breast and colorectal cancer, cervical cancer is the 3rd leading cancer site worldwide irrespective of gender and second among women. In 2008, there were an estimated 530,000 cases and 270,000 deaths attributed to cervical cancer, with 86% of cases and 88% of deaths occurring in developing countries [38]. In these developing countries, the age-standardized incidence rate (ASIR) and age-standardized mortality rate (ASMR) were 18 and 10 per 100,000 women, respectively; whereas in more developed countries, the ASIR and ASMR were 9 and 3 per 100,000 women, respectively. Globally, incidence of ICC ranges from < 3 to > 50 cases per 100,000 women for low- and high-burden countries, respectively. These differences between countries are believed to reflect protection from screening, and variance in exposure to HPV and other cofactors like smoking and oral contraceptive use, and other sexually transmitted infections such as human immunodeficiency virus [38].

The global burden of other HPV related cancers is also substantial. Worldwide, approximately 97,215 cases of non-cervical cancers for which HPV infection may be an etiologic factor are diagnosed annually; roughly 50,780 in men (520 penile, 26,775 oropharyngeal and 13,485 anal cancers) and 46,435 in women (25,600 vaginal/vulvar, 6048 oropharyngeal and 14,787 anal cancers) [39]. However, it is important to recognize that not all of these cases are attributable to HPV and that these estimates represent the upper limit for the annual burden of cancers caused by HPV. only a quarter of oropharyngeal cancers are attributable to HPV; meanwhile approximately 90% of anal cancers, and 40% of penile, vaginal or vulvar cancers are attributable to the virus. Although there is some evidence implicating HPV with several other cancers (e.g., lung, colon, ovary, breast, prostate, urinary bladder, esophageal and nasal/sinonasal cancers), current molecular and epidemiological data are sparse and do not yet support a causal role for HPV in the etiology of these cancers [30, 40-42]. The role of HPV in the causation of esophageal squamous cell carcinoma is unclear.

Globally, HPV accounts for roughly 5.2% of the total cancer burden — the highest among all infectious agents. However, as may be expected, the distribution varies considerably according to country development status, where HPV accounts for approximately 7.7% and 2.2% of all cancer cases in developing and developed countries, respectively [42].

3. Screening methods for detect HPV infection

HPV cannot be cultured in conventional cell cultures. Other classical direct virological diagnostic techniques, such as immunohistochemistry, lack the sensitivity as well as specificity for the routine detection of HPV. Serological assays for the detection of anti-HPV antibodies have only limited analytical accuracy and their possible clinical utility is currently unresolved. Consequently, all HPV tests currently in diagnostic use rely, on the detection of HPV nucleic acids in clinical specimens.

Having relied on cervical cytology effectively for several decades, primary human papillomavirus (HPV) testing is increasingly and widely recognised as the means to deliver effective cervical screening and the prevention of cervical cancer. Despite differences in the interventions amongst the main primary screening studies [43-46], the key message seems to be clear and consistent: a primary HPV test will increase the sensitivity for detecting *cervical intraepithelial neoplasia, grade 2+* (CIN2+), compared with cytology, and will allow the screening interval to be extended with fewer life-time tests for women. Conventional cytology-based screening is very effective in reducing cervical cancer when delivered in well-managed programmes with high population coverage and robust quality assurance, but is costly in terms of workforce, finance and infrastructure. These programmes will be more difficult to sustain with lower detection rates of abnormalities in HPV-immunised populations. Yet cervical screening needs to sit alongside HPV immunisation to optimise cancer prevention. Screening programmes will differ between different resource settings: e.g. introducing basic screening where no previous programme has existed in low- or medium-resource settings, or providing more clinically effective prevention in highly resourced countries with organised or opportunistic screening. In protocols of prevention and treatment of cervical cancer involved, in addition to cytology and HPV detection, other diagnostic tools such as colposcopy, histological categorization and use of new biomarkers, with the correct risk stratification parameter that must be used to choose the appropriate procedures in the different phases of the clinical process: screening, triage, diagnosis and treatment [47].

Screening, defined as the preventive activity that can diagnose the disease in healthy population a priori, should have as target detecting cervical intraepithelial neoplasia grade 3 (CIN3), or being even stricter CIN2, histological stages of the disease are even preventable. Screening by cervical cytology detects only 50-60% of cases of CIN3, including cytological revisions very close in time. The analytical sensitivity of the detection of HPV DNA in exfoliated cells is much higher, above 90%, but the clinical specificity is low because of virological diagnostic predicts non persistence, necessary to cause the development of cancer. This limitation is accentuated in young women with a good chance of getting an HPV infection self-limited. However, the negative predictive value of HPV testing is very high and would, in patients free of viruses could increase the periods between two revisions in years. Using both techniques simultaneously (cytology + HPV), as has been done in some trial cohort (Northern California Kaiser Permanent), increases the control intervals to three years with good results. Implementation of HPV DNA testing in cervical screening leads to earlier detection of clinically relevant CIN grade 2 or worse, which when adequately treated, improves protection against CIN grade 3 or worse and cervical cancer. Early detection of high-grade cervical legions caused by HPV16 was a major component of this benefit [48].

The costs are reduced in the triage by using a technique followed by another in accordance with the results of the first. The cytology followed by HPV testing has been used but as already discussed the problems of the low sensitivity of cytology and uncertain cytology triage (ASCUS) or low-risk lesions (LSIL) can lead to positive HPV tests with unknown clinical significance. However, the benefits of the HPV test result prior cytology have been demonstrated [49]. Currently there are proposals to make the detection of HPV followed by cytology, which has the best results of clinical sensitivity, reducing costs to distance the negative control women but also may increase if performed in populations with a high incidence of infection, as in young women [50]. Hence, several protocols established older than 30-35 years for a suitable cost-effectiveness. It remains to determine the usefulness of combining HPV screening combined with a new biomarkers triage as detection of HPV mRNA, p16-INK, and other histological progression markers (Ki-67, MCM2 and TOP2A).

This scenario has increased the range of methods and technologies for the diagnosis of HPV in clinical samples, whether exfoliated cells or biopsy, even paraffin. Extraction procedures of nucleic acids, methods of viral genome detection and automation necessary for a determination which is becoming routine laboratories have acquired high levels of complexity for the most suitable choice [51]. The commercially available tests can be systematized in five groups [52]: 1) screening assays based on the detection of HPV DNA of high risk, which includes hybrid capture as the reference method because of the enormous experience gathered in previous studies, amplification using probes invader and PCR procedures, 2) similar screening tests for the detection of DNA of high-risk HPV concurrent determinations of genotypes or reflex HPV-16 and HPV-18 genotypes whose infection is a risk of developing cancer than other genotypes too, 3) genotyping assays based on HPV PCR using various technologies: reverse hybridization, microarray, array and RFLP suspension, which joins the pyrosequencing and other methods of mass sequencing, 4) based screening assays for the quantification of mRNA expression of E6/E7 high-risk HPVs, with the added value of its utility as a marker of progression, and 5) in situ hybridization, available but with limitations because of lower sensitivity.

4. HPV-DNA screening methods

High-risk HPV-DNA-based screening assays represent a group of qualitative or semi-quantitative multiplex assays in which the DNA of the targeted HPV types is detected using mixtures of probes (probe cocktails) for several HPV types with similar clinical characteristics. None of the assays from this group allow the exact determination of HPV type(s) present in a clinical specimen, but rather express the results of the tested group of HPV types as positive or negative. Until recently, such an approach has been widely accepted by the HPV community as the best way to present the results of hr-HPV testing to clinicians involved in primary screening for cervical carcinoma and management of patients with cervical intraepithelial neoplasia (CIN). The Hybrid Capture 2 (HC2) HPV DNA Test, originally developed by Digene Corporation (Gaithersburg, MD, USA) in 1997 and currently marketed by Qiagen, has been the most important HPV diagnostic assay for the last decade and is still the most frequently used diagnostic HPV test worldwide [53]. The main problems of the current version of HC2 are: analytical inaccuracy due to the cross-reactivity of its probe cocktails with untargeted HPV types; and lack of internal control to evaluate specimen adequacy or the presence of potentially interfering substances. In order to resolve the current problems of analytical inaccuracy and to improve HC2 throughput, a next-generation diagnostic system has been developed [54]. Significant improvements have been engineered into the next-generation hybrid-capture system, which builds on the current advantages of the FDA-approved HPV screening technology, HC2. Central to the improved chemistry in the NextGen assay on the QIAensemble automated system is the new collection medium, DCM [54].

The Amplicor HPV Test (Amplicor; Roche Molecular Systems, Branchburg, NJ, USA), launched on the European market in 2004, is a qualitative PCR-based test designed to detect the same 13 HPV types as HC2: HPV-16, HPV-18, HPV-31, HPV-33, HPV-35, HPV-39, HPV-45, HPV-51, HPV-52, HPV-56, HPV-58, HPV-59 and HPV-68. Similarly to HC2, Amplicor expresses the results of the tested group of hr-HPV types as positive or negative. Amplicor is based on standard PCR amplification and detection of PCR products on microwell plates [55]. The Cervista HPV HR Test (Cervista; Hologic) is another FDA-approved signal amplification-based qualitative test for the routine detection of 14 HPVs. In March 2009, the FDA approved Cervista for two indications: to screen patients with ASC-US cervical cytology results to determine the need for referral to colposcopy; and to be used adjunctively with cervical cytology to screen women 30 years of age and older to assess the presence or absence of hr-HPV types [56]. In contrast to HC2, Cervista is based on the Invader chemistry, a signal amplification method for detecting specific nucleic acid sequences. With support from the Bill and Melinda Gates Foundation, a careHPV Test (Qiagen), based on simplified HC2 technology, has been recently developed to detect the 13 HPV types included in the original HC2 plus HPV-66, in approximately 3 h. Such rapid, simple and affordable HPV tests, whereby results can be given to a patient within the same visit, are anticipated to have the greatest impact in countries in which cervical cancer screening programs do not exist or in countries in which substantial loss to follow-up impairs the effectiveness of cervical cancer screening programs [57].

5. HPV-DNA screening methods with concurrent or reflex HPV-16 & HPV-18 genotyping

Reflex HR HPV DNA testing is now recognized as a cost-effective strategy to refer women with an ASC-US cytology for colposcopy [58, 59]. High-risk HPV-DNA-based screening assays with individual or pooled HPV-16 and HPV-18 genotyping are a group of novel HPV assays in which qualitative detection of 13–14 HPV types is combined with concurrent or reflex HPV-16 and HPV-18 genotyping. The Abbott RealTime High Risk HPV test (RealTime; Abbott Molecular, Des Plaines, IL, USA) is a real-time PCR assay based on concurrent individual genotyping for HPV-16 and HPV-18 and pooled detection of 12 other HPVs: HPV-31, HPV-33, HPV-35, HPV-39, HPV-45, HPV-51, HPV-52, HPV-56, HPV-58, HPV-59, HPV-66 and HPV-68. Amplification of human β-globin is used as an internal control. The assay was launched on the European market in January 2009. RealTime is performed on the m2000rt real-time PCR instrument (Abbott Molecular) using a modified GP5+/GP6+ primer mix consisting of three forward and two reverse primers [60]. Analytical sensitivity of RealTime was comparable to that of HC2 (97.6% vs 95.1%), whereas RealTime demonstrated significantly higher analytical specificity compared with HC2 [61, 62].

The cobas 4800 HPV Test (Roche Molecular Diagnostics, Pleasanton, CA, USA) is a real-time PCR assay based on concurrent individual genotyping for HPV-16 and HPV-18 and pooled detection of 12 other HPVs: HPV-31, HPV-33, HPV-35, HPV-39, HPV-45, HPV-51, HPV-52, HPV-56, HPV-58, HPV-59, HPV-66 and HPV-68 [63-65]. An excellent agreement (>93%) was obtained between cobas 4800 HPV and HC2 or Linear Array (LA) for the detection of HR HPV DNA in CIN [66]. The cobas 4800 HPV test will refer fewer women to colposcopy than automatic referral of all women with ASC-US. It will also distinguish women infected with HPV16 or HPV18 from those infected with other HR HPV genotypes, although this feature is not yet included in clinical guidelines for the management of women with ASC-US. When the cobas 4800 HPV was utilized by a diagnostic laboratory, its performance was equivalent to that of HC2 and show comparable levels of performance including results for women >30 years old with ASCUS cytology [67]. Gage et al found agreement between Cobas and LA to be very good, better than that between Cobas and HC2 [68].

The Cervista HPV 16/18 Test (Hologic) is a signal amplification qualitative test based on the Invader chemistry specifically designed to detect HPV-16 and HPV-18 [69].

6. HPV-DNA genotyping methods

HPV DNA-based genotyping as says, which allow exact determination of several alpha-HPV types present in a clinical sample, are the largest group of currently available HPV commercial assays. In contrast to the previously described two groups of commercial HPV assays, the clinical value of HPV DNA-based genotyping assays has still not been finally determined [70-72]. Currently, HPV genotyping methods are indispensable as research tools for the study of the natural history, transmission, pathogenesis and prevention of HPV infection. However, it is highly likely that genotyping methods will also have a role in clinical management in the near future [70, 73, 74]. As the use of prophylactic HPV vaccines becomes more widespread, surveillance for population-level effectiveness will become an increasingly important activity, which will require the use of a HPV genotyping method. If HPV genotyping is to be used for diagnostic applications and not just as a research tool, it will require standardized and validated methods for the specific detection and identification of a defined spectrum of HPV types.

Although DNA sequencing is still considered to be the 'gold standard' for HPV genotyping, it is costly, time-consuming and difficult to apply in routine diagnostic settings. Thus, in daily practice, the majority of laboratories use nonsequencing based methods for HPV genotyping, However the next generation sequencing can be implemented in the HPV detection [75]. This methodology also provides a tumor genomic copy number karyogram, and in the samples analyzed here, a lower level of chromosome instability was detected in HPV-positive tumors compared to HPV-negative tumors, as observed in previous studies. Thus, the use of next-generation sequencing for the detection of HPV provides a multiplicity of data with clinical significance in a single test.

The most frequently used HPV genotyping assays today utilize the principle of reverse line-blot (RLB) hybridization. In these assays a fragment of the HPV genome is first PCR-amplified using biotinylated HPV-specific primers and the resulting amplicons are then denatured and hybridized with HPV-specific oligonucleotide probes immobilized as parallel lines on nylon or a nitrocellulose membrane strip. After hybridization, streptavidin-conjugated alkaline phosphatase or horseradish peroxidase is added, which binds to any biotinylated hybrid previously formed. Incubation with chromogenic substrates (e.g., BCIP/NBT for alkaline phosphatase) yields a colored precipitate at the probe positions where hybridization occurs. The genotyping strip is then read and interpreted visually by comparing the pattern of HPV-positive probes to the test reference guide for each of the targeted HPV types. In addition to the in-house GP5+/GP6+ RLB Genotyping Assay which has been used in several important HPV trials [76, 77]. INNO-LiPA HPV Genotyping is one of the most widely used HPV genotyping tests. Several versions of this assay have been developed. In all versions, amplification of a 65 bp region of the HPV *L1* gene using biotinylated SPF10 primers is followed by hybridization of the resulting amplicons with 17–28 (depending on the assay version) HPV-specific oligonucleotide probes immobilized on a nitrocellulose strip [78]. An evaluation of INNO-LiPA *Extra*, performed on 70 HC2-positive samples, showed comparable genotyping results to the *digene* HPV Genotyping RH Test RUO (*digene* RH Test; Qiagen) and a significantly higher sensitivity of INNO-LiPA *Extra* for the detection of multiple infections [79]. Recently is described this method with realtime PCR [80]. The Linear Array HPV Genotyping Test (Linear Array) is one of the most commonly used HPV genotyping assays, which combines PCR amplification and reverse line-blot hybridization for the identification of 36 alpha-HPV types. Linear Array is based on the co-amplification of a 450 bp region of the HPV *L1* gene and a 268 bp region of the human β-globin gene, using biotinylated primer sets PGM09/PGMY11 and PC04/GH20 [81]. Steinau et al [82] compared the performance of three line blot assays (LBAs), the Linear Array HPV genotyping assay (LA) (Roche Diagnostics), INNO-LiPA HPV Genotyping Extra (LiPA) (Innogenetics), and the reverse hybridization assay (RH) (Qiagen). Although the assays had good concordance in the clinical samples, the greater accuracy and specificity in the plasmid panel suggest that LA has an advantage for internationally comparable genotyping studies.

Similar to reverse line-blot assays, microarray-based HPV genotyping assays also employ the principle of reverse hybridization. Following PCR amplification of a fragment of a viral genome with HPV-specific primers, the resulting amplicons are denatured and hybridized with a number of HPV-specific oligonucleotide probes attached on the surface of an insoluble supporter or DNA chip (also known as microchip, biochip and gene chip). DNA chips can consist of one to several DNA microarrays, thus enabling simultaneous analysis of multiple samples in a single experiment. After hybridization, fluorescence light from the bound PCR amplicon is detected by excitation with monochromatic light. Currently, laser scanners are used for the highly sensitive fluorescence microarray readout systems. The fluorescence label of the hybridizing amplicons can be introduced during PCR and/or during the hybridization step. Some of the microarray-based HPV genotyping tests utilize the principle of chromogenic precipitation instead of fluorescence detection. The PapilloCheck HPV-Screening Test (PapilloCheck; Greiner Bio-One GmbH, Frickenhausen, Germany) is currently one of the two most frequently used PCR-microarray-based assays. The assay allows identification of 24 alpha-HPV types. [83]. Clart HPV 2 – papillomavirus clinical arrays (Clart HPV 2; Genomica, Coslada, Spain) combine PCR amplification and an oligonucleotide microarray-based detection system for the identification of 35 alpha-HPVs. The assay consists of pre-aliquoted, ready to use amplification mix tubes and allows amplification of a 450 bp region of the HPV *L1* gene together with an internal control template and the human *CFTR* gene using three different sets of biotinylated primers [84].

The suspension array that uses bead-based xMAP or Luminex technology is based on the use of polystyrene beads with a diameter of 5.6 µm, which are internally dyed with various ratios of two spectrally distinct fluorophores (red and infrared). Different bead sets with specific absorption spectra can be mixed and used for the multiplexed detection of different analytes; currently, an array of 100 bead sets (bead mix) can be generated. For HPV genotyping purposes, each bead set in the bead mix is usually coupled to a single oligonucleotide probe specific for one HPV type. HPV genotyping is done by reverse hybridization technique using biotinylated PCR amplicons. After denaturation and hybridization of target HPV sequences to the bead-bound probes, labeling of the hybridized biotinylated amplicons is done using R-phycoery-thrin-labeled streptavidin, serving as a reporter fluorophore. The bead sets are then read and analyzed on a Luminex analyzer; the HPV types are discerned according to the unique bead signature, whereas the presence of specific PCR amplicons is determined by R-phycoerythrin fluorescence. The Luminex readouts are expressed as the median fluorescent intensity of the reporter fluorescence for each HPV type. Positivity for the relevant types is calculated from the median fluorescent intensity over a defined threshold level, and can provide a semi-quantitative numerical output. Several in-house genotyping protocols based on xMAP technology have been developed in the last 5 years [85-91]; some of them are considered to be the most sensitive HPV detection methods currently available [85]. In addition, at least two commercial assays based on this technology are available at present.

Gel electrophoresis-based HPV genotyping assays utilize general primer-mediated PCR, type-specific or group-specific PCR, to screen for a broad spectrum of HPVs, followed by agarose gel electrophoresis. Restriction fragment length polymorphism (RFLP) is consequently applied to identify HPV type-specific restriction patterns. In addition to several in-house genotyping protocols based on RFLP, one commercial assay based on this technology is currently available.

Yi et al [92] report the development of a highly sensitive, highly automated assay based on the MALDI-TOF-MS platform for the detection and individual genotyping of 14 different HR-HPV types. The use of the MassARRAY technique and combination of automated DNA extraction/ PCR pipetting procedures increased the detection throughput, which consequently decreased the cost per case of the assay. Now we can deal with 3,000 samples within 2 working days, and the current total cost per sample is about $2 (US). The MS HPV genotyping assay is potentially suitable for routine HPV detection, especially in large-scale cervical cancer screening programs owing to its high throughput and low cost per case. Proper population-based clinical validation is needed to establish the clinical relevance of this highly analytically sensitive assay.

7. HPV E6/E7 mRNA screening methods

Several recent studies have clearly shown that testing for HPV mRNA instead of HPV DNA can be clinically useful [70, 93, 94]. The most relevant transcripts for diagnostic purposes are those encoding viral oncoproteins E6 and E7. The detection of viral mRNA can be done by reverse transcriptase real time PCR [95] or by nucleic acid sequence-based amplification (NASBA). For the latter, three commercially available assays that detect E6/E7 transcripts are currently available. PreTect HPV-Proofer (HPV-Proofer; NorChIp, Klokkarstua, Norway) is an assay based on NASBA technology, which allows qualitative determination of E6/E7 mRNA transcripts of the five most frequently identified hr-HPV types in cervical cancer worldwide: HPV-16, HPV-18, HPV-31, HPV-33 and HPV-45 [96]. The NucliSENS EasyQ HPV V1 assay (NucliSENS; bioMérieux) was launched in 2007 and is based on the original HPV-Proofer assay, except for the proprietary hardware platform and the software for NASBA measurements and data analysis [97]. APTIMA HPV Assay (APTIMA; Gen-Probe, San Diego, CA, USA) is a transcription-mediated amplification-based assay, which allows the detection of E6/E7 mRNA transcripts of 14 HPV types: HPV-16, HPV-18, HPV-31, HPV-33, HPV-35, HPV-39, HPV-45, HPV-51, HPV-52, HPV-56, HPV-58, HPV-59, HPV-66 and HPV-68. The assay generates a qualitative result for the presence/absence of 14 targeted HPVs and does not allow the exact determination of HPV type(s) present in a clinical specimen [98]. APTIMA yielded similar sensitivity for CIN2+ compared with hc2, Amplicor and Linear Array (95.2 vs 99.6%, 98.9% and 98.2%, respectively), but a significantly higher specificity (42.2 vs 28.4%, 21.7% and 32.8%, respectively) [55]. In a comparative evaluation of APTIMA and hc2 on PreservCyt specimens collected from 800 women referred to colposcopy, APTIMA showed comparable sensitivity to hc2 for the detection of CIN2+ (91 vs 95%), as well as CIN3+ (98 vs 99%), but had higher clinical specificity (>55 vs 47% for CIN2+; 53 vs 44% for CIN3+) [99]. APTIMA had the best sensitivity/specificity balance measured by AUC (area under ROC curve) comparison test (significant for CIN2+), and the colposcopy referral rate (9.2%) comparable to that of liquid citology (8.7%) [100].

8. In situ hybridization metods

In situ hybridization (ISH) is the only molecular method allowing reliable detection and identification of HPVs in topographical relation to their pathological lesions. Unlike other molecular methods, in ISH the whole HPV detection procedure occurs within the nuclei of infected cells and not on solid supports or in solutions. The result of the hybridization reaction is evaluated microscopically and the appearance of an appropriate precipitate within the nuclei of epithelial cells is indicative of the presence of HPVs in the specimen being tested. In addition, the physical state of the virus can be evaluated by the presence of punctuate signals for integrated virus and diffuse signals for episomal virus. Although commercially available HPV assays based on ISH have been validated technically, they are insufficiently clinically validated. In addition, current ISH-based assays are considered by many experts in the field to be too laborious and to have insufficient clinical sensitivity to be used in routine screening [52].

9. Progression markers

9.1. HPV viral load

HPV viral load is a product of the number of cells infected and number of viruses per infected cell and is therefore influenced by two main factors: (i) the extent of an HPV infection on the cervical surface and (ii) the level of viral production in the area of infection. Viral load has been suggested to be a potential biomarker for cervical intraepithelial neoplasia grade 2 (CIN2) or greater, but currently there is no consistent evidence that a one-time measurement of viral load is a useful marker of prevalent disease or disease progression [101]. A widespread productive infection might be associated with high viral load, while a small incipient CIN3 with low-level virus production might be associated with low viral load. Furthermore, viral load in a cytological sample is subject to sampling variation in which there are varying proportions of lesional cells, normal epithelial cells, inflammatory exudate, and blood. A further complication in using viral load to predict neoplasia of CIN2 or greater is the high prevalence of multiple carcinogenic HPV infections detected in cervical samples. The current paradigm is that cervical lesions clonally expand following infection with one specific genotype (one virus-one lesion concept). On the cervical surface, multiple independent infections or lesions may occur that are caused by different genotypes. Without specific genotyping conducted *in situ*, assigning a causal HPV genotype to a specific lesion can only be based on assumptions [102]. HPV16 is the only genotype for which there is some indication that viral load may predict viral persistence and progression to precancer [103-105].

Quantitating HPV viral load seems to be a rational strategy of identifying women at risk for persistent HPV infection and progression to high-grade dysplasia. Accordingly, a high viral load could represent many cells with few virions each or a few cells containing many virions. An inaccurate description of the viral biology and the possible implications for the host could result from this discrepancy. Recently, studies have focused on longitudinal observations of viral load to predict viral clearance or lesion progression [106, 107]. Initial data indicate that repeated measurements can improve prediction of persistence or clearance, but these data are, so far, limited to HPV16 only. Although signal intensities from HC2 or various endpoint PCR-based assays have been proposed and partly used as surrogates for viral load, these approaches have limitations [108, 109]. HC2 only gives aggregate signal strength for a pool of 13 carcinogenic types, and commercial genotyping assays, such as the Roche Linear Array (LA) or Innogenetics InnoLiPA (line probe assay), do not formally report quantitative results. Overestimation of the presence of oncogenic HPV may result. Despite these caveats, the development of HPV viral load assays that may reliably be used as an adjunct screening tool to identify women at increased risk of progression to CIN 2+ and cervical cancer remains a promising tool in cervical cancer screening. Recently, Wentzensen et al [110] measuring signal intensities on LA HPV genotyping strips provides quantitative information comparable to viral load measurements based on Q-PCR. This approach offers the potential for viral load assessment for 37 types in parallel, simplifying conducting repeated measurements of viral load in epidemiologic studies and addressing the problems of multiple HPV genotype infections in studies of HPV load.

Screening for HPV integration into the host genome is a subcategory of HPV diagnostics. HPV integration is a key molecular event in the transition from an innocuous HPV infection to one that has oncogenic potential. Human papilloma virus integration results in increased expression of the viral E6 and E7 proteins. Increased expression of these proteins ultimately results in the disruption of host cell proteins, p53 and retinoblastoma protein [111]. Tests that detect the integration of HPV into the host cell and corresponding risk of CIN 2+ or cancer are in development, and may provide a useful way of screening women at risk for cervical cancer. Studies have shown that viral integrants are detected in 100% of HPV-18-positive and 70–80% of HPV-16-positive cases of cervical carcinoma [112, 113]. A smaller subset of HSIL (15%) and 0% of LSIL contain transcriptionally active viral integrants [111].

Detection of p16(INK4a) correlates tightly with viral integration. In a normal cell, p16 blocks cyclindependent kinases (CDK) 4/6. Increased expression of the E6 and E7 oncogenes disrupt cell–cycle regulation, resulting in cell–cycle progression. In the normal cell, cell–cycle progression is activated by CDK 4/6 and in part regulated by p16. Because in HPV-transformed cells, cell–cycle activation is caused by E7 and not by CDK 4/6, p16 has no effect on the cell–cycle activation. Increased expression of p16 in cells driven by viral oncogene-mediated cell–cycle dysregulation can be detected through cellular immunostaining [114].

Because the correlation between HPV mRNA and high-grade dysplasia is a biologically plausible biomarker of risk, HPV mRNA detection may improve the specificity in the evaluation of women with ASCUS and LSIL Pap smears [115]. Many women have lesions that will not progress to CIN3 or invasive cancer, and these women currently present a treatment dilemma. No reliable methods can identify those lesions that are likely to regress. As a result, these women are monitored with serial colposcopic examinations at great expense to patients and the healthcare community. Detection and quantification of mRNA transcripts in these women may further refine current broad-spectrum, high-risk HPV DNA typing by allowing clinicians to know whether or not the virus is actively replicating E6 and E7 oncogenes. Messenger RNA transcript assays show great promise for being able to stratify the risk of progression to high-grade dysplasia in women with abnormal cytology.

The E6 strip test is also a biomarker that indicates viral integration. Schweizer et al. [116] evaluated the correlation of the HPV E6 test (Arbor Vita Corporation, Fremont, CA), which takes an hour to carry out and detects the HPV-E6 oncoprotein of HPV types 16,18 and 45, with detection of oncogenic HPV DNA in cytologic samples.

9.2. Screening methods identifying epigenetic changes

Many genes are currently being evaluated as potential methylation biomarkers for cervical cancer, but assay reliability for these methylation markers is highly variable. Within the human genome, methylation of cytosines in the CpG dinucleotides (also known as CpG sites) clustered into islands associated with transcriptional promoters is an important cellular mechanism to regulate gene expression. Methylation of HPV DNA by infected cells may alter the expression patterns of viral genes that are relevant for infection and transformation [117]. Increased methylation of CpG sites within the HPV16 genome before diagnosis and at the time of diagnosis was associated with cervical precancer [118]. Some promising candidate genes include DAPK1, CADM1, and RARB [119].

Another area of biomarker research is in the use of telomerase RNA component (TERC) identification by fluorescence in-situ hybridisation. Most cervical cancers have an extra copy of the long arm of chromosome 3, and consequently show amplification of TERC (present on chromosome band 3q26), which seems to play a key role in progression from low-grade dysplasia to cancer [120]. Many studies indicate that TERC identification may become a useful screening tool for cervical cancer. A prospective study by Andersson et al. [121] found a correlation between increasing TERC detection in cytology specimens and higher grade of dysplasia. They showed that progression to cervical cancer is never seen without TERC amplification and that, conversely, specimens without extra copies of TERC were likely to undergo spontaneous regression of HPV infection.

Other biomarkers under early evaluation for cervical cancer screening include CDC6 and MCM5. These proteins are present in normal cells only during the activation of the cell cycle and help form prereplicative DNA complexes during the G1 phase. They are absent from the cell during quiescence and differentiation. Dysplastic cells have unregulated cell cycles and, as a result, CDC6 and MCM5 reflect cell proliferation [122]. Studies indicate that CDC6 may be a biomarker of high-grade and invasive lesions of the cervix, with limited use in low-grade dysplasia. MCM5 seems to be a biomarker that is expressed independent of high-risk HPV infection, and may in the future serve as a useful marker for both HPV dependent and HPV-independent cervical dysplasia [122].

General markers of cell proliferation like MIB-1, MCMs or ProEx C, and surrogate markers of high risk HPV infection like p16 INK4A have shown promising results. Other potential candidates need to be tested until we find an ideal combination. Following the example of the p16 INK4A /MIB-1 dual staining combination and the MCM2/TOP2A combination (ProEx C), combinations are often superior to any single marker and should be tested. A critical determinant for the success of future investigations will be the standardization of sample preparation and interpretation. Furthermore, before reaching the point of routine application, this ideal 'biomolecular' or 'immune-enhanced Papanicolaou test' needs to be evaluated in large prospective clinical trials with appropriate colposcopic, histological, and clinical endpoints as well as adequate follow-up [123].

9.3. Screening methods for detect HPV infection

In order to facilitate the acceptance of novel HPV assays, mainly for cervical screening purposes, several recommendations have recently been published [70, 124, 125]. Meijer *et al.* proposed that before a new HPV assay can be used for cervical screening purposes, it should demonstrate at least similar if not better clinical characteristics (sensitivity, specificity, reproducibility, and so on) for the detection of CIN2+ as hc2 [125]. Other experts believe that large-scale clinical trials, with an assessment of prospective disease outcomes, are required to validate any proposed HPV screening test and that cross-sectional comparisons of new HPV assay to HC2 using several hundred specimens are not an acceptable form of assay validation [70]. Stoler *et al.* recently proposed that any novel HPV assay aiming to be used for cervical screening should have a clinical sensitivity of 92% ± 3% for CIN3+ to render a high NPV or the capacity to predict the future detection of a CIN3+ outcome that might occur during a recommended screening interval [124]. The HPV assay aiming to be used for cervical screening should also have a clinical specificity of at least 85% to achieve an adequate PPV for CIN3. The common idea behind all proposed recommendations is that a clinically useful HPV assay should achieve an optimal balance between clinical sensitivity and clinical specificity for detection of CIN2+/CIN3+ in order to minimize redundant or excessive follow-up procedures for hr-HPV-positive women with transient hr-HPV infections and/or without cervical lesions. Thus, as an example, a HPV assay with very high analytical sensitivity can yield a large number of clinically insignificant positive results, which will cause unnecessary clinical follow-up, unnecessary diagnostic procedures and unnecessary treatment of healthy women [126].

In forthcoming years, self-sampling may become increasingly important in cervical screening since self-collection for HPV testing (HPV self-sampling) has shown to persuade a subset of non-attendees to participate [127-129]. Targeting non-attendees is important, because they are at higher risk of developing cervical cancer. Additionally, self-sampling may make cervical screening accessible to women in developing regions [130].

An accurate and internationally comparable HPV DNA detection and genotyping methodology is an essential component both in the evaluation of HPV vaccines and in the effective implementation and monitoring of HPV vaccination programs. Genotyping assays used today differ in their analytical performance with regard to type-specific sensitivity and specificity [131]. The evaluation of assay performance needs to be performed in a standardized manner, where different assay performances can be evaluated and results can be compared against a known and accepted standard over time.

In 2008, the WHO HPV LabNet conducted a proficiency study based on HPV DNA plasmids containing the genomes from 14 oncogenic HPV types and 2 benign HPV types and open for participation to laboratories worldwide [132]. This study demonstrated that it is possible to perform global proficiency studies with unitage traceable to ISs based on plasmid DNA and that such studies can provide an overview of the status of the HPV detection and typing methodology worldwide. More recently, based on a proficiency panel composed of the same HPV DNA plasmid material used in 2008, with the amount of DNA titrated in amounts traceable to the IS. The use of the same panel material allowed a reproducible, standardized evaluation of assay sensitivity over time. Specificity was defined as absence of incorrect typing. The sample preprocessing was evaluated with extraction controls of cervical cancer cell lines. The panel was distributed to 105 laboratories worldwide and analyzed using a range of HPV DNA typing assays in a blinded manner [133]. Among laboratories that used the same assay in both years, 27% were proficient in 2008, whereas 30% were proficient in 2010. They also saw a strong trend toward increased sensitivity of assays. For example, among the laboratories using the same assay in 2008 and 2010, 50 IU of HPV-16 could be detected by all (100%) laboratories in 2010, whereas 86% of laboratories could detect 50 IU of HPV-16 in 2008. However, for several laboratories, the increased sensitivity was accompanied by increased amounts of false-positive results, resulting in nonproficiency, suggesting that recommendations for HPV laboratory testing include an increased emphasis on the use of negative controls in the assays.

The demands on sensitivity of HPV typing assays vary depending on the purpose of the testing. The WHO HPV LabNet proficiency panels are designed to evaluate the performance of HPV typing tests used in HPV vaccinology and HPV surveillance. In vaccinology, high analytical sensitivity is needed, as failure to detect prevalent infections at trial entry may result in false vaccine failures in vaccination trials. It should be noted that the HPV tests used in cervical cancer screening programs have different requirements for evaluation, since for that purpose, only HPV infections associated with high-grade cervical intraepithelial neoplasia or cancer and not those transient HPV infections that do not give rise to clinically meaningful disease are relevant. Since the latter are characterized by low viral loads, HPV screening assays do not have demands on analytical sensitivity that are as high [125].

10. Measuring the immune response to vaccine

HPV serology is an essential technology for both HPV vaccinology and HPV epidemiology. Definitions of HPV-naïve subjects eligible for HPV vaccination trials include seronegativity for HPV. Immunogenicity of HPV vaccines has been used to bridge results from efficacy trials in adolescents to children and to evaluate different batches of HPV vaccines. Antibody measurements are also important in vaccinology research, e.g. for characterizing the immune response with respect to studies of seroconversion and antibody increases, cross-reactions, immune memory and immune persistence as well as kinetics of antibody responses and establishment of correlates of protection. Finally, HPV seroepidemiology is also useful for understanding the epidemiology of HPV infections in populations to be targeted by HPV vaccination programs. The lack of a standardized assay to measure HPV antibody levels has hindered both epidemiological studies of HPV infection and comparison of results from different HPV vaccine trials [134]. WHO Guidelines for HPV vaccines suggest that "initial assessment of immune responses to HPV VLP vaccines should be based on measurement of neutralizing antibodies in serum". The available data [134-136] suggest that neutralizing and ELISA antibody titres are usually highly correlated when the ELISA antigen target is confor-mationally intact VLPs. Due to the complexity and labour-intensiveness of neutralization assays, VLP-based ELISAs have been preferred in large epidemiological studies. E.g., a study of HPV seroprevalences was conducted by measuring HPV 16 antibodies with an HPV16 L1 VLP-based ELISA to estimate the public-health impact of HPV vaccination strategies [137].

WHO has been coordinating work to develop standard assays that will help in assessing vaccine quality and monitoring impact after vaccination [138]. In 2006, WHO established a global HPV laboratory network (LabNet) with a main focus being the harmonization and standardization of laboratory testing procedures to support consistent laboratory evaluation of regional disease burden and monitoring of the performance of HPV vaccines. At a WHO consultation in January 2008, a group of experts recommended that the HPV LabNet should develop or identify standardized assays for general use and that efforts towards standardiza-tion on VLP-ELISA should be a high priority of the WHO HPV LabNet [139]. Following the recommendation, the WHO HPV LabNet launched a serology standardization program encompassing: (i) an international collaborative study to evaluate and refine a direct HPV 16 VLP-ELISA suggested Standard Operating Procedure (SOP), (ii) an international request for donations of VLPs to be used as international reference reagents for serology, followed by characterization and selection of optimal reagents, and (iii) an international collaborative proficiency study on HPV 16 serology, where participating laboratories used the same standardized SOP and the same VLP reference reagent [140].

Serologic assays for the evaluation of HPV vaccine responses are currently limited to an enzyme-linked immunosorbent assay (ELISA) [141], three multiplex assay systems [142-144], and a pseudovirus neutralization assay [145], and emerging data suggest that each system has some utility for characterizing HPV vaccine antibody specificity [136, 146]. Protection against vaccine types is thought to be mediated by neutralizing antibodies [147], and while the mechanism of vaccine-induced cross-protection is uncertain, the measurement of antibodies against nonvaccine types may be useful as a potential correlate or surrogate of cross-protection [148, 149]. Recently, Bissett et al [150] obtain a sera panel. These plasma pools could be useful as reference reagents. They are currently available as 250-µl aliquots of liquid plasma archived at −80°C and can be obtained from the National Institute for Biological Standards and Control.

Type-specific L1 VLP-antibodies reach maximum titres at month 7, i.e. 1 month after administration of the third dose. Titres decline until month 24 and remain rather stable thereafter [151, 152]. At 3 years, antibody titres remain two- to 20-fold higher than in placebo controls [152]. Complete protection against HPV16 associated CIN lesions was observed over the whole follow-up duration of two Phase IIb trials: 6 years for the monovalent HPV16 vaccine, 5 5 years for the bivalent HPV16/18 vaccine [153, 154] and 4 years for the quadrivalent vaccine. Follow-up is continuing, and continued protection against HPV 16/18-associated disease end-points has been shown for the entire available observation time, even when specific antibody titres fall.

HPV infection is the most prevalent soon after sexual debut of a girl [155]. The current HPV vaccines, being prophylactic in nature, should be used before exposure of girls to HPV infection. National mass vaccination programs targeting adolescent girls between 12 and 17 years of age are available in most of the developed countries. The vaccine coverage varies greatly between countries, but school-based schemes have thus far demonstrated the highest coverage rate of 80% or higher [1, 156-158]. Australia is the first country to implement a school-based mass vaccination program with Gardasil in April 2007 and, within 3 years, has already witnessed a reduced incidence of high-grade abnormalities (HGAs) among women below 18 years of age [1].

High coverage rates of adolescent vaccination with rubella and hepatitis B suggest that, with appropriate parental and public education, adequate HPV vaccine uptake rate of 50% or more is achievable. This coverage rate is critical for mass vaccination to attain cost-effectiveness as a public measure in controlling cervical cancer burden [159]. It will also remove the imbalance in accessing screening and effectively diminish the unequal distribution of cervical cancer burden among women in the metropolitan and rural areas, among women of different ethnic groups, and among women of various socio-economic status in developed countries. Adolescent HPV infection protects women from the first exposure to HPV infection at sexual debut and abolishes the opportunity for latent infection to occur with a resultant reduction of cervical cancer in old age. The current HPV vaccines induce very high levels of anti-HPV-16 and anti-HPV-18 antibody levels to sustain protection from infection by these aggressive oncogenic HPV subtypes for at least 20 years to cover the average age period of sexual debut [160].

A measure to address the concern of vaccination efficacy for older women is to consider vaccinating women at middle ages. Undoubtedly, vaccinating mid-adult women misses the most at-risk period of a woman's life for contracting HPV infection at sexual debut. It is, however, shown that one must not dismiss lightly a mid-adult woman who wants to take the vaccination to prevent new or repeat HPV infection [161]. The vaccines have been shown to be immunogenic in adult women and significant prevention of persistent HPV-16 and HPV-18 infection has been demonstrated in a randomized control trial [162]. The effectiveness of the vaccines among these women in reducing the incidence of HGAs is being awaited with great interest. The shifting burden of cervical cancer to the young and the old in the screened population should disappear in the HPV vaccination era [163].

Immunization of boys with VLPs elicits a serum immune response similar to that in girls. Because genital HPV infection is sexually transmitted, immunization of men may help to prevent infection of women. Modeling studies on herd immunity, i.e. indirect protection of those who remain susceptible, owing to a reduced prevalence of infections in the risk group for disease, have been published [164]. The utility of immunization of males depends upon the assumed population coverage of vaccination, with successively smaller additional benefits seen in scenarios with high population coverage [165]. Modeling of programs with high population coverage (90%) have found that addition of male vaccination gives a more rapid infection control and have suggested that both sex vaccination programs may be required to achieve an ultimate eradication of the infection [137].

Limitations of the current HPV vaccines include the need for multiple parenteral doses, the lack of protection against some HPV types that cause cervical cancer, and a relatively high cost. The opportunity to overcome 1 or more of these limitations provides a rationale for developing candidate second-generation vaccines. Low-cost second-generation vaccines that could induce long-term protective immunity with fewer doses would be especially attractive for the developing world. Vaccines with activity against a broader range of the HPV types that cause cervical cancer could increase their effectiveness throughout the world, and Merck has indicated that a nonavalent (9 HPV targets) VLP vaccine is currently in clinical trials [166]. If successful, such a vaccine might reduce the frequency of potentially oncogenic infections to a degree that would permit a drastic reduction in cervical cancer screening, which accounts for most of the cost of HPV-associated disease in developed countries [167].

11. Future prospects and conclusions

HPV differs from most other vaccine-preventable diseases in that the major diseases to be prevented occur many decades after infection. Whereas clinical trials have documented prevention of infection and intermediate disease end-points (condylomas and precancers), surveillance following vaccine implementation will be required to document the expected gains in cancer prevention if there is appropriate population coverage. Surveillance will also provide data to indicate if type replacement or escape mutants occur. Other important tasks for the HPV surveillance include monitoring of the duration of protection, long-term safety and actual effects on health-care cost consumption. Monitoring the impact of vaccination on type-specific infection could be important as it is the earliest change that could be anticipated, and failure to detect protection from infection will indicate failure to impact cancer in the decades that follow and allow appropriate changes in strategy to be introduced. As countries differ in their health-care priorities and infrastructure as well as in their incidence and prevalence of various HPV infections, their HPV vaccination strategies are also likely to differ [168]. As has been mentioned, the waning in the levels of HPV antibodies post-vaccination appears to plateau after 5 years. It is not known whether waning of HPV antibody levels in the longer term will require a vaccine booster. In addition, antibody correlates of protection have not been defined because there have so far been almost no cases of vaccination failure. If a reliable immunological correlate of protection can be identified, this will help in assessing the requirement for booster vaccinations and greatly facilitate the evaluation of second-generation vaccines.

As the type-specific prevalence of HPV infection is very high in young sexually active populations, the effect of a successful HPV vaccination programme should be detected quite rapidly by sentinel surveillance in these populations. The specific design of these sentinel studies will vary, but selecting clinics offering sexual counselling may be more efficient than school-based sampling. Reduction in the prevalence of types targeted by the vaccines as well as no increase in the prevalence of non-vaccine types are important end-points. Baseline data are needed to establish prevaccine prevalence as well as to determine the sample size required to observe impact beyond confidence intervals of sampling and testing errors. It is imperative that all HPV DNA prevalence surveys are performed using testing methodology that has been subjected to an international quality assurance, as comparability of data between countries or even before *versus* after will otherwise not be possible.

Screening remains an important strategy in cervical cancer control in the HPV vaccination era. Women who have received HPV vaccination should continue regular screening, as cases of HGAs and invasive cervical cancer among vaccinated women have been reported [169]. There is also a concern whether the protective effect of adolescent vaccination has an impact on the incidence of cervical cancer when the vaccinated cohort reaches older age. It is reassuring to see evidence that, in well informed communities, there appears to be no change in women's attitude toward continual screening [170]. Furthermore, screening remains the only effective method for cervical cancer prevention for women who opt out of vaccination. However, reduction in the incidence of HGAs in young women following adolescent mass HPV vaccination supports a strategy to delay screening to a later age than the current practice of starting screening once the girl becomes sexually active.

Evidence from meta-analysis has overwhelmingly demonstrated the superiority in sensitivity of HPV DNA test over cytology in cervical cancer screening. Indeed, retrospective analysis of invasive cervical cancer tissues in well screened populations showed that more than 80% of cases were related to HPV-16 or HPV-18 [171]. With elimination of HPV-16 and HPV-18 with mass vaccination, the remaining oncogenic subtypes of HPV, which have low neoplastic transformation rates, should significantly lower the incidence of HGAs. The sensitivity and positive predictive value of cytologic screening will be further compromised [172]. The recently available HPV-16-specific and HPV-18-specific screening technology further enhances the technical advances that makes the HPV DNA screening test even more attractive in the vaccination era than before. The high sensitivity of the HPV DNA test should allow the screening interval to be increased to a longer period [173].

The reduction in background risk of cervical cancer by elimination of the most important HPV types will affect cost-effectiveness of screening programs and may, in the long term, allow increasing screening intervals. Co-ordinated quality assurance/monitoring of HPV vaccination and cervical screening is advisable for finding the most efficient strategies for cervical cancer control. Data on vaccination coverage will be essential for every country performing HPV vaccinations. HPV vaccination registries are preferable, but sales statistics and serosurveys may be alternatives.

For rapid assessment of vaccine program efficacy, the continuous monitoring of which HPV types are spreading in the population will become necessary for early monitoring of 'type replacement' phenomena, inappropriate vaccination strategies or other reasons for vaccination failure. Surveys in sexually active teenagers and/or in younger participants of cervical screening programs should be contemplated.

Author details

Fátima Galán-Sánchez and Manuel Rodríguez-Iglesias

Department of Microbiology, School of Medicine and Clinical Microbiology Laboratory, Puerta del Mar Univ. Hosp. University of Cádiz, Spain

References

[1] Brotherton JM, Fridman M, May CL, Chappell G, Saville AM, Gertig DM. Early effect of the HPV vaccination programme on cervical abnormalities in Victoria, Australia: an ecological study. Lancet 2011;377:2085-92.

[2] Parkin DM, Bray F. Chapter 2: The burden of HPV-related cancers. Vaccine 2006;24 Suppl 3:11-25.

[3] Moscicki AB, Burt VG, Kanowitz S, Darragh T, Shiboski S. The significance of squamous metaplasia in the development of low grade squamous intraepithelial lesions in young women. Cancer 1999;85:1139-44.

[4] Doorbar J. Molecular biology of human papillomavirus infection and cervical cancer. Clin Sci (Lond) 2006;110:525-41.

[5]   Bruni L, Diaz M, Castellsague X, Ferrer E, Bosch FX, de Sanjose S. Cervical human papillomavirus prevalence in 5 continents: meta-analysis of 1 million women with normal cytological findings. J Infect Dis 2010;202:1789-99.

[6]   de Sanjose S, Diaz M, Castellsague X, Clifford G, Bruni L, Munoz N, et al. Worldwide prevalence and genotype distribution of cervical human papillomavirus DNA in women with normal cytology: a meta-analysis. Lancet Infect Dis 2007;7:453-9.

[7]   Gonzalez P, Hildesheim A, Rodriguez AC, Schiffman M, Porras C, Wacholder S, et al. Behavioral/lifestyle and immunologic factors associated with HPV infection among women older than 45 years. Cancer Epidemiol Biomarkers Prev 2010;19:3044-54.

[8]   Maglennon GA, McIntosh P, Doorbar J. Persistence of viral DNA in the epithelial basal layer suggests a model for papillomavirus latency following immune regression. Virology 2011;414:153-63.

[9]   Chow LT, Broker TR, Steinberg BM. The natural history of human papillomavirus infections of the mucosal epithelia. APMIS 2010;118:422-49.

[10] Strickler HD, Burk RD, Fazzari M, Anastos K, Minkoff H, Massad LS, et al. Natural history and possible reactivation of human papillomavirus in human immunodeficiency virus-positive women. J Natl Cancer Inst 2005;97:577-86.

[11] Nowak RG, Gravitt PE, Morrison CS, Gange SJ, Kwok C, Oliver AE, et al. Increases in human papillomavirus detection during early HIV infection among women in Zimbabwe. J Infect Dis 2011;203:1182-91.

[12] Gravitt PE. The known unknowns of HPV natural history. J Clin Invest 2011;121:4593-9.

[13] Dunne EF, Unger ER, Sternberg M, McQuillan G, Swan DC, Patel SS, et al. Prevalence of HPV infection among females in the United States. JAMA 2007;297:813-9.

[14] Partridge JM, Hughes JP, Feng Q, Winer RL, Weaver BA, Xi LF, et al. Genital human papillomavirus infection in men: incidence and risk factors in a cohort of university students. J Infect Dis 2007;196:1128-36.

[15] Smith JS, Gilbert PA, Melendy A, Rana RK, Pimenta JM. Age-specific prevalence of human papillomavirus infection in males: a global review. J Adolesc Health 2011;48:540-52.

[16] Machalek DA, Poynten M, Jin F, Fairley CK, Farnsworth A, Garland SM, et al. Anal human papillomavirus infection and associated neoplastic lesions in men who have sex with men: a systematic review and meta-analysis. Lancet Oncol 2012;13:487-500.

[17] Schiffman M, Clifford G, Buonaguro FM. Classification of weakly carcinogenic human papillomavirus types: addressing the limits of epidemiology at the borderline. Infect Agent Cancer 2009;4:8.

[18] Giuliano AR, Tortolero-Luna G, Ferrer E, Burchell AN, de Sanjose S, Kjaer SK, et al. Epidemiology of human papillomavirus infection in men, cancers other than cervical and benign conditions. Vaccine 2008;26 Suppl 10:K17-28.

[19] Abramowitz L, Jacquard AC, Jaroud F, Haesebaert J, Siproudhis L, Pradat P, et al. Human papillomavirus genotype distribution in anal cancer in France: the EDiTH V study. Int J Cancer 2011;129:433-9.

[20] Bosch FX, Manos MM, Munoz N, Sherman M, Jansen AM, Peto J, et al. Prevalence of human papillomavirus in cervical cancer: a worldwide perspective. International biological study on cervical cancer (IBSCC) Study Group. J Natl Cancer Inst 1995;87:796-802.

[21] Li N, Franceschi S, Howell-Jones R, Snijders PJ, Clifford GM. Human papillomavirus type distribution in 30,848 invasive cervical cancers worldwide: Variation by geographical region, histological type and year of publication. Int J Cancer 2011;128:927-35.

[22] de Sanjose S, Quint WG, Alemany L, Geraets DT, Klaustermeier JE, Lloveras B, et al. Human papillomavirus genotype attribution in invasive cervical cancer: a retrospective cross-sectional worldwide study. Lancet Oncol 2010;11:1048-56.

[23] Mendez F, Munoz N, Posso H, Molano M, Moreno V, van den Brule AJ, et al. Cervical coinfection with human papillomavirus (HPV) types and possible implications for the prevention of cervical cancer by HPV vaccines. J Infect Dis 2005;192:1158-65.

[24] Plummer M, Schiffman M, Castle PE, Maucort-Boulch D, Wheeler CM. A 2-year prospective study of human papillomavirus persistence among women with a cytological diagnosis of atypical squamous cells of undetermined significance or low-grade squamous intraepithelial lesion. J Infect Dis 2007;195:1582-9.

[25] Vaccarella S, Franceschi S, Snijders PJ, Herrero R, Meijer CJ, Plummer M. Concurrent infection with multiple human papillomavirus types: pooled analysis of the IARC HPV Prevalence Surveys. Cancer Epidemiol Biomarkers Prev 2010;19:503-10.

[26] Jenkins D. A review of cross-protection against oncogenic HPV by an HPV-16/18 AS04-adjuvanted cervical cancer vaccine: importance of virological and clinical endpoints and implications for mass vaccination in cervical cancer prevention. Gynecol Oncol 2008;110(Suppl 1):S18-25.

[27] Brown DR, Kjaer SK, Sigurdsson K, Iversen OE, Hernandez-Avila M, Wheeler CM, et al. The impact of quadrivalent human papillomavirus (HPV; types 6, 11, 16, and 18) L1 virus-like particle vaccine on infection and disease due to oncogenic nonvaccine HPV types in generally HPV-naive women aged 16-26 years. J Infect Dis 2009;199:926-35.

[28] Paavonen J, Naud P, Salmeron J, Wheeler CM, Chow SN, Apter D, et al. Efficacy of human papillomavirus (HPV)-16/18 AS04-adjuvanted vaccine against cervical infec-

tion and precancer caused by oncogenic HPV types (PATRICIA): final analysis of a double-blind, randomised study in young women. Lancet 2009;374:301-14

[29] Gillison ML. Human papillomavirus-related diseases: oropharynx cancers and potential implications for adolescent HPV vaccination. J Adolesc Health 2008;43(4 Suppl):S52-60.

[30] Kreimer AR, Clifford GM, Boyle P, Franceschi S. Human papillomavirus types in head and neck squamous cell carcinomas worldwide: a systematic review. Cancer Epidemiol Biomarkers Prev 2005;14:467-75.

[31] Herrero R, Castellsague X, Pawlita M, Lissowska J, Kee F, Balaram P, et al. Human papillomavirus and oral cancer: the International Agency for Research on Cancer multicenter study. J Natl Cancer Inst 2003;95:1772-83.

[32] D'Souza G, Kreimer AR, Viscidi R, Pawlita M, Fakhry C, Koch WM, et al. Case-control study of human papillomavirus and oropharyngeal cancer. N Engl J Med 2007;356:1944-56.

[33] Gillison ML, D'Souza G, Westra W, Sugar E, Xiao W, Begum S, et al. Distinct risk factor profiles for human papillomavirus type 16-positive and human papillomavirus type 16-negative head and neck cancers. J Natl Cancer Inst 2008;100:407-20.

[34] Pow-Sang MR, Ferreira U, Pow-Sang JM, Nardi AC, Destefano V. Epidemiology and natural history of penile cancer. Urology 2010;76(2 Suppl 1):S2-6.

[35] Moscicki AB, Widdice L, Ma Y, Farhat S, Miller-Benningfield S, Jonte J, et al. Comparison of natural histories of human papillomavirus detected by clinician- and self-sampling. Int J Cancer 2010;127:1882-92.

[36] Markowitz LE, Sternberg M, Dunne EF, McQuillan G, Unger ER. Seroprevalence of human papillomavirus types 6, 11, 16, and 18 in the United States: National Health and Nutrition Examination Survey 2003-2004. J Infect Dis 2009;200:1059-67.

[37] Kahn JA, Brown DR, Ding L, Widdice LE, Shew ML, Glynn S, et al. Vaccine-type human papillomavirus and evidence of herd protection after vaccine introduction. Pediatrics 2011; 30:e249-56.

[38] Arbyn M, Castellsague X, de Sanjose S, Bruni L, Saraiya M, Bray F, et al. Worldwide burden of cervical cancer in 2008. Ann Oncol 2012;22:2675-86.

[39] Gillison ML, Chaturvedi AK, Lowy DR. HPV prophylactic vaccines and the potential prevention of noncervical cancers in both men and women. Cancer 2008;113(10 Suppl):3036-46.

[40] Sitas F, Egger S, Urban MI, Taylor PR, Abnet CC, Boffetta P, et al. InterSCOPE study: Associations between esophageal squamous cell carcinoma and human papillomavirus serological markers. J Natl Cancer Inst 2012;104:147-58.

[41] Chaturvedi AK. Beyond cervical cancer: burden of other HPV-related cancers among men and women. J Adolesc Health 2010;46(4 Suppl):S20-6.

[42] Parkin DM. The global health burden of infection-associated cancers in the year 2002. Int J Cancer 2006;118:3030-44.

[43] Kitchener HC, Gilham C, Sargent A, Bailey A, Albrow R, Roberts C, et al. A comparison of HPV DNA testing and liquid based cytology over three rounds of primary cervical screening: extended follow up in the ARTISTIC trial. Eur J Cancer 2011;47:864-71.

[44] Bulkmans NW, Berkhof J, Rozendaal L, van Kemenade FJ, Boeke AJ, Bulk S, et al. Human papillomavirus DNA testing for the detection of cervical intraepithelial neoplasia grade 3 and cancer: 5-year follow-up of a randomised controlled implementation trial. Lancet 2007;370:1764-72.

[45] Naucler P, Ryd W, Tornberg S, Strand A, Wadell G, Elfgren K, et al. Efficacy of HPV DNA testing with cytology triage and/or repeat HPV DNA testing in primary cervical cancer screening. J Natl Cancer Inst 2009;101:88-99.

[46] Anttila A, Kotaniemi-Talonen L, Leinonen M, Hakama M, Laurila P, Tarkkanen J, et al. Rate of cervical cancer, severe intraepithelial neoplasia, and adenocarcinoma in situ in primary HPV DNA screening with cytology triage: randomised study within organised screening programme. BMJ 2010;340:c1804.

[47] Schiffman M, Wentzensen N, Wacholder S, Kinney W, Gage JC, Castle PE. Human papillomavirus testing in the prevention of cervical cancer. J Natl Cancer Inst 2011;103:368-83.

[48] Rijkaart DC, Berkhof J, Rozendaal L, van Kemenade FJ, Bulkmans NW, Heideman DA, et al. Human papillomavirus testing for the detection of high-grade cervical intraepithelial neoplasia and cancer: final results of the POBASCAM randomised controlled trial. Lancet Oncol 2012;13:78-88.

[49] Benoy IH, Vanden Broeck D, Ruymbeke MJ, Sahebali S, Arbyn M, Bogers JJ, et al. Prior knowledge of HPV status improves detection of CIN2+ by cytology screening. Am J Obstet Gynecol 2011;205:569.e1-7.

[50] Franceschi S, Denny L, Irwin KL, Jeronimo J, Lopalco PL, Monsonego J, et al. Eurogin 2010 roadmap on cervical cancer prevention. Int J Cancer 2011;128:2765-74.

[51] Szarewski A, Mesher D, Cadman L, Austin J, Ashdown-Barr L, Ho L, et al. Comparison of seven tests for high-grade cervical intraepithelial neoplasia in women with abnormal smears: the Predictors 2 study. J Clin Microbiol 2012;50:1867-73.

[52] Poljak M, Kocjan BJ. Commercially available assays for multiplex detection of alpha human papillomaviruses. Expert Rev Anti Infect Ther 2010;8:1139-62.

[53] Arbyn M, Ronco G, Cuzick J, Wentzensen N, Castle PE. How to evaluate emerging technologies in cervical cancer screening? Int J Cancer 2009;125:2489-96.

[54] Eder PS, Lou J, Huff J, Macioszek J. The next-generation Hybrid Capture High-Risk HPV DNA assay on a fully automated platform. J Clin Virol 2009;45 Suppl 1:S85-92.

[55] Szarewski A, Ambroisine L, Cadman L, Austin J, Ho L, Terry G, et al. Comparison of predictors for high-grade cervical intraepithelial neoplasia in women with abnormal smears. Cancer Epidemiol Biomarkers Prev 2008;17:3033-42.

[56] Day SP, Hudson A, Mast A, Sander T, Curtis M, Olson S, et al. Analytical performance of the Investigational Use Only Cervista HPV HR test as determined by a multicenter study. J Clin Virol 2009;45 Suppl 1:S63-72.

[57] Qiao YL, Sellors JW, Eder PS, Bao YP, Lim JM, Zhao FH, et al. A new HPV-DNA test for cervical-cancer screening in developing regions: a cross-sectional study of clinical accuracy in rural China. Lancet Oncol 2008;9:929-36.

[58] Kim JJ, Wright TC, Goldie SJ. Cost-effectiveness of alternative triage strategies for atypical squamous cells of undetermined significance. JAMA 2002;287:2382-90.

[59] Solomon D, Schiffman M, Tarone R. Comparison of three management strategies for patients with atypical squamous cells of undetermined significance: baseline results from a randomized trial. J Natl Cancer Inst 2001;93:293-9.

[60] Huang S, Tang N, Mak WB, Erickson B, Salituro J, Li Y, et al. Principles and analytical performance of Abbott RealTime High Risk HPV test. J Clin Virol 2009;45 Suppl 1:S13-7.

[61] Venturoli S, Leo E, Nocera M, Barbieri D, Cricca M, Costa S, et al. Comparison of Abbott RealTime High Risk HPV and Hybrid Capture 2 for the detection of high-risk HPV DNA in a referral population setting. J Clin Virol 2012;53:121-4.

[62] Jentschke M, Soergel P, Lange V, Kocjan B, Doerk T, Luyten A, et al. Evaluation of a new multiplex real-time polymerase chain reaction assay for the detection of human papillomavirus infections in a referral population. Int J Gynecol Cancer 2012;22:1050-6.

[63] Castle PE, Sadorra M, Lau T, Aldrich C, Garcia FA, Kornegay J. Evaluation of a prototype real-time PCR assay for carcinogenic human papillomavirus (HPV) detection and simultaneous HPV genotype 16 (HPV16) and HPV18 genotyping. J Clin Microbiol 2009;47:3344-7.

[64] Castle PE, Stoler MH, Wright TC, Jr., Sharma A, Wright TL, Behrens CM. Performance of carcinogenic human papillomavirus (HPV) testing and HPV16 or HPV18 genotyping for cervical cancer screening of women aged 25 years and older: a subanalysis of the ATHENA study. Lancet Oncol 2011;12:880-90.

[65] Heideman DA, Hesselink AT, Berkhof J, van Kemenade F, Melchers WJ, Daalmeijer NF, et al. Clinical validation of the cobas 4800 HPV test for cervical screening purposes. J Clin Microbiol 2011;49:3983-5.

[66] Lapierre SG, Sauthier P, Mayrand MH, Dufresne S, Petignat P, Provencher D, et al. Human papillomavirus (HPV) DNA triage of women with atypical squamous cells of undetermined significance with cobas 4800 HPV and Hybrid Capture 2 tests for detection of high-grade lesions of the uterine cervix. J Clin Microbiol 2012;50:1240-4.

[67] Wong AA, Fuller J, Pabbaraju K, Wong S, Zahariadis G. Comparison of the Hybrid Capture 2 and cobas 4800 Tests for Detection of High-Risk Human Papillomavirus in Specimens Collected in PreservCyt Medium. J Clin Microbiol 2011;50:25-9.

[68] Gage JC, Sadorra M, Lamere BJ, Kail R, Aldrich C, Kinney W, et al. Comparison of the cobas Human Papillomavirus (HPV) Test with the Hybrid Capture 2 and Linear Array HPV DNA Tests. J Clin Microbiol 2012;50:61-5.

[69] Einstein MH, Martens MG, Garcia FA, Ferris DG, Mitchell AL, Day SP, et al. Clinical validation of the Cervista HPV HR and 16/18 genotyping tests for use in women with ASC-US cytology. Gynecol Oncol 2010;118:116-22.

[70] Gravitt PE, Coutlee F, Iftner T, Sellors JW, Quint WG, Wheeler CM. New technologies in cervical cancer screening. Vaccine 2008;26 Suppl 10:K42-52.

[71] Cox JT. History of the use of HPV testing in cervical screening and in the management of abnormal cervical screening results. J Clin Virol 2009;45 Suppl 1:S3-S12.

[72] Cuzick J, Arbyn M, Sankaranarayanan R, Tsu V, Ronco G, Mayrand MH, et al. Overview of human papillomavirus-based and other novel options for cervical cancer screening in developed and developing countries. Vaccine 2008;26 Suppl 10:K29-41.

[73] Feng Q, Cherne S, Winer RL, Balasubramanian A, Lee SK, Hawes SE, et al. Development and evaluation of a liquid bead microarray assay for genotyping genital human papillomaviruses. J Clin Microbiol 2009;47:547-53.

[74] van Hamont D, van Ham MA, Bakkers JM, Massuger LF, Melchers WJ. Evaluation of the SPF10-INNO LiPA human papillomavirus (HPV) genotyping test and the roche linear array HPV genotyping test. J Clin Microbiol 2006;44:3122-9.

[75] Conway C, Chalkley R, High A, Maclennan K, Berri S, Chengot P, et al. Next-generation sequencing for simultaneous determination of human papillomavirus load, subtype, and associated genomic copy number changes in tumors. J Mol Diagn 2012;14:104-11.

[76] Meijer CJ, Berkhof H, Heideman DA, Hesselink AT, Snijders PJ. Validation of high-risk HPV tests for primary cervical screening. J Clin Virol 2009;46 Suppl 3:S1-4.

[77] van den Brule AJ, Pol R, Fransen-Daalmeijer N, Schouls LM, Meijer CJ, Snijders PJ. GP5+/6+ PCR followed by reverse line blot analysis enables rapid and high-through-

put identification of human papillomavirus genotypes. J Clin Microbiol 2002;40:779-87.

[78] Kleter B, van Doorn LJ, Schrauwen L, Molijn A, Sastrowijoto S, ter Schegget J, et al. Development and clinical evaluation of a highly sensitive PCR-reverse hybridization line probe assay for detection and identification of anogenital human papillomavirus. J Clin Microbiol 1999;37:2508-17.

[79] Seme K, Lepej SZ, Lunar MM, Iscic-Bes J, Planinic A, Kocjan BJ, et al. Digene HPV Genotyping RH Test RUO: comparative evaluation with INNO-LiPA HPV Genotyping Extra Test for detection of 18 high-risk and probable high-risk human papillomavirus genotypes. J Clin Virol 2009;46:176-9.

[80] Micalessi MI, Boulet GA, Vorsters A, De Wit K, Jannes G, Mijs W, et al. A real-time PCR approach based on SPF10 primers and the INNO-LiPA HPV Genotyping Extra assay for the detection and typing of human papillomavirus. J Virol Methods 2013;187:66-71.

[81] Gravitt PE, Peyton CL, Alessi TQ, Wheeler CM, Coutlee F, Hildesheim A, et al. Improved amplification of genital human papillomaviruses. J Clin Microbiol 2000;38:357-61.

[82] Steinau M, Onyekwuluje JM, Scarbrough MZ, Unger ER, Dillner J, Zhou T. Performance of commercial reverse line blot assays for human papillomavirus genotyping. J Clin Microbiol 2012;50:1539-44.

[83] Dalstein V, Merlin S, Bali C, Saunier M, Dachez R, Ronsin C. Analytical evaluation of the PapilloCheck test, a new commercial DNA chip for detection and genotyping of human papillomavirus. J Virol Methods 2009;156:77-83.

[84] Galan-Sanchez F, Rodriguez-Iglesias MA. Comparison of human papillomavirus genotyping using commercial assays based on PCR and reverse hybridization methods. APMIS 2009;117:708-15.

[85] Schmitt M, Dondog B, Waterboer T, Pawlita M, Tommasino M, Gheit T. Abundance of multiple high-risk human papillomavirus (HPV) infections found in cervical cells analyzed by use of an ultrasensitive HPV genotyping assay. J Clin Microbiol 2010;48:143-9.

[86] Jiang HL, Zhu HH, Zhou LF, Chen F, Chen Z. Genotyping of human papillomavirus in cervical lesions by L1 consensus PCR and the Luminex xMAP system. J Med Microbiol 2006;55:715-20.

[87] Oh Y, Bae SM, Kim YW, Choi HS, Nam GH, Han SJ, et al. Polymerase chain reaction-based fluorescent Luminex assay to detect the presence of human papillomavirus types. Cancer Sci 2007;98:549-54.

[88] Wallace J, Woda BA, Pihan G. Facile, comprehensive, high-throughput genotyping of human genital papillomaviruses using spectrally addressable liquid bead microarrays. J Mol Diagn 2005;7:72-80.

[89] Nazarenko I, Kobayashi L, Giles J, Fishman C, Chen G, Lorincz A. A novel method of HPV genotyping using Hybrid Capture sample preparation method combined with GP5+/6+ PCR and multiplex detection on Luminex XMAP. J Virol Methods 2008;154:76-81.

[90] Schmitt M, Dondog B, Waterboer T, Pawlita M. Homogeneous amplification of genital human alpha papillomaviruses by PCR using novel broad-spectrum GP5+ and GP6+ primers. J Clin Microbiol 2008;46:1050-9.

[91] Schmitt M, Bravo IG, Snijders PJ, Gissmann L, Pawlita M, Waterboer T. Bead-based multiplex genotyping of human papillomaviruses. J Clin Microbiol 2006;44:504-12.

[92] Yi X, Li J, Yu S, Zhang A, Xu J, Yi J, et al. A new PCR-based mass spectrometry system for high-risk HPV, part I: methods. Am J Clin Pathol 2011;136:913-9.

[93] Lie AK, Kristensen G. Human papillomavirus E6/E7 mRNA testing as a predictive marker for cervical carcinoma. Expert Rev Mol Diagn 2008;8:405-15.

[94] Cuschieri K, Wentzensen N. Human papillomavirus mRNA and p16 detection as biomarkers for the improved diagnosis of cervical neoplasia. Cancer Epidemiol Biomarkers Prev 2008;17:2536-45.

[95] Depuydt CE, Benoy IH, Beert JF, Criel AM, Bogers JJ, Arbyn M. Clinical validation of a type-specific real-time quantitative human papillomavirus PCR against the performance of hybrid capture 2 for the purpose of cervical cancer screening. J Clin Microbiol 2012;50: 4073-7.

[96] Molden T, Kraus I, Skomedal H, Nordstrom T, Karlsen F. PreTect HPV-Proofer: real-time detection and typing of E6/E7 mRNA from carcinogenic human papillomaviruses. J Virol Methods 2007;142:204-12.

[97] Jeantet D, Schwarzmann F, Tromp J, Melchers WJ, van der Wurff AA, Oosterlaken T, et al. NucliSENS EasyQ HPV v1 test - Testing for oncogenic activity of human papillomaviruses. J Clin Virol 2009;45 Suppl 1:S29-37.

[98] Dockter J, Schroder A, Eaton B, Wang A, Sikhamsay N, Morales L, et al. Analytical characterization of the APTIMA HPV Assay. J Clin Virol 2009;45 Suppl 1:S39-47.

[99] Dockter J, Schroder A, Hill C, Guzenski L, Monsonego J, Giachetti C. Clinical performance of the APTIMA HPV Assay for the detection of high-risk HPV and high-grade cervical lesions. J Clin Virol 2009;45 Suppl 1:S55-61.

[100] Monsonego J, Hudgens MG, Zerat L, Zerat JC, Syrjanen K, Smith JS. Risk assessment and clinical impact of liquid-based cytology, oncogenic human papillomavirus

(HPV) DNA and mRNA testing in primary cervical cancer screening (the FASE study). Gynecol Oncol 2012;125:175-80.

[101] Lorincz AT, Castle PE, Sherman ME, Scott DR, Glass AG, Wacholder S, et al. Viral load of human papillomavirus and risk of CIN3 or cervical cancer. Lancet 2002;360:228-9.

[102] Wentzensen N, Schiffman M, Dunn T, Zuna RE, Gold MA, Allen RA, et al. Multiple human papillomavirus genotype infections in cervical cancer progression in the study to understand cervical cancer early endpoints and determinants. Int J Cancer 2009;125:2151-8.

[103] Boulet GA, Benoy IH, Depuydt CE, Horvath CA, Aerts M, Hens N, et al. Human papillomavirus 16 load and E2/E6 ratio in HPV16-positive women: biomarkers for cervical intraepithelial neoplasia >or=2 in a liquid-based cytology setting? Cancer Epidemiol Biomarkers Prev 2009;18:2992-9.

[104] Gravitt PE, Kovacic MB, Herrero R, Schiffman M, Bratti C, Hildesheim A, et al. High load for most high risk human papillomavirus genotypes is associated with prevalent cervical cancer precursors but only HPV16 load predicts the development of incident disease. Int J Cancer 2007;121:2787-93.

[105] Xi LF, Hughes JP, Castle PE, Edelstein ZR, Wang C, Galloway DA, et al. Viral load in the natural history of human papillomavirus type 16 infection: a nested case-control study. J Infect Dis 2011;203:1425-33.

[106] Marks M, Gravitt PE, Utaipat U, Gupta SB, Liaw K, Kim E, et al. Kinetics of DNA load predict HPV 16 viral clearance. J Clin Virol 2011;5:44-9.

[107] Monnier-Benoit S, Dalstein V, Riethmuller D, Lalaoui N, Mougin C, Pretet JL. Dynamics of HPV16 DNA load reflect the natural history of cervical HPV-associated lesions. J Clin Virol 2006;35:270-7.

[108] Gravitt PE, van Doorn LJ, Quint W, Schiffman M, Hildesheim A, Glass AG, et al. Human papillomavirus (HPV) genotyping using paired exfoliated cervicovaginal cells and paraffin-embedded tissues to highlight difficulties in attributing HPV types to specific lesions. J Clin Microbiol 2007;45:3245-50.

[109] Pretet JL, Dalstein V, Monnier-Benoit S, Delpeut S, Mougin C. High risk HPV load estimated by Hybrid Capture II correlates with HPV16 load measured by real-time PCR in cervical smears of HPV16-infected women. J Clin Virol 2004;31:140-7.

[110] Wentzensen N, Gravitt PE, Long R, Schiffman M, Dunn ST, Carreon JD, et al. Human papillomavirus load measured by Linear Array correlates with quantitative PCR in cervical cytology specimens. J Clin Microbiol 2012;50:1564-70.

[111] Pett M, Coleman N. Integration of high-risk human papillomavirus: a key event in cervical carcinogenesis? J Pathol 2007;212:356-67.

[112] Cullen AP, Reid R, Campion M, Lorincz AT. Analysis of the physical state of different human papillomavirus DNAs in intraepithelial and invasive cervical neoplasm. J Virol 1991;65:606-12.

[113] Pirami L, Giache V, Becciolini A. Analysis of HPV16, 18, 31, and 35 DNA in pre-invasive and invasive lesions of the uterine cervix. J Clin Pathol 1997;50:600-4.

[114] Tsoumpou I, Arbyn M, Kyrgiou M, Wentzensen N, Koliopoulos G, Martin-Hirsch P, et al. p16(INK4a) immunostaining in cytological and histological specimens from the uterine cervix: a systematic review and meta-analysis. Cancer Treat Rev 2009;35:210-20.

[115] Molden T, Nygard JF, Kraus I, Karlsen F, Nygard M, Skare GB, et al. Predicting CIN2+ when detecting HPV mRNA and DNA by PreTect HPV-proofer and consensus PCR: A 2-year follow up of women with ASCUS or LSIL Pap smear. Int J Cancer 2005;114:973-6.

[116] Schweizer J, Lu PS, Mahoney CW, Berard-Bergery M, Ho M, Ramasamy V, et al. Feasibility study of a human papillomavirus E6 oncoprotein test for diagnosis of cervical precancer and cancer. J Clin Microbiol 2010;48:4646-8.

[117] Fernandez AF, Rosales C, Lopez-Nieva P, Grana O, Ballestar E, Ropero S, et al. The dynamic DNA methylomes of double-stranded DNA viruses associated with human cancer. Genome Res 2009;19:438-51.

[118] Mirabello L, Sun C, Ghosh A, Rodriguez AC, Schiffman M, Wentzensen N, et al. Methylation of human papillomavirus type 16 genome and risk of cervical precancer in a Costa Rican population. J Natl Cancer Inst 2012;104:556-65.

[119] Wentzensen N, Sherman ME, Schiffman M, Wang SS. Utility of methylation markers in cervical cancer early detection: appraisal of the state-of-the-science. Gynecol Oncol 2009;112:293-9.

[120] Feng Q, Hawes SE, Stern JE, Dem A, Sow PS, Dembele B, et al. Promoter hypermethylation of tumor suppressor genes in urine from patients with cervical neoplasia. Cancer Epidemiol Biomarkers Prev 2007;16:1178-84.

[121] Andersson S, Sowjanya P, Wangsa D, Hjerpe A, Johansson B, Auer G, et al. Detection of genomic amplification of the human telomerase gene TERC, a potential marker for triage of women with HPV-positive, abnormal Pap smears. Am J Pathol 2009;175:1831-47.

[122] Murphy N, Ring M, Heffron CC, King B, Killalea AG, Hughes C, et al. p16INK4A, CDC6, and MCM5: predictive biomarkers in cervical preinvasive neoplasia and cervical cancer. J Clin Pathol 2005;58:525-34.

[123] Pinto AP, Degen M, Villa LL, Cibas ES. Immunomarkers in gynecologic cytology: the search for the ideal 'biomolecular Papanicolaou test'. Acta Cytol 2012;56:109-21.

[124] Stoler MH, Castle PE, Solomon D, Schiffman M. The expanded use of HPV testing in gynecologic practice per ASCCP-guided management requires the use of well-validated assays. Am J Clin Pathol 2007;127:335-7.

[125] Meijer CJ, Berkhof J, Castle PE, Hesselink AT, Franco EL, Ronco G, et al. Guidelines for human papillomavirus DNA test requirements for primary cervical cancer screening in women 30 years and older. Int J Cancer 2009;124:516-20.

[126] Kinney W, Stoler MH, Castle PE. Special commentary: patient safety and the next generation of HPV DNA tests. Am J Clin Pathol 2010;134:193-9.

[127] Gok M, van Kemenade FJ, Heideman DA, Berkhof J, Rozendaal L, Spruyt JW, et al. Experience with high-risk human papillomavirus testing on vaginal brush-based self-samples of non-attendees of the cervical screening program. Int J Cancer 2011;130:1128-35.

[128] Szarewski A, Cadman L, Mesher D, Austin J, Ashdown-Barr L, Edwards R, et al. HPV self-sampling as an alternative strategy in non-attenders for cervical screening - a randomised controlled trial. Br J Cancer 2011;104:915-20.

[129] Lindell M, Sanner K, Wikstrom I, Wilander E. Self-sampling of vaginal fluid and high-risk human papillomavirus testing in women aged 50 years or older not attending Papanicolaou smear screening. BJOG 2011;119:245-8.

[130] Lazcano-Ponce E, Lorincz AT, Cruz-Valdez A, Salmeron J, Uribe P, Velasco-Mondragon E, et al. Self-collection of vaginal specimens for human papillomavirus testing in cervical cancer prevention (MARCH): a community-based randomised controlled trial. Lancet 2011;378:1868-73.

[131] Klug SJ, Molijn A, Schopp B, Holz B, Iftner A, Quint W, et al. Comparison of the performance of different HPV genotyping methods for detecting genital HPV types. J Med Virol 2008;80:1264-74.

[132] Eklund C, Zhou T, Dillner J. Global proficiency study of human papillomavirus genotyping. J Clin Microbiol 2010;48:4147-55.

[133] Eklund C, Forslund O, Wallin KL, Zhou T, Dillner J. The 2010 global proficiency study of human papillomavirus genotyping in vaccinology. J Clin Microbiol 2012;50:2289-98.

[134] Ferguson M, Heath A, Johnes S, Pagliusi S, Dillner J. Results of the first WHO international collaborative study on the standardization of the detection of antibodies to human papillomaviruses. Int J Cancer 2006;118:1508-14.

[135] Einstein MH, Baron M, Levin MJ, Chatterjee A, Edwards RP, Zepp F, et al. Comparison of the immunogenicity and safety of Cervarix and Gardasil human papillomavirus (HPV) cervical cancer vaccines in healthy women aged 18-45 years. Hum Vaccine 2009;5:705-19.

[136] Dessy FJ, Giannini SL, Bougelet CA, Kemp TJ, David MP, Poncelet SM, et al. Correlation between direct ELISA, single epitope-based inhibition ELISA and pseudovirion-based neutralization assay for measuring anti-HPV-16 and anti-HPV-18 antibody response after vaccination with the AS04-adjuvanted HPV-16/18 cervical cancer vaccine. Hum Vaccines 2008;4:425-34.

[137] Ryding J, French KM, Naucler P, Barnabas RV, Garnett GP, Dillner J. Seroepidemiology as basis for design of a human papillomavirus vaccination program. Vaccine 2008;26:5263-8.

[138] Pagliusi SR, Dillner J, Pawlita M, Quint WG, Wheeler CM, Ferguson M. Chapter 23: International Standard reagents for harmonization of HPV serology and DNA assays--an update. Vaccine 2006;24 Suppl 3:S3/193-200.

[139] Ferguson M, Wilkinson DE, Zhou T. WHO meeting on the standardization of HPV assays and the role of the WHO HPV Laboratory Network in supporting vaccine introduction held on 24-25 January 2008, Geneva, Switzerland. Vaccine 2009;27:337-47.

[140] Eklund C, Unger ER, Nardelli-Haefliger D, Zhou T, Dillner J. International collaborative proficiency study of Human Papillomavirus type 16 serology. Vaccine 2012;30:294-9.

[141] Harper DM, Franco EL, Wheeler C, Ferris DG, Jenkins D, Schuind A, et al. Efficacy of a bivalent L1 virus-like particle vaccine in prevention of infection with human papillomavirus types 16 and 18 in young women: a randomised controlled trial. Lancet 2004;364:1757-65.

[142] Dias D, Van Doren J, Schlottmann S, Kelly S, Puchalski D, Ruiz W, et al. Optimization and validation of a multiplexed luminex assay to quantify antibodies to neutralizing epitopes on human papillomaviruses 6, 11, 16, and 18. Clin Diagn Lab Immunol 2005;12:959-69.

[143] Faust H, Knekt P, Forslund O, Dillner J. Validation of multiplexed human papillomavirus serology using pseudovirions bound to heparin-coated beads. J Gen Virol 2010;91:1840-8.

[144] Michael KM, Waterboer T, Sehr P, Rother A, Reidel U, Boeing H, et al. Seroprevalence of 34 human papillomavirus types in the German general population. PLoS Pathog 2008;4:e1000091.

[145] Buck CB, Pastrana DV, Lowy DR, Schiller JT. Generation of HPV pseudovirions using transfection and their use in neutralization assays. Methods Mol Med 2005;119:445-62.

[146] Schiller JT, Lowy DR. Immunogenicity testing in human papillomavirus virus-like-particle vaccine trials. J Infect Dis 2009;200:166-71.

[147] Schiller JT, Day PM, Kines RC. Current understanding of the mechanism of HPV infection. Gynecol Oncol 2010;118(1 Suppl):S12-7.

[148] Draper E, Bissett SL, Howell-Jones R, Edwards D, Munslow G, Soldan K, et al. Neu-
       tralization of non-vaccine human papillomavirus pseudoviruses from the A7 and A9
       species groups by bivalent HPV vaccine sera. Vaccine 2011;29:8585-90.

[149] Kemp TJ, Hildesheim A, Safaeian M, Dauner JG, Pan Y, Porras C, et al. HPV16/18 L1
       VLP vaccine induces cross-neutralizing antibodies that may mediate cross-protec-
       tion. Vaccine 2011;29:2011-4.

[150] Bissett SL, Wilkinson D, Tettmar KI, Jones N, Stanford E, Panicker G, et al. Human
       papillomavirus antibody reference reagents for use in postvaccination surveillance
       serology. Clin Vaccine Immunol 2012;19:449-51.

[151] Villa LL, Costa RL, Petta CA, Andrade RP, Ault KA, Giuliano AR, et al. Prophylactic
       quadrivalent human papillomavirus (types 6, 11, 16, and 18) L1 virus-like particle
       vaccine in young women: a randomised double-blind placebo-controlled multicentre
       phase II efficacy trial. Lancet Oncol 2005;6:271-8.

[152] Villa LL, Ault KA, Giuliano AR, Costa RL, Petta CA, Andrade RP, et al. Immunologic
       responses following administration of a vaccine targeting human papillomavirus
       Types 6, 11, 16, and 18. Vaccine 2006;24:5571-83.

[153] Harper DM. Impact of vaccination with Cervarix (trade mark) on subsequent
       HPV-16/18 infection and cervical disease in women 15-25 years of age. Gynecol On-
       col 2008;110(3 Suppl 1):S11-7.

[154] Joura EA, Kjaer SK, Wheeler CM, Sigurdsson K, Iversen OE, Hernandez-Avila M, et
       al. HPV antibody levels and clinical efficacy following administration of a prophylac-
       tic quadrivalent HPV vaccine. Vaccine 2008;26:6844-51.

[155] Collins S, Mazloomzadeh S, Winter H, Blomfield P, Bailey A, Young LS, et al. High
       incidence of cervical human papillomavirus infection in women during their first
       sexual relationship. BJOG 2002;109:96-8.

[156] Fagot JP, Boutrelle A, Ricordeau P, Weill A, Allemand H. HPV vaccination in France:
       uptake, costs and issues for the National Health Insurance. Vaccine 2011;29:3610-6.

[157] Smith LM, Brassard P, Kwong JC, Deeks SL, Ellis AK, Levesque LE. Factors associat-
       ed with initiation and completion of the quadrivalent human papillomavirus vaccine
       series in an ontario cohort of grade 8 girls. BMC Public Health 2011;11:645.

[158] Kale AR, Snape MD. Immunisation of adolescents in the UK. Arch Dis Child
       2011;96:492-5.

[159] Lee VJ, Tay SK, Teoh YL, Tok MY. Cost-effectiveness of different human papilloma-
       virus vaccines in Singapore. BMC Public Health 2011;11:203.

[160] David MP, Van Herck K, Hardt K, Tibaldi F, Dubin G, Descamps D, et al. Long-term
       persistence of anti-HPV-16 and -18 antibodies induced by vaccination with the AS04-

adjuvanted cervical cancer vaccine: modeling of sustained antibody responses. Gynecol Oncol 2009;115(3 Suppl):S1-6.

[161] Olsson SE, Kjaer SK, Sigurdsson K, Iversen OE, Hernandez-Avila M, Wheeler CM, et al. Evaluation of quadrivalent HPV 6/11/16/18 vaccine efficacy against cervical and anogenital disease in subjects with serological evidence of prior vaccine type HPV infection. Hum Vaccin 2009;5:696-704.

[162] Castellsague X, Munoz N, Pitisuttithum P, Ferris D, Monsonego J, Ault K, et al. End-of-study safety, immunogenicity, and efficacy of quadrivalent HPV (types 6, 11, 16, 18) recombinant vaccine in adult women 24-45 years of age. Br J Cancer 2011;105:28-37.

[163] Tay SK. Cervical cancer in the human papillomavirus vaccination era. Curr Opin Obstet Gynecol 2011;24:3-7.

[164] Garnett GP. Role of herd immunity in determining the effect of vaccines against sexually transmitted disease. J Infect Dis 2005;191 Suppl 1:S97-106.

[165] Garnett GP, Kim JJ, French K, Goldie SJ. Chapter 21: Modelling the impact of HPV vaccines on cervical cancer and screening programmes. Vaccine 2006;24 Suppl 3:178-86.

[166] Peres J. For cancers caused by HPV, two vaccines were just the beginning. J Natl Cancer Inst 2011;103:360-2.

[167] Lowy DR, Schiller JT. Reducing HPV-Associated Cancer Globally. Cancer Prev Res (Phila) 2012;5:18-23.

[168] Dillner J, Arbyn M, Unger E, Dillner L. Monitoring of human papillomavirus vaccination. Clin Exp Immunol 2011;163:17-25.

[169] Wong C, Krashin J, Rue-Cover A, Saraiya M, Unger E, Calugar A, et al. Invasive and in situ cervical cancer reported to the vaccine adverse event reporting system (VAERS). J Womens Health (Larchmt) 2010;19:365-70.

[170] Anhang Price R, Koshiol J, Kobrin S, Tiro JA. Knowledge and intention to participate in cervical cancer screening after the human papillomavirus vaccine. Vaccine 2011;29:4238-43.

[171] Powell N, Boyde A, Tristram A, Hibbitts S, Fiander A. The potential impact of human papillomavirus vaccination in contemporary cytologically screened populations may be underestimated: an observational retrospective analysis of invasive cervical cancers. Int J Cancer 2009;125:2425-7.

[172] Lynge E, Antilla A, Arbyn M, Segnan N, Ronco G. What's next? Perspectives and future needs of cervical screening in Europe in the era of molecular testing and vaccination. Eur J Cancer 2009;45:2714-21.

[173] Franco EL, Mahmud SM, Tota J, Ferenczy A, Coutlee F. The expected impact of HPV vaccination on the accuracy of cervical cancer screening: the need for a paradigm change. Arch Med Res 2009;40:478-85.

Chapter 4

Ancillary Techniques in the Histopathologic Diagnosis of Squamous and Glandular Intraepithelial Lesions of the Uterine Cervix

Evanthia Kostopoulou and George Koukoulis

Additional information is available at the end of the chapter

1. Introduction

Squamous cell carcinoma, adenocarcinoma and adenosquamous carcinoma comprise the most common cancers of the uterine cervix. Cervical cancer is one of the common cancers in women, especially in certain parts of the world, as Sub-Saharan Africa, Central America, South Central Asia and Melanesia [1]. In several countries the incidence of cervical cancer was reduced after the introduction of effective screening methods and prevention programs, initially based on the Papanicolaou smear (Pap test), and it is expected to diminish much further with the introduction of vaccination against human papilloma virus (HPV) [2-4].

In recent years papilloma virus has been linked to these cancers through a significant amount of scientific data, derived from epidemiologic, clinical, experimental and molecular studies [5-10]. A. large number of scientific reports during the last three decades led to an explosion of information regarding the role of HPV in lower genital tract carcinogenesis, thus paving the way for the introduction of effective vaccines against the virus, expected to diminish the incidence of both HPV-related carcinomas and precursor lesions in forthcoming years [2,3,5]. This has affected in several ways the histopathologic diagnostic approach to cervical carcinomas and their precursor lesions, including the classification and terminology of the latter. Although several important questions remain, we are now able to examine HPV-related morphologic alterations from a different perspective that encompasses parts -although limited- of this new information, in an effort to achieve more efficient and precise recognition of precancerous lesions.

In the field of cervical squamous precursor lesions the basic concept underlying the Cervical Intraepithelial Neoplasia (CIN) terminology, which refers to a single disease spectrum, has been questioned and gradually replaced by various approaches trying to face the whole group of HPV-related histopathologic abnormalities. In the field of glandular precursor lesions adenocarcinoma in situ is considered the precursor to most invasive cervical adenocarcinomas, while the concept of glandular "dysplasia" is being evaluated [11-15].

Morphology represents a gold standard for lesion diagnosis, since histologic and/or cytologic examination allows in most cases the recognition of viral cytopathic effects and precancerous epithelial alterations; however it can be hampered by inter- and intra-observer variability. In this context, several biomarkers have been investigated for their potential utility in assisting the histopathologic classification of preinvasive lesions and facilitating their distinction from non-HPV induced alterations [16-21]. Human papillomavirus-related intracellular interactions formed the basis for the identification of markers that may assist in this distinction, including cellular proteins targeted directly by viral oncoproteins, and markers related to the cell cycle, which is disturbed by multiple actions of the virus. Additionally, it is expected that the correlation of slight cellular alterations with new sensitive methods of HPV-detection might lead to the identification of different groups of lesions of clinical significance, as well as to the correct application of current morphologic criteria [21-23].

The application of immunohistochemistry and in situ hybridization techniques in the histopathologic diagnosis of cervical intraepithelial alterations of both squamous and glandular epithelium will be presented in this chapter. The immunohistochemical markers that are currently in use in several laboratories worldwide, as well as some new promising biomarkers will be included. Scientific background for each of these markers and special indications for their application will be summarized. A synoptic review of the pertinent literature will be presented, in an effort to summarize the existing data and the remaining questions at both the practical and the theoretical level.

2. Precursor lesions of cervical carcinoma

Precursor lesions of both squamous cell carcinoma and adenocarcinoma are well defined, according to our current understanding of cervical neoplasia. However, years of scientific observations and research preceded the recognition of these lesions. Observations concerning spatial and/or temporal relationship between invasive carcinomas and non-invasive, intraepithelial alterations of the uterine cervix had been repeatedly reported in the past, as early as the end of the 19th century [24-27]. These observations resulted in the recognition of precancerous alterations of cervical epithelium, for which different terms and definitions have been used in the following years.

The terms carcinoma in situ and dysplasia have been in use for several decades, in order to describe non-invasive, intraepithelial lesions showing cytologic abnormalities akin to those of invasive carcinoma. In the late 1960's the concept of one disease spectrum was introduced, based on observed similarities between groups of lesions, which were considered as different grades of the same disease process, termed cervical intraepithelial neoplasia / CIN [28,29]. This

Ancillary Techniques in the Histopathologic Diagnosis of Squamous and Glandular Intraepithelial
Lesions of the Uterine Cervix

95

terminology became the most widely used for the next decades and is currently in use in many laboratories worldwide.

The recognition of the important role[s] of human papillomavirus in cervical carcinogenesis gradually led to different approaches, concerning the whole group of HPV-related lesions and their classification, based on more recent biologic and molecular data [11,13,30,31]. Among them the distinction between two basic biological entities was included: specifically, between a productive viral infection and an intraepithelial neoplastic process. Several questions remain to be answered; however, on a practical level, patient management remains an important basis that influences and often guides choices of terminology.

In the last decades a binary system of classification based on The Bethesda System [TBS] has been mainly in use by cytopathologists; however, several histopathology laboratories world-wide have also adopted similar terminology. A binary system is more consistent with the current knowledge concerning HPV-related disease and is considered to form a basis for improved communication between gynaecologists and pathologists [31]. Moreover, the intermediate group (IN2) has not been shown to comprise a reproducible diagnostic category among pathologists.

2.1. Precursor lesions of squamous cell carcinoma

The terms squamous intraepithelial lesion (SIL) of the uterine cervix or cervical intraepithelial neoplasia (CIN) encompass a group of alterations of squamous epithelium that usually occur in or close to the transformation zone and are related to HPV.

Abnormal proliferation and maturation of squamous cells and nuclear atypia, including enlargement, pleomorphism, irregular nuclear borders, and change in chromatin texture, are the characteristics of these intraepithelial lesions. In one group of lesions the observed cellular alterations reflect mainly viral cytopathic effect, corresponding to koilocytic atypia. This is characterized by an abnormal appearing nucleus surrounded by an irregularly shaped cytoplasmic halo with a sharp edge. In these lesions atypia is more conspicuous in the maturing squamous cells, with mild alterations of the basal-parabasal cell morphology. In other groups of lesions cellular atypia is conspicuous in all cell layers: both middle/upper and lower epithelial layers (Fig.1)

Low-grade squamous intraepithelial lesions (LSILs) exhibit differences in density, size and staining of the maturing squamous cells, often accompanied by binucleated cells, cytoplasmic halos, and/or changes in epithelial thickness (Fig.1a) [14]. High-grade squamous intraepithelial lesions (HSILs) exhibit conspicuous nuclear atypia in all epithelial layers, with nuclear crowding, high nuclear:cytoplasmic ratio, loss of normal polarity, irregular nuclear membranes, and increased mitoses, which can be atypical [32]. In these lesions koilocytosis may be identified or not. There is significant basal/parabasal atypia, with little or no cytoplasmic maturation in the middle-upper layers of the epithelium, and mitotic activity extends to these epithelial layers (Fig.1c).

The differential diagnosis includes mainly: (a) reactive epithelial changes, (b) immature metaplastic changes, and (c) postmenopausal/atrophic epithelia, which may all mimic squamous intraepithelial lesions. The distinction of these alterations from HPV-related lesions is based on well-defined morphologic criteria; however, in certain lesions the distinction is less straightforward, and ancillary techniques can be of help, leading to a more precise diagnosis and increased diagnostic reproducibility. Regressing LSILs may also cause a diagnostic problem [33]. On the other hand, ruling out invasion can be difficult in certain high-grade lesions. The next parts of the present chapter are going to describe the ancillary techniques, which allow for a more precise diagnosis in some of the problematic cases.

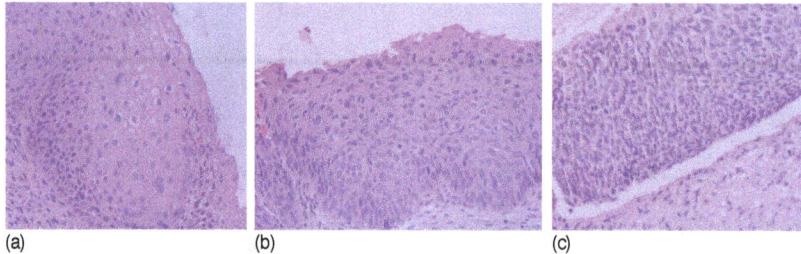

(a)   (b)   (c)

Figure 1. a-c). The above lesions represent a spectrum of alterations in cervical biopsies, ranging from low-grade to high-grade lesions.

2.2. Precursor lesions of cervical adenocarcinoma

The precursor lesion of cervical adenocarcinoma, that is adenocarcinoma in situ (AIS), was introduced as a concept in 1953 and is now acknowledged to be the precursor to most invasive cervical adenocarcinomas [34]. AIS is less common than SIL, with a ratio of AIS/HSIL ranging in most series between 1:26 and 1:237 [33].

Adenocarcinoma in situ is characterized by glands with nuclear hyperchromasia and atypia, increased nuclear:cytoplasmic ratio, pseudostratification or stratification, mitoses and apoptotic bodies (Fig.2). It may coexist with SIL and can also be multifocal. It may show a variety of cellular differentiation, and several subtypes have been described, including endocervical, endometrioid, intestinal, tubal, and stratified [34].

The diagnosis of glandular dysplasia has been used for intraepithelial alterations of glandular epithelium less pronounced than AIS. However, it has low reproducibility, and it has been suggested that this term should no longer be used in the clinical setting [35], especially since glandular epithelium does not support a productive infection by HPV [33]. It has been suggested that problematic endocervical glandular atypias should be evaluated with special studies [34,35]. The term cervical glandular intraepithelial neoplasia (CGIN), with high grade CGIN equating to AIS, is being used in several laboratories [20].

Cervical endometriosis, tubal and endometrioid metaplasia, and reparative changes have to be distinguished from AIS. Arias-Stella reaction, atypia due to irradiation, atypical forms of microglandular hyperplasia, as well as other viral infections, specifically Cytomegalovirus and

Herpesvirus, may occasionally pose problems of differential diagnosis. Ancillary techniques can be of help in these cases, as described in the next parts of the present chapter.

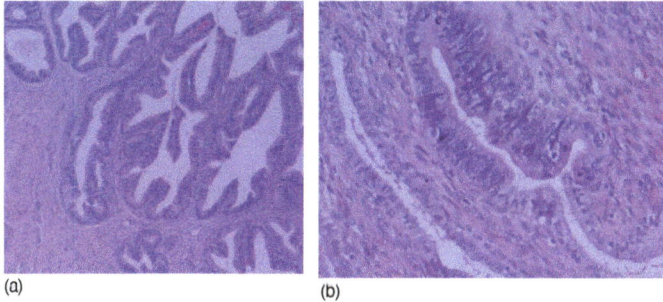

(a)   (b)

Figure 2. a-b). AIS. Continuity with benign cervical epthelium is obvious in [b].

3. HPV in carcinogenesis

Human papillomavirus is estimated to comprise a causal agent in 5% of human cancers and is associated with more human cancers than any other virus [36]. Among them, it is associated with the vast majority of cervical cancer cases. In contrast to several other infectious agents, which act as indirect carcinogens by inducing immunosuppression or by preventing apoptosis, high-risk HPVs (HR-HPVs) act mainly as direct carcinogenic factors [3]. Persistent infection by HR-HPVs correlates with increased risk of cervical cancer. However, infection by low-risk HPV types (LR-HPVs), carries a negligible risk of malignant progression. Additionally, other factors, related to the host or the environment, contribute to the development of neoplasia.

Several studies have revealed the complex intracellular interactions, which take place among oncoproteins encoded by human papillomaviruses and their cellular target proteins [3,37-39]. Their complexity is reflected in the long interval between infection and invasive carcinoma detection, often spanning a period of 15 to 25 years [3]. These interactions have offered to investigators the opportunity to study important cellular pathways related to the carcinogenic process, while several participating proteins have been studied for their possible use as markers of HPV infection in biopsy or cytology specimens. These biomarkers are presented in the next part of the present chapter.

3.1. HPV in carcinomas of the anogenital tract

Cervical cancer represents today a relatively well-studied prototype of a human tumor related to a viral infection, as well as a model for multi-step carcinogenesis. The revealed strong association led to the suggestion that human papillomavirus is not only the main cause of cervical cancer, but also a necessary cause [6].

In addition to cervical cancers, a significant percentage of vaginal, vulvar, penile, anal and perianal carcinomas are HPV-positive [7,40-42], while a fraction of carcinomas in other sites of the human body has also been linked to high-risk [HR] HPV infections. Percentages of HPV positivity observed in carcinomas of the anogenital area are presented in Table 1.

Vaginal carcinomas	60-91%
Vulvar carcinomas	50%
Penile carcinomas	30-50%
Anal and perianal carcinomas	60-94%

Table 1. Percentage of HPV detection in carcinomas of the anogenital region other than cervical carcinoma [4,7].

The distinction of HPV types into low- and high-risk is based on their association with carcinomas, and this distinction is sometimes challenging, especially in the case of rare/weakly carcinogenic viral types. The most common HPV types detected in cervical carcinomas include HPV 16, 18, 45, 31, 33, 52, 58, and 35, belonging to the high-risk group [43-45]. Low-risk viral types may confer risk reflecting an "at risk behavior" [14].

The fraction of cervical squamous cell carcinomas attributable to HPV16 and HPV18, which comprise the two most common high-risk viral types, is estimated at about 70%, while the respective fraction of cervical adenocarcinomas is 86%. As expected, in low-grade squamous intraepithelial alterations the respective percentages differ, since a significant number of these lesions contain HPVs which do not belong to the most common high-risk types.

3.2. Human papillomavirus oncoproteins and their main interactions with cellular pathways

HPVs are epitheliotropic double-stranded DNA viruses, whose replication is dependent on the terminally differentiating epithelial tissue. Their circular genome includes several open reading frames (ORFs) encoding for proteins which control early (E) and late (L) viral functions (E1, E2, E4, E5, E6, E7, L1, and L2) [46].

High-risk mucosal HPVs encode three transforming proteins: E5, E6 and E7, which exhibit multiple biological activities. These have been extensively studied in the last few decades; however, several aspects remain to be elucidated [47-48].

HPV E5 is able to transform mouse fibroblasts and keratinocytes in culture [49]. It is believed to contribute to early stages of carcinogenesis and works in concert with E6 and E7 [50-51]. These latter proteins, which often act synergistically, are necessary for the induction and maintenance of the transformed phenotype. They inhibit the function of tumor suppressors p53 and pRb, respectively, whereas their expression enables cells to bypass normal cell cycle checkpoints.

E6 and E7 are required for both the development of precursor lesions of cervical carcinoma, and for maintaining the malignant phenotype of cervical cancer cells [3]. E6 and E7 proteins play critical roles, being able to immortalize human keratinocytes and induce cell proliferation and transformation. High-risk HPV E6 proteins target p53 for proteasomal degradation through association with the cellular ubiquitin ligase E6AP [48,52]. Low-risk HPV E6 proteins can also associate with E6AP; however, high-risk HPV proteins target p53 for ubiquitination. Activation of telomerase is another important facet of E6 functions, which is augmented by E7-induced interactions.

HPV E7 proteins interact with the retinoblastoma tumor suppressor protein, pRB, which controls S-phase entry through association with E2F transcription factor family members. They also interact with the related pocket proteins, p107 and p130. High-risk HPV E7 targets pRB for proteasomal degradation, while low-risk HPV E7 binds pRB with lower efficiency (approximately 10-fold lower) than the former [47,53]. E7 proteins cause aberrant activation of cdk2 (cyclin-dependent kinase 2), which is associated with cyclins E and A, as well as cdk inhibitors, mainly $p21^{CIP1}$ and $p27^{KIP1}$. E7 expression results in dysregulated expression of cyclins E and A [48,54]. Through its multiple interactions, E7 can uncouple keratinocyte differentiation from cell cycle progression and retain differentiating keratinocytes in a DNA synthesis competent state.

The above interactions form the basis for the application of some important biomarkers used nowadays in many laboratories worldwide. These include p16, a cyclin-dependent kinase inhibitor, often exhibiting increased expression in HPV-related intraepithelial lesions, as well as cyclin E, as will be discussed in the following. Furthermore, proliferation markers, like Ki67, show increased/altered expression, in comparison to non-HPV-infected epithelium of the uterine cervix.

In addition, HR-HPV E6 and E7 proteins cooperate to generate mitotic defects and aneuploidy through induction of supernumerary centrosomes and multipolar mitoses in epithelial cells [55], while genomic instability results in the addition of molecular alterations. The detection of abnormal mitoses is a useful morphologic indicator of high-risk HPV-associated lesions [32].

Finally, integration of HPV genome into host chromosomes is an important event in cervical carcinogenesis [56,57]. Integration occurs frequently during malignant progression and may result in dysregulation of E6/E7 expression due to disruption of E2, with associated loss of the inhibitory E2 action.

Except for the above interactions, several other factors contribute to the development of neoplasia, and these are related to the host or the environment. Smoking, the use of oral contraceptives, high parity and Chlamydia are associated with a relative risk of 2 to 4 [7,9,58-60]. Immunity plays an important role, and this is reflected in data concerning cervical lesions in HIV-infected individuals and in transplant-recipients.

4. Immunohistochemical stains in the diagnosis of cervical intraepithelial lesions

The role of the pathologist examining a cervical biopsy suspicious for an intraepithelial lesion consists of: a) confirming or excluding the presence of a lesion, b) excluding other entities entering the differential diagnosis, and, c) if the diagnosis of an intraepithelial lesion is confirmed, distinguishing a low-grade from a high-grade alteration. Histopathological diagnosis of intraepithelial lesions is based on well-defined criteria, as discussed above. However, in certain cases distinguishing both low- and high-grade lesions from their mimics may pose problems [14,61], even to experienced gynecologic pathologists. Florid reactive changes and metaplastic patterns may present histopathologic features, which may cause difficulties in the distinction from HPV-induced alterations. Attempts have been made to redefine the traditional criteria for lesion diagnosis, while other efforts aimed at the adoption of new, more objective methods, which might support the former [22,23,62-64]. However, studies attempting to correlate HPV presence and replication to certain cytohistologic alterations are becoming less frequent and/or fruitful.

In recent years immunohistochemistry (IHC) is an important adjunct in many diagnoses of surgical pathology, since it may reveal certain characteristics of cells and tissues, which cannot be evaluated by morphology alone. Cervical biopsies are not an exception. Molecular studies have revealed markers that might be of utility in the diagnosis of squamous and glandular intraepithelial alterations, including cellular proteins targeted directly by viral oncoproteins, and markers related to the cell cycle, which is disturbed by multiple actions of the virus, as summarized in the above paragraphs.

4.1. Immunohistochemical stains in the diagnosis of squamous intraepithelial lesions (SILs)

The immunohistochemical stains that are currently in use in several laboratories worldwide, as well as some new promising markers are presented in the following paragraphs. The terms low grade squamous intraepithelial lesion (LSIL) and high grade squamous intraepithelial lesion (HSIL) will be used interchangeably with CIN1 and CIN2/3, respectively.

4.1.1. p16

One extensively studied marker is p16 [INK4A] (hereafter referred to as p16), a cyclin-dependent kinase inhibitor, which decelerates the cell cycle and functions as a tumor suppressor, while having a role in cellular senescence. p16 affects pRb-mediated regulation of the G1/S transition [65-68]. The expression of p16 is altered in several human tumors by deletions, mutations, or methylation. Germ-line mutation carriers are predisposed to a high risk of pancreatic and breast cancers [69].

Increased expression of p16 is often observed in HPV-related intraepithelial lesions and this is mainly attributed to the presence of a feedback loop, which depends on the status of retinoblastoma protein (pRb) and the potential of high-risk HPV E7 protein to inactivate the latter [48,65,70]. Thus, it could be regarded as a marker of E7 activity. Despite the presence of high levels of p16 in SILs, its suppressor function is not normally exerted.

Several groups of investigators have examined immunohistochemically the expression of p16 in cervical squamous intraepithelial lesions and its possible correlations with lesion grade, HPV types and/or lesion "progression" (reviewed by Kostopoulou et al. [17]). Indeed, p16 is one of the best studied markers in gynaecologic pathology. However, percentages of immu-

Ancillary Techniques in the Histopathologic Diagnosis of Squamous and Glandular Intraepithelial
Lesions of the Uterine Cervix

101

nohistochemical positivity vary among different studies, as presented in Table 2. In the latter, studies published in the last ten years and including more than 100 cases of squamous intraepithelial lesions in histopathologic specimens are summarized [71-85], and the reported percentages of p16 immunopositivity are presented, together with the criteria and the antibodies used by the authors. As shown in the Table, different criteria have been used for p16 immunoreactivity evaluation, with some authors focusing only on diffuse immunopositivity, some reporting any type of immunostaining, and others reporting nuclear and cytoplasmic staining separately. Importantly, some authors interpret focal positivity as a false-positive reaction. Positivity in the studies presented below varied from 5.6% to 100% for LSIL and from 45.2% to 100% for HSIL (Table 2). The percentage of immunopositivity observed in negative for SIL (NS) epithelia also varied between 0% and 32.7%.

In one recent study [17] the two basic patterns of immunoreactivity, that is focal and diffuse, were further subdivided into groups as following: Focal positivity was subdivided into cases with occasional positive cells, dispersed or in small groups, observed either (a) mainly in the lower epithelial layers, or (b) above the basal/parabasal layer. Diffuse positivity in the horizontal plane involved either (a) all epithelial layers, or (b) only the basal, parabasal and intermediate layers, without extending to the upper third of the epithelium. In HSIL only diffuse positivity was encountered, observed in 24/25 cases (96%) (Figure 3a). In LSIL 41/55 cases (74.5%) showed some type of positivity, most commonly focal/sporadic (Figure 3b). Interestingly, a difference in HPV type distribution was observed between the two patterns of sporadic/focal positivity, involving lower vs intermediate/upper epithelial layers, and probably reflecting an earlier sporadic expression of E7 in certain lesions [17]. LSILs associated with high-risk or probable high-risk HPV types showed positivity for p16 in 25/35 cases (71.4%). Study of the pertinent literature revealed that a percentage of LSILs testing positive for HR-HPV by PCR or HC2 does not exhibit any p16 immunopositivity. Indeed, the percentage of p16 positivity reported for HR-HPV positive LSILs varied from 32.4% to 94.4% [17,78,86]. Furthermore, strong p16 positivity in LSIL cases appeared to be independent of HPV punctate signal pattern by ISH, in a study by Kalof et al [86].

Additionally, as shown in the Table, in several studies often appears a small group of HSILs that do not show any p16 immunoreactivity. The above observations lead to the conclusion that a negative or equivocal p16 immunostain should be carefully evaluated in conjunction with the histopathologic findings and should not be used as the main criterion for diagnosis.

In three large series of the literature reporting more than 200 cases (SILs and controls) each [71,79,81], as summarized in [17], sensitivity of p16 for the detection of SIL varied from 76.6% to 94.8%, with a value of 83.7% calculated in the total number of their cases, while specificity varied from 77.1% to 92.1%, with a value of 84.6% calculated for the total number of cases. In the same studies the positive predictive value varied from 75.7% to 94.1%. In the study by Kostopoulou et al. [17] sensitivity of p16 immunopositivity for the detection of SIL was 81.2% and specificity 85%, while the positive predictive value was 95.6%. In the study by van Niekerk et al. sensitivity and specificity for HSIL were estimated at 90% and 85%, respectively.

Reference	LSIL	HSIL	NS	Evaluation	Antibody
[71]	56.6%	84.5%	11.5%	N and C ≥5% cells	E6H4 (MTM)
[72]	35%	81.2%	0%	N and/or C	Polyclonal (Abcam)
[73]	74.7	100%	ND	N and C ≥5% cells in lower third	CINtec p16 Kit (DakoCytomation)
[74]	37.2%	45.2%	3.2%	N and/or C	E6H4 (MTM)
[75]	72%	94.7%	32.7%	Any reactivity	E6H4 (MTM)
[76]	74.1%	96.1%	7.0%	N and/or C	JC8 (Biocare Medical)
[77]	100%	98.7%	0%	N or C	p16 (Pharmingen)
[78]	24.5%	87.5%	0%	Moderate and strong	E6H4 (MTM)
[79]	90.9%	100%	7.9%	C and N ≥5% cells	Ab7 16PO7 (Neomarkers)
[80]	71.4%	100%	6%	Continuous basal and parabasal	p16 Histology Kit (Dako)
[81]	57.1%	96.9%	22.9%	N and C ≥5% cells in each layer	E6H4 (DakoCytomation)
[82]	50%	96.2%	0%	C and N	CINtec p16 Kit (Dako)
[83]	5.6%	96.7%	ND	Diffuse, >1/3 of epithelium	Ab-4, 16P04 (Lab Vision)
[84]	26.7%	79.7%	0%	N and C ≥5% cells	p16 (NeoMarkers)
[85]	44%	99%	11%	Lower ¼ of epithelium	E6H4 (DakoCytomation)

LSIL: low-grade squamous intraepithelial lesion; HSIL: high-grade squamous intraepithelial lesion; NS: negative for SIL; N: nuclear; C: cytoplasmic; ND: no data

[a] Only studies including more than 100 cases of squamous intraepithelial lesions in histopathologic specimens are presented.

Table 2. Percentages of immunopositivity for p16 in studies reported in the last ten years[a]

In conclusion, the results of the above mentioned studies point towards the use of p16 immunostain in conjunction with histopathologic evaluation, since the latter remains the "gold standard" in lesion diagnosis. Addition of a consecutive p16-stained slide to the hematoxylin-eosin (HE) stained slides has been shown to improve significantly interobserver agreement for both punch and cone biopsies [18,83,87]. It is of note that a high level of agreement has been observed among pathologists in calling a staining pattern diffusely positive [18]. Moreover, p16 immunostaining may help in the identification of occult lesions [88] and of unusual high-grade lesions not easily recognized in hematoxylin-eosin stained slides [89]. The differential diagnosis from non-neoplastic alterations can be facilitated, especially in conjunction with other immunostains, as presented below. Lesion grading can be more accurate, especially concerning aggressive-appearing low-grade lesions, which could easily be upgraded [83]. p16 IHC may also be of use in evaluating cauterized cervical resection margins, since the positive staining pattern of HGSIL is not affected by diathermy in LLETZ biopsies [76]. Awareness of the different patterns of immunoreactivity and its limitations might allow for a most proper use in certain clinicopathological settings. However, significant variability remains in the reported percentage of cases that stain positively for p16, and the need for standardization of sample preparation and evaluation protocols cannot be overemphasized [90].

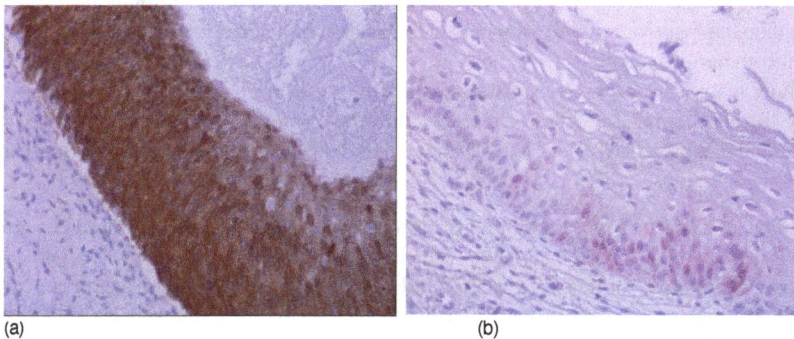

(a)   (b)

Figure 3. a – b). Diffuse p16 positivity in a HSIL (a) and focal positivity in a LSIL (b).

In the recent consensus recommendations of the College of American Pathologists and the American Society for Colposcopy and Cervical Pathology [31], p16 was considered as the only biomarker with sufficient evidence on which to make recommendations regarding use in squamous lesions of the lower anogenital tract in the context of HPV biology. p16 immunohistochemical evaluation was recommended for the distinction of high grade lesions from their mimics, as well as for diagnosis clarification of a lesion falling in the CIN2 group. However, p16 IHC is not indicated for the distinction of low grade lesions from non-HPV induced alterations or as a routine adjunct to histologic assessment of biopsy specimens with HSIL/CIN3 or LSIL morphology. An exception to the latter concerns cases interpreted as ≤LSIL that are at high risk for missed high-grade disease, in relation to previous cytology results or HPV-

test [31]. The estimated magnitude of p16 IHC utilization, according to these recommendations, is for <25% of cervical biopsy specimens.

Finally, another aspect of p16 immunostaining is the possibility of correlation with lesion
"progression". It has been suggested that certain phases of a given HR-HPV-associated
neoplastic process may have different indices of p16 expression [16]. Although the detailed
examination of this subject is not included in the aim of the present text, it should be mentioned
that, in an interesting study by Hariri and Oster, 25/26 low-grade lesions with negative p16
staining (concerning diffuse staining) and a minimum follow-up period of five years had a
benign or normal outcome, revealing a negative predictive value of p16 in predicting the
outcome of CIN 1 cases as high as 96% [80]. In a study including conization specimens with
coexisting CIN1 and CIN3 areas, all CIN1 were p16 positive [91], while p16 staining did not
predict persistence or clearance of HR-HPV after treatment for CIN in a study by Branca et al.
[72]. In a recent report by Ozaki et al. [85] including 99 patients with CIN1 and follow-up data,
26/76 cases in the regression group showed p16 immunopositivity vs 17/23 in the persistence/
progression groups.

4.1.2. Cyclins

Cyclins along with cyclin-dependent kinases and their inhibitors are important molecules for
the orderly progression of cells through phases of the cell cycle. Their immunohistochemical
evaluation has been reported to be of help in the diagnosis of SIL in cervical specimens. Cyclin
E is uncommonly expressed in epithelia not infected by HPV and its conspicuous immunopositivity may facilitate the recognition of SIL [16]. In addition, cyclin B1 immunoreactivity
above the basal/parabasal cells correlates significantly with HPV detection and could be a
marker of HPV presence [21]. Cyclins D and A have been also studied as possible markers of
HPV-related lesions.

Cyclin B1. It has been reported that E6/E7 oncoproteins of HPV type 18 induced changes in
the expression of cell cycle regulatory proteins before immortalization [92]. Significantly
increased expression was noted for cyclin B and its transcriptional activation was documented.
In 2000, Southern et al. demonstrated increased cyclin B1 expression in HGSILs [93]. In their
study cyclin B protein was up-regulated and persisted into the upper epithelial layers in
parallel with cyclin A expression in high-grade squamous intraepithelial lesions.

In a study performed in our laboratory, cyclin B1 immunopositivity above the basal/parabasal
cells correlated significantly with HPV detection (p<0.001) (Figure 4). In all cases of HSIL
immunopositivity for cyclin B1 extended above the basal/parabasal layers, most often
involving the superficial layers as well [21]. Furthermore, increased cyclin B1 immunoreactivity was observed in 51/52 low-grade lesions (98.07%), and in seven of 15 biopsies (46.6%)
characterized as atypia of unknown significance (AUS). Six of these seven cases tested HPV-
positive by PCR.

The main staining pattern observed in low-grade lesions and non-diagnostic atypias in the
above study consisted of sporadic cyclin B1 staining in mature squamous polygonal cells often
just above the basal layers, with slight differences between flat and elevated lesions. Immu-

nopositivity was seen in 52 of 55 cases with HPV infection detected by PCR, whereas it was seen in only 5 cases without PCR-proven HPV infection. In 4 of the latter cases, however, p16 immunoreactivity was observed, suggesting that HPV could be present though not detected by PCR.

The pattern of immunoreactivity observed in low-grade lesions and AUS cases could be perceived as cytoplasmic accumulation or retention of cyclin B1 in suprabasal squamous cells, which might reflect early events in the inhibition of G2-to-M transition, a well-known phenomenon during HPV infection in vitro. The possibility was suggested that these cyclin B1-positive cells could be viewed as a type of "prekoilocytes", whose eventual progression to koilocytes would depend on several parameters related to the intricacies of HPV infection.

In conclusion, cyclin B1 positivity above the basal/parabasal layers correlates significantly with HPV detection and could be a marker of HPV presence. Thus, it might constitute a helpful finding in difficult to diagnose cases. Immunopositivity in a specimen showing non-diagnostic atypia should prompt reevaluation and/or HPV testing, as it is likely that the case could represent a genuine low-grade intraepithelial lesion. Thus, a search for "pre-koilocytes" with B1 immunostaining might be useful in certain cases.

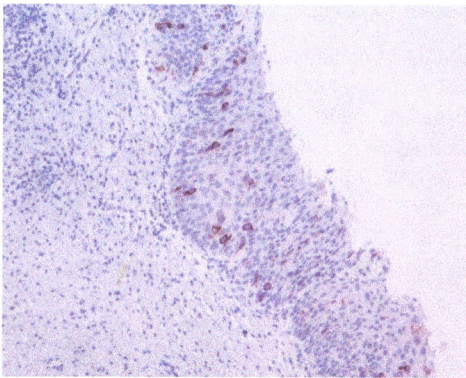

Figure 4. Cyclin B1 immunopositivity above the basal/parabasal cells correlates significantly with HPV detection.

Cyclin E. Cyclin E is another important cell cycle regulator, promoting G1 transition, which has been reported to exhibit increased expression in squamous intraepithelial lesions and invasive cervical carcinomas, although the exact mechanisms are not clear [16].

Moderate to strong immunopositivity for cyclin E was observed in 92.6% and in 91.6% of LSIL and HSIL, respectively, in a study by Keating et al., being positive in 38/41 HR-HPV positive cases. In a group of nondiagnostic squamous atypias cyclin E positivity was associated with HPV positivity [16]. In a study by Bahnassy et al. cyclin E staining increased from CIN1 to invasive carcinoma (from 16.7% to 88.4%, respectively), while gene amplification was detected in 11.1% of CIN1 cases, in 45.5% of CINII, in 55.3% of CINIII, and in 88.4% of carcinoma cases [94].

In conclusion, cyclin E immunostaining could be used to discriminate reactive from neoplastic epithelium [14] especially in conjunction with other markers, discussed in other parts of the present text. However, it is not useful in the distinction of low-grade from high-grade lesions.

4.1.3. Ki67

Ki-67 is an antigen expressed in the nuclei of proliferating cells during the whole cell cycle, except for the G0 and G1 early phases. MIB-1 is a monoclonal antibody that detects this antigen in paraffin tissue sections. Although positivity is observed under normal conditions in the lower compartments of the multilayered squamous epithelium, staining of the middle and upper layers is indicative of an intraepithelial lesion (Figure -5).

Immunopositivity for Ki-67 increases as a function of increasing lesion grade [16,19,95-98]. HSIL/CIN3 lesions usually show nuclear positivity scattered throughout all epithelial layers, while lower grade lesions show less diffuse immunoreaction. However, immunostains should be interpreted with caution. It is well-known to pathologists that reactive and reparative changes may pose a problem in the examination of cell proliferation, and, in the case of Ki-67, immunostaining may extend through the upper layers of the epithelium. In addition, tangential sectioning may sometimes result in the false impression that positive parabasal cells are more superficially placed, thus leading to a SIL diagnosis [99].

It should be noted that Ki-67 immunohistochemical stain may be especially helpful in differentiating atrophic epithelial changes from high-grade lesions [14]. It can also be used in the evaluation of cauterized margins, which often pose diagnostic problems [20]. In addition, Ki-67 immunostaining can be used as an adjunct to other markers. In one study of metaplastic cervical epithelia, addition of Ki67 positivity in >50% of lesional cells to p16 "band" positivity increased specificity (from 92.5 to 96%) and positive predictive value (from 85.7 to 91.7%) for the diagnosis of high-grade CIN [100]. Dual IHC stain with evaluation of colocalization of antibodies represents an interesting approach to this theme [101].

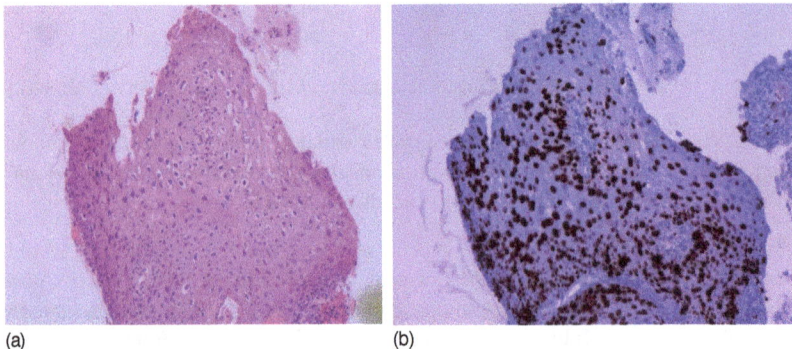

(a)   (b)

Figure 5. Ki-67 positivity in a low-grade SIL.

4.1.4. ProEx C

ProEx C is a recently developed biomarker reagent that targets two proteins having a significant role in the regulation of DNA replication during S-phase: the minichromosome maintenance protein 2 (MCM2) and DNA topoisomerase IIa (TOP2A). TOP2A is a nuclear enzyme that regulates the enzymatic unlinking of DNA strands during chromosome replication. MCM2 functions also during DNA replication by loading the pre-replication complex onto DNA and unwinding the latter through helicase activity to permit synthesis. These proteins are overexpressed in aberrant S-phase induction and have been shown to be overexpressed in CINs and cervical carcinomas [98,99,102,103]. ProEx C appears to be efficient in distinguishing reactive epithelial changes from squamous lesions. The stain can be used alone or in conjunction with p16.

The staining pattern of ProEx C in histologic sections is evaluated in a way reminiscent of MIB-1, since only nuclear positivity above the basal one-third layer is considered positive [99]. ProEx C has been reported to stain reactive epithelial cell nuclei less and LSIL nuclei more than MIB-1 [99]. Strong positive staining for ProEx C involving the lower and upper halves of the epithelium was observed in 92% of high-grade squamous intraepithelial lesions in a study by Badr et al. [102]. Condylomas and CIN I showed greater variability in patterns of staining, with immunopositivity extending into the upper half of the epithelium in 48% of cases. According to the authors, the stain can be applied to confirm the diagnosis of HSIL and to triage cases of atypical squamous metaplasia. According to Shi et al. [103], ProEx C is a better marker than p16 for the detection of LSILs, showing positivity in 94% of the cases in a series of 34 LSILs.

One study by Pinto et al. [98] examined cases with the differential diagnosis of HSIL vs reactive epithelial changes. ProEx C showed 87% sensitivity and 71% specificity for SIL in biopsy material. The authors reported a larger number of cells stained by ProEx C in comparison to MIB-1 in both HSIL and LSIL cases. In addition, the combination of p16 and ProEx C predicted more NoSIL (including normal, reactive, and/or atrophic epithelia) than p16 and MiB-1 (61% vs 43%). These observations suggested that ProEx C could be more useful in the distinction of reactive epithelial changes from SILs than MiB-1.

Sanati et al. reported a sensitivity and specificity of 89% and 100%, respectively, for ProExC immunostain in distinguishing high-grade squamous intraepithelial lesions from squamous metaplasia, while positive and negative predictive values were 100% and 82%, respectively [104]. In a recent study by Guo et al., diffuse positivity for ProExC significantly increased from benign cervix/CIN 1 to CIN 2 or 3/carcinoma, while the highest specificity for CIN 2+ and CIN3+ (100% and 93%, respectively) was achieved when immunostaining was positive for both ProExC and p16, suggesting that it is advantageous to use these two markers together in order to distinguish high-grade lesions from their mimics [105]. The use of the same two markers, p16 and ProExC, as a first step, followed by Ki-67 immunostaining in discordant cases, has been suggested as cost saving strategy by Walts and Bose [106]. According to these authors, performing the two above stains initially and adding Ki-67 only when p16 and ProExC yield discordant results provided the same diagnostic accuracy while reducing the cost, since only one third of the cases required performance of the third stain.

4.1.5. L1 capsid protein

HPV L1 capsid protein is the major structural protein of human papillomavirus. In the last few years L1 immunoreactivity has been examined repeatedly in cytologic material. Nuclear positivity is mainly observed in productive lesions and is gradually lost in high grade lesions and carcinomas.

It has been suggested that combined L1/p16 IHC may be helpful for clinical management, especially in cases in which the grade of the lesion is difficult to assess [91]. In a study by Negri et al. L1 was expressed in 34.85% of CIN1 cases, including 12/38 (31.56%) cases with coexisting CIN3 in conization specimens and 11 of 28 (39.29%) biopsy specimens from women with cytologically proven regression [91]. In the latter group a high staining score was often observed. The authors suggested that combining p16 and L1 immunostaining might allow for a distinction between different risk patterns of LSIL.

In a study by Galgano et al. immunohistochemical staining of HPV L1 was negatively associated with the increasing severity of their consensus diagnosis (p_{trend}<0.001) and decreased with increasing intensity of p16INK4a (p_{trend}<0.001) and Ki-67 (p_{trend}<0.001) [107]. Positivity for L1 was observed in 32%, 32.2%, and 16.5% of CIN1, CIN2, and CIN3/AIS, respectively, and was also observed in 3.3% of negative specimens. It was negatively associated with having a CIN2+ or CIN3+ diagnosis (OR=0.62, and 0.18, respectively). The authors reported that L1 IHC detection was neither sensitive nor specific for any group of cervical neoplasia in biopsy material and this was attributed to the complexity of the temporal evolution of the HPV virion production which may be quite transient. It is interesting that L1 positive cases with a negative consensus diagnosis in this study commonly had at least 1 reviewer diagnosis of CIN1, revealing once again the difficulties in the distinction of SIL vs negative for SIL.

In a recent study by Gatta et al. L1 was expressed in the nuclei of superficial cells of dysplastic epithelia, often with characteristics of koilocytes [108]. L1 positivity was observed in 8/32 CIN1 biopsies (25%) and in 1/10 CIN2 cases (10%), but it was not observed in CIN3 and carcinoma cases examined. Their only case which showed a punctate signal with catalyzed signal-amplified colorimetric DNA in situ hybridization, suggestive of viral integration, belonged to the L1-negative/p16-positive group.

4.1.6. Other markers

In the above paragraphs some of the most important markers used in the histopathologic diagnosis of SIL have been presented. Ki67 and p16 have been used for several years in many laboratories worldwide, while ProEx C and L1 have only been in use for the last few years. However, several other markers have been tested in cervical biopsies for their potential utility in diagnosis. It should be noted that in recent years development of high-throughput technol-ogies, as gene expression profiling, has increased the potential for biomarker discovery. However, although some of these markers showed promising results, in most cases they did not present any specific advantages in comparison to the already existing biomarkers from a diagnostic point of view.

4.2. Immunohistochemical stains in the diagnosis of glandular intraepithelial lesions

Several entities have to be distinguished from AIS, including cervical endometriosis, tubal metaplasia, reparative changes, Arias-Stella reaction, atypia due to irradiation, atypical forms of microglandular hyperplasia, as well as other viral infections, specifically Cytomegalovirus and Herpesvirus. Biomarkers can be of help in these cases.

4.2.1. p16

Already discussed in the paragraphs concerning squamous intraepithelial lesions, p16 has also emerged as a potentially useful marker in the evaluation of glandular cervical alterations [20, 109-111]. Most AIS lesions show diffuse nuclear and/or cytoplasmic immunopositivity (Figure 6). Microglandular hyperplasia and reactive lesions are usually negative for p16. Positivity can be observed in tubal metaplasia; however, it is commonly focal/weak.

p16 was diffusely and strongly expressed (3+) in 29/29 AIS in a study by Negri et al [110], while patchy positivity was observed in tubal metaplasias, endometriosis and endometrial samples. Likewise, all 19 AIS cases showed diffuse nuclear and cytoplasmic reactivity in a study by Little and Stewart [111], while rare single cells were positive in normal endocervical epithelium. Staining was focal in most cases of tubo-endometrioid metaplasia in this study; however, eight of these latter cases included glands that were diffusely p16 positive and/or showed Ki-67 labeling in >25% of cells.

These results emphasize the importance of using panels of antibodies in some of these problematic cases in conjunction with careful morphologic examination.

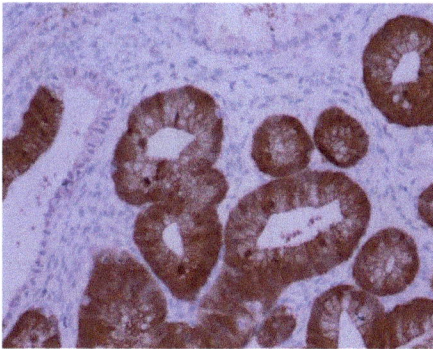

Figure 6. p16 immunopositivity in AIS. Compare with adjacent normal glands. Abrupt transition is focally observed between normal and neoplastic epithelium.

4.2.2. Ki-67

Nuclear positivity for Ki-67 is usually observed in >30% of cells in adenocarcinoma in situ, and often in the majority of the cells. In the contrary, only a small percentage of cells (<10%) stain positively in tubal metaplasia. In practice, it is not usually necessary to undertake a count of positive cells, as there are typically only scattered positive nuclei in tubal metaplasia, while the majority of nuclei are positive in AIS [20].

All cases of adenocarcinoma in situ showed markedly increased Ki-67 labeling together with diffuse nuclear and cytoplasmic reactivity for p16 in the study by Little and Stewart [111], and typically the positive cells were sharply demarcated from the adjacent normal, unstained endocervical epithelium.

However, AIS may occasionally exhibit a low proliferation index [110]. Additionally, some benign lesions, like endometriosis, may show a high proliferation index. Thus, a combination of different markers is more useful than isolated stains in the evaluation of glandular intraepithelial alterations.

4.2.3. bcl-2

Bcl-2 is a member of a large family of proteins, some inhibiting and others favoring apoptosis.

Lesions of adenocarcinoma in situ with significant apoptosis show negative or focally positive bcl-2 immunostains [109]. In the contrary, tubal metaplasia and endometriosis typically exhibit diffuse cytoplasmic positivity, reminiscent of normal fallopian tube epithelium and proliferative endometrium [20]. However, normal endocervical glands are also negative. Consequently, immunostaining for bcl-2 can comprise part of a panel of antibodies, including p16 and Ki-67 [20,112]. It can also be used in the evaluation of cauterized margins [20], as already discussed for p16 and Ki-67 in squamous lesions.

4.2.4. Other markers

Except for the above discussed markers, several other immunostains have been reported to be of help in the diagnosis of glandular lesions. Vimentin can be useful in distinguishing AIS from endometriosis and tuboendometrial metaplasia, since the latter two entities exhibit cytoplasmic positivity. They also show positivity for estrogen receptor, while AIS is negative or focally positive [20]. One additional marker is carcinoembryonic antigen (CEA), which is observed cytoplasmically in a significant percentage of AIS cases, whereas normal endocervical epithelium shows only luminal or no staining.

Interestingly, complete negativity for cyclin D1 was commonly observed in AIS in a study by Little and Stewart [111], in contrast to tuboendometrial metaplasia and normal endocervical epithelia, although staining was typically focal in the latter. Microglandular hyperplasia and mesonephric duct elements were also cyclin D1 positive although relatively few cases were examined in that study.

It should be also noted that the intestinal type of AIS has been reported to show CK7 positivity and CK20 negativity or extremely focal positivity, in spite of the presence of morphological intestinal differentiation in a few cases examined, as reported by McCluggage [20].

Finally, immunohistochemical stains for cytomegalovirus and herpesvirus can be of use for confirmation of these infections, although they are not usually likely to be confused with AIS [34].

5. In Situ Hybridization (ISH)

Detection of HPV nucleic acids is performed by methods that can be broadly subdivided into: a) methods based on target amplification, and b) those based on signal amplification [113]. In addition to several existing liquid phase techniques, in situ hybridization (ISH) methods have been developed for the detection of nucleic acids in cytological and histological specimens. Efforts at improving ISH performance have focused both on amplifying nucleic acid targets before hybridization or on amplifying signals afterwards (e.g. by using in situ PCR, or tyramide signal amplification). Both fluorescent detection and coloured substrate deposition followed by bright-field microscopy can be used, and can be combined with tyramide signal amplification. In addition, ISH assays can be automated along the same lines as immunohistochemistry.

Issues concerning sensitivity of ISH techniques in comparison to PCR have been repeatedly raised. However, these techniques are becoming increasingly sensitive [114,115]. One main contribution of ISH to HPV research is the fact that it permits concurrent morphological evaluation of the cells examined, especially in the case of histological specimens, which is a significant advantage in comparison to liquid phase techniques. In addition, the signal patterns observed in HPV in situ hybridization have been reported to be associated with the physical status of viral DNA in the cell, that is episomal or integrated. Specifically, the punctate pattern of positivity has been linked to viral forms integrated in the host genome [86,116-118].

In a study by Kalof et al. punctate signals were detected in 17/17 (100%) CIN 2/3 lesions, but in only 13.6% of high-risk HPV-positive CIN 1 lesions [86]. In cytology material Ho et al. reported a punctate pattern in 8.7% of CIN1 lesions vs 34.0% of CIN3 lesions [119].

ISH and PCR had fair to good agreement in detecting HPV DNA across CIN categories in a study by Guo et al.; however, ISH detected significantly fewer HPV-positive cases in carcinomas than PCR did, probably as a result of lower copy numbers of episomal HPV DNA in the latter [120]. In addition, although the pure punctate pattern of HPV indicated a high level of viral integration, in cases with mixed signal patterns the level of HPV integration could not be accurately determined, probably due to a variation in the percentage of the two patterns in these cases.

According to Kong et al., in cases of atypical squamous metaplasia, p16 reactivity (focal strong and diffuse strong) was significantly more sensitive than ISH in correlating with the presence of human papillomavirus as detected by PCR [121]. Voss et al. compared a fluorescence in situ hybridization (FISH) HR-HPV assay to Hybrid Capture 2 (HC2) and PCR for the detection of HR-HPV subtypes in cervical cytology specimens [122]. FISH was concordant with HC2 and PCR in 85% and 82% of the specimens, respectively, while HC2 and PCR were concordant in 84% of the specimens. In a more recent study by Kelesidis et al., ISH exhibited a sensitivity of 89.5% for the detection of CIN2+ lesions, while PCR showed sensitivity of 94.7% for these lesions. Importantly, a percentage of ISH-positive cases was not detected by polymerase chain reaction (performed on liquid-based sample media), emphasizing the technical problems and limitations of the techniques [114].

As is apparent from the above results, the applications of HPV DNA ISH are partly dependent on the sensitivity of the assay and its sufficiency to carry a high negative predictive value [14]. This is especially important if clinical decisions are based on a negative result. However, ISH represents a useful tool for ancillary molecular HPV testing when concurrent morphological evaluation of the area examined is necessary.

Except for HPV nucleic acids, there are also other applications of in situ hybridization techniques in cervical specimens, including the detection of amplification of the gene coding for the telomerase RNA component (TERC) at 3q26 [56,123,124]. TERC amplification has been reported to increase with severity of dysplasia and it has been suggested that this might serve as a marker in the distinction between low- and high-grade lesions.

Except for DNA ISH, in situ RNA detection shows promising results in certain applications. RNA markers have emerged as an important group of biomarkers after the widespread use of genome-wide gene expression profiling techniques. New sensitive RNA in situ hybridization methods can detect more than one target simultaneously, can be applied on formalin-fixed paraffin-embedded tissue, and they allow for simultaneous evaluation of morphology [125]. As expected, preanalytical variables related to fixation can affect biomarker measurements and should be considered in the application of these techniques.

Both cellular and viral proteins related to lesion prognosis, previously examined at the mRNA level with PCR techniques, might prove to be important markers for RNA ISH applications. Recently, transcriptional analysis of HPV16 genes by in situ hybridization in histological sections of cervical dysplasia revealed transcription patterns that bring into question some of the current beliefs on the mechanism of HPV-16 infection in the progression to cervical cancer [126]. The detection of HPV E6/E7 mRNA expression appears also promising in the case of multiple infections [127].

In addition, the polymerase chain reaction has been used for target amplification before hybridization, with promising results. *In situ* PCR combines increased sensitivity with the anatomical localization provided by in-situ hybridization, and allows the examination of the specific genetic material at a specific cellular level. Although the method is subject to both false positive and negative outcomes, it allows correlation of viral DNA localization with relevant target proteins, thus providing important information concerning the development of cervical neoplasia [128,129], which cannot be obtained by polymerase chain reaction-based methods alone.

6. Other techniques

Finally, it should be noted that new techniques continue to emerge in the field of cervical lesion detection. Of particular interest in the context of biopsy processing is the development of a water-soluble protein-saving biopsy processing method, which is followed by analysis of proteins of the supernatant samples. This method resulted in the identification of proteins that discriminate between grades of cervical neoplasia, while preserving the tissue for conventional microscopic analysis [130,131].

Ancillary Techniques in the Histopathologic Diagnosis of Squamous and Glandular Intraepithelial
Lesions of the Uterine Cervix

113

7. Conclusions

In the above text important ancillary techniques currently in use in several laboratories worldwide for the evaluation of cervical biopsies have been presented, along with their main applications in diagnosis. Suggested panels of antibodies for specific diagnostic dilemmas have been discussed. Furthermore, the significance of certain negative stains has been presented. It should be noted that histopathologic examination remains the "gold standard" for the diagnosis of low- and high-grade SIL and AIS; however, certain biomarkers have emerged as helpful adjuncts, assisting in a more precise diagnosis of cervical precursor lesions.

It is obvious from the above presented data that the diagnosis of a lesion in a diagnostically challenging case cannot at present be based solely on any particular marker, but rather on a combination of markers with careful morphologic evaluation. Important requirements for the proper use of the presented markers include standardization of protocols and familiarity with the patterns of immunostaining. Finally, an important issue, not specifically analyzed, which may emerge in the next few years and merits further study, is the exact performance of these markers in the detection of lesions related to uncommon HPV types, other than those addressed by the current vaccines.

Author details

Evanthia Kostopoulou and George Koukoulis

Pathology Department, Faculty of Medicine, University of Thessaly, Greece

References

[1] Wells M, Ostor A, Crum C, Franceschi S et al. Tumours of the uterine cervix. Epithelial tumours. In: Tavassoli FA, Devilee P, eds. WHO Classification of tumors: Tumors of the breast and female genital organs. Lyon, France: IARC; 2003

[2] Crum CP, Abbott DW, Quade BJ. Cervical cancer screening: from the Papanicolaou smear to the vaccine era. J. Clin. Oncol. 2003;21(10 Suppl): 224–30.

[3] zur Hausen H. Papillomaviruses—to Vaccination and Beyond. Biochemistry (Moscow), 2008;73(5): 498-503.

[4] zur Hausen H. Papillomaviruses in the causation of human cancers — a brief historical account. Virology 2009;384: 260–265.

[5] zur Hausen, H.. Human papilloma viruses and their possible role in squamous cell carcinomas. Curr. Top. Microbiol. Immunol. 1977;78: 1–30.

[6] Walboomers JMM, Jacobs MV, Manos MM, Bosch FX, Kummer JA, Shah KV, Snijders PJF, Peto J, Meijer CJLM, Munoz N: Human papillomavirus is a necessary cause of invasive cervical cancer worldwide. J. Pathol. 1999;189: 12–19.

[7] Munoz N, Castellsague X, Berrington de Gonzalez A, Gissmann L. Chapter 1: HPV in the etiology of human cancer. Vaccine 2006;24S3: S3/1–S3/10.

[8] Bosch FX, Lorincz A, Munoz N, Meijer CJ, Shah KV. The causal relation between human papillomavirus and cervical cancer. J. Clin. Pathol. 2002;55: 244 – 65.

[9] Bosch FX, Qiao Y, Castellsague X. The epidemiology of human papillomavirus infection and its association with cervical cancer. International Journal of Gynecology and Obstetrics 2006;94 (Supplement 1): S8---S21.

[10] Schiffman M, Wentzensen N, Wacholder S, Kinney W, Gage J, Castle P. Human Papillomavirus Testing in the Prevention of Cervical Cancer J. Natl. Cancer Inst. 2011;103(5): 368-83.

[11] Nucci MR, Crum CP. Redefining early cervical neoplasia: recent progress. Adv. Anat. Pathol. 2007;14(1): 1-10.

[12] Crum CP. Contemporary theories of cervical carcinogenesis: the virus, the host, and the stem cell. Mod. Pathol.. 2000;13: 243–251.

[13] Wright TC. Pathology of HPV infection at the cytologic and histologic levels: basis for a 2-tiered morphologic classification system. Int. J. Gynecol. Obstet. 2006;94(Suppl 1): 22–31.

[14] Crum CP, Rose P. Cervical squamous neoplasia. In: Crum CP, Lee KR, eds. Diagnostic Gynecologic and Obstetric Pathology. Elsevier; 2006; 267-354.

[15] Park K, Soslow R. Current concepts in cervical pathology. Arch. Pathol. Lab. Med. 2009;133: 729–37.

[16] Keating JT, Cviko A, Riethdorf S, Riethdorf L, Quade BJ, Sun D, et al. Ki-67, cyclin E, and p16INK4 are complimentary surrogate biomarkers for human papilloma virus-related cervical neoplasia. Am. J. Surg. Pathol. 2001;25: 884–91.

[17] Kostopoulou E, Samara M, Kollia P, Zacharouli K, Mademtzis I, Daponte A, Messinis IE, Koukoulis G. Different patterns of p16 immunoreactivity in cervical biopsies: Correlation to lesion grade and HPV detection, with review of the literature. Eur. J. Gynaecol. Oncol. 2011;32: 54-61.

[18] Bergeron C, Ordi J, Schmidt D, Trunk M, Keller T, Ridder R, for the European CINtec Histology Study Group. Conjunctive p16INK4a Testing Significantly Increases Accuracy in Diagnosing High-Grade Cervical Intraepithelial Neoplasia. Am. J. Clin. Pathol. 2010;133: 395-406.

[19] Conesa-Zamora P, Doménech-Peris A, Orantes-Casado FJ, et al. Effect of human papillomavirus on cell cycle-related proteins p16, Ki-67, cyclin D1, p53, and ProEx C in

Ancillary Techniques in the Histopathologic Diagnosis of Squamous and Glandular Intraepithelial
Lesions of the Uterine Cervix

115

precursor lesions of cervical carcinoma: a tissue microarray study. American Journal of Clinical Pathology 2009;132(3): 378–90.

[20] McCluggage G. Immunohistochemistry as a diagnostic aid in cervical pathology. Pathology 2007;39(1): 97–111.

[21] Kostopoulou E, Samara M, Kollia P, Zacharouli K, Mademtzis I, Daponte A, Messinis IE, Koukoulis G. Correlation Between Cyclin B1 Immunostaining in Cervical Biopsies and HPV Detection by PCR. Appl. Immunohistochem. Mol. Morphol. 2009;17(2): 115-120. Epub Oct 28; 2008.

[22] Guillaud M, Adler-Storthz K,Malpica A, Staerkel G, Matisic J, Van Niekirk D, Cox D, Poulin N, Follen M, MacAulay C. Subvisual chromatin changes in cervical epithelium measured by texture image analysis and correlated with HPV. Gynecol. Oncol. 2005;99(3 suppl 1): 16 23.

[23] Bollmann M, Bankfalvi A, Trosic A, et al. Can we detect cervical human papillomavirus (HPV) infection by cytomorphology alone? Diagnostic value of non-classic cytological signs of HPV effect in minimally abnormal Pap tests. Cytopathology. 2005;16: 13–21.

[24] Williams J. Cancer of the uterus. Harveian lectures for 1886. Lewis, London; 1888.

[25] Pemberton F, Smith G. The early diagnosis and prevention of carcinoma of the cervix: a clinical pathologic study of borderline cases treated at the Free Hospital for women. Am. J. Obstet. Gynecol. 1929;17: 165.

[26] Papanicolaou GN, and Traut HF. Diagnosis of Uterine Cancer by the Vaginal Smear. Commonwealth Fund, New York; 1943.

[27] Friedell G, McKay D. Adenocarcinoma in situ of endocervix. Cancer 1953;6: 887-97.

[28] Richart RM. Cervical intraepithelial neoplasia. Pathol. Annu.. 1973;8: 301-28.

[29] Richart RM. A theory of cervical carcinogenesis. Obstet. Gynecol. Surv. 1969;24(7 Pt 2): 874-79.

[30] Crum CP. Symposium part 1: Should the Bethesda System terminology be used in diagnostic surgical pathology?: Point. Int J Gynecol Pathol. 2003;22(1): 5-12.

[31] Darragh TM, Colgan TJ, Cox JT, Heller DS, Henry MR, Luff RD, McCalmont T, Nayar R, Palefsky JM, Stoler MH, Wilkinson EJ, Zaino RJ, Wilbur DC; Members of LAST Project Work Groups. The Lower Anogenital Squamous Terminology Standardization Project for HPV-Associated Lesions: background and consensus recommendations from the College of American Pathologists and the American Society for Colposcopy and Cervical Pathology. J. Low Genit Tract Dis. 2012 Jul;16(3): 205-42.

[32] Crum CP, Ikenberg H, Richart RM, Gissmann L. Human papillomavirus type 16 and early cervical neoplasia. N. Engl. J. Med. 1984;310: 880–883.

[33] Wright T, Ronnett B, Kurman R, Ferenczy A. Precancerous lesions of the cervix. In: Kurman R, Ellenson L, Ronnett B, eds. Blaustein's pathology of the female genital tract. Springer; 2011.

[34] Lee K, Rose P. Glandular neoplasia of the cervix. In: Crum CP, Lee KR, eds. Diagnostic Gynecologic and Obstetric Pathology. Elsevier; 2006.

[35] Ioffe OB, Sagae S, Moritani S, Dahmoush L, Chen TT, Silverberg SG. Proposal of a new scoring scheme for the diagnosis of noninvasive endocervical glandular lesions. Am. J. Surg. Pathol. 2003 Apr;27(4): 452-60.

[36] Bergonzini V, Salata C, Calistri A, Parolin C, Palu G. View and review on viral oncology research. Infectious Agents and Cancer 2010;5: 11.

[37] Munger K, Howley P. Human papillomavirus immortalization and transformation functions. Virus Research 2002;89: 213-228.

[38] Pim D, Banks L. Interaction of viral oncoproteins with cellular target molecules: infection with high-risk vs low-risk human papillomaviruses. APMIS 2010 Jun;118(6-7): 471-93.

[39] Yugawa T, Kiyono T. Molecular mechanisms of cervical carcinogenesis by high-risk human papillomaviruses: novel functions of E6 and E7 oncoproteins. Rev. Med. Virol. 2009;19(2): 97-113.

[40] Fuste V, del Pino M, Perez A, Garcia A, Torne A, Pahisa J & Ordi J. Primary squamous cell carcinoma of the vagina: human papillomavirus detection, p16INK4A overexpression and clinicopathological correlations. Histopathology 2010;57: 907–916.

[41] Gross G, Pfister H. Role of human papillomavirus in penile cancer, penile intraepithelial squamous cell neoplasias and in genital warts. Med. Microbiol. Immunol. 2004;193: 35–44.

[42] Insinga R, Liaw K, Johnson L, and Madeleine M. A Systematic Review of the Prevalence and Attribution of Human Papillomavirus Types Among Cervical, Vaginal and Vulvar Precancers and Cancers in the United States. Cancer Epidemiol. Biomarkers Prev. 2008;17(7): 1611–22.

[43] Clifford GM, Smith JS, Plummer M, Munoz N, Franceschi S. Human papillomavirus types in invasive cervical cancer worldwide: a metaanalysis. Br. J. Cancer 2003;88(1): 63–73.

[44] Munoz N, Bosch FX, de Sanjose S, Herrero R, Castellsague X, Shah KV, et al. Epidemiologic classification of human papillomavirus types associated with cervical cancer. N. Engl. J. Med. 2003;348: 518–27.

[45] Schiffman M, Clifford G, Buonaguro FM. Classification of weakly carcinogenic human papillomavirus types: addressing the limits of epidemiology at the borderline. Infect. Agent Cancer 2009;4: 8.

[46] Zheng ZM, Baker CC. Papillomavirus genome structure, expression, and post-transcriptional regulation. Front. Biosci. 2006;11: 2286-302.

[47] McLaughlin-Drubin M and Münger K. The Human Papillomavirus E7 Oncoprotein. Virology. 2009; 384(2): 335–344.

[48] McLaughlin-Drubin M and Münger K. Oncogenic Activities of Human Papillomaviruses. Virus Res. 2009;143(2): 195–208.

[49] Straight SW, Hinkle PM, Jewers RJ, McCance DJ. The E5 Oncoprotein of Human Papillomavirus Type 16 Transforms Fibroblasts and Effects the Downregulation of the Epidermal Growth Factor Receptor in Keratinocytes. J. Virol. 1993;67(8): 4521–32.

[50] Talbert-Slagle K, DiMaio D. The bovine papillomavirus E5 protein and the PDGF beta receptor: it takes two to tango. Virology 2009;384(2): 345–51.

[51] Hu L, Plafker K, Vorozhoko V, Zuna R, Hanigan M, Gorbsky G, Plafker S, Angeletti P, and Ceresa B. Human Papillomavirus 16 E5 Induces Bi-Nucleated Cell Formation By Cell-Cell Fusion. Virology. 2009;384(1): 125–34.

[52] Scheffner M, Werness BA, Huibregtse JM, Levine AJ, Howley PM. The E6 oncoprotein encoded by human papillomavirus types 16 and 18 promotes the degradation of p53. Cell 1990;63: 1129–36.

[53] Münger K, Yee CL, Phelps WC, Pietenpol JA, Moses HL, Howley PM. Biochemical and biological differences between E7 oncoproteins of the high- and low risk human papillomavirus types are determined by amino-terminal sequences. Journal of Virology 1991;65: 3943–48.

[54] Zerfass K, Schulze A, Spitkovsky D, Friedman V, Henglein B, Jansendurr P. Sequential activation of cyclin E and cyclin A gene expression by human papillomavirus type 16 E7 through sequences necessary for transformation. Journal of General Virology 1995;69: 6389–99.

[55] Duensing S, Lee LY, Duensing A, Basile J, Piboonniyom S, Gonzalez S, Crum CP, Scheffner K. The human papillomavirus type 16 E6 and E7 oncoproteins cooperate to induce mitotic defects and genomic instability by uncoupling centrosome duplication from the cell division cycle. Proc. Natl. Acad. Sci. U S A 2000;97: 10002-07.

[56] Hopman AH, Theelen W, Hommelberg PP, Kamps MA, Herrington CS, Morrison LE, Speel EJ, Smedts F, Ramaekers FC. Genomic integration of oncogenic HPV and gain of the human telomerase gene TERC at 3q26 are strongly associated events in the progression of uterine cervical dysplasia to invasive cancer. J. Pathol.. 2006;210(4): 412-19.

[57] Pett M, Coleman N. Integration of high-risk human papillomavirus: a key event in cervical carcinogenesis? J. Pathol. 2007;212: 356–67.

[58] Collins S, Rollason T, Young L, and Woodman C. Cigarette smoking is an independent risk factor for cervical intraepithelial neoplasia in young women: A longitudinal study. Eur. J. Cancer. 2010;46(2): 405–11.

[59] Louie KS, Castellsague X, de Sanjose S, Herrero R, Meijer CJ, Shah K, Munoz N, Bosch FX; for the International Agency for Research on Cancer Multicenter Cervical Cancer Study Group. Smoking and Passive Smoking in Cervical Cancer Risk: Pooled Analysis of Couples from the IARC Multicentric Case-Control Studies. Cancer Epidemiol. Biomarkers Prev. 2011;20(7): 1379-90. Epub 2011 May 24.

[60] Frazer I. Interaction of human papillomaviruses with the host immune system: A well evolved relationship. Virology 2009;384: 410–14.

[61] Kostopoulou E, Keating JT, Crum CP. Pathology. In: Eifel PJ, Levenback C, eds. American Cancer Society Atlas of Clinical Oncology. Cancer of the female lower genital tract. BC Decker, Hamilton, London; 2001.

[62] Cho NH, Kang S, Hong S, et al. Multinucleation of koilocytes is in fact multilobation and is related to aberration of the G2 checkpoint. J. Clin. Pathol. 2005;58: 576–82.

[63] Prasad C, Genest D, Crum CP. Nondiagnostic squamous atypia of the cervix (atypical squamous epithelium of undetermined significance): histologic and molecular correlates. Int. J. Gynecol. Pathol. 1994;13: 220–227.

[64] Salvia P, Bergo S, Bonesso-Sabadini P, Tagliarini E, Hackel C, De Angelo Andrade L. Correlation between histological criteria and human papillomavirus presence based on PCR assay in cervical biopsies. Int. J. Gynecol. Cancer. 2004;14: 126–32.

[65] Lukas J, Parry D, Aagaard L, Mann, D J, Bartkova J, Strauss M, et al. Retinoblastoma-protein-dependent cell-cycle inhibition by the tumour suppressor p16. Nature 1995;375: 503–06.

[66] Ohtani N, Yamakoshi K, Takahashi A, Hara E. The p16INK4A-RB pathway: molecular link between cellular senescence and tumor suppression. J. Med. Invest. 2004;51: 146-53.

[67] Serrano M. The Tumor Suppressor Protein p16INK4a. Exp. Cell Res. 1997;237: 7–13.

[68] Sano T, Oyama T, Kashiwabara K, Fukuda T, Nakajima T. Expression status of p16 protein is associated with human papillomavirus oncogenic potential in cervical and genital lesions. Am. J. Pathol. 1998;153: 1741–48.

[69] Borg A, Sandberg T, Nilsson K, Johannsson O, Klinker M, Måsbäck A, Westerdahl J, Olsson H, Ingvar C. High frequency of multiple melanomas and breast and pancreas carcinomas in CDKN2A mutation-positive melanoma families.J. Natl. Cancer Inst. 200092(15): 1260-66.

[70] Giarrè M, Caldeira S, Malanchi I, Ciccolini F, Leão MJ, Tommasino M. Induction of pRb degradation by the human papillomavirus type 16 E7 protein is essential to efficiently overcome p16INK4a-imposed G1 cell cycle arrest. J. Virol. 2001;75(10): 4705-12.

[71] Agoff SN, Lin P, Morihara J, Mao C, Kiviat NB, Koutsky LA. p 16(INK4a) expression correlates with degree of cervical neoplasia: a comparison with Ki-67 expression and detection of high-risk HPV types. Mod. Pathol. 2003;16: 665-73

[72] Branca M, Ciotti M, Santini D, Di Bonito L, Giorgi C, Benedetto A, et al. p16INK4a expression is related to grade of CIN and high-risk human papillomavirus but does not predict virus clearance after conization or disease outcome. Int. J. Gynecol. Pathol. 2004;23: 354-65.

[73] Negri G, Vittadello F, Romano F, Kasal A, Rivasi F, Girlando S, et al. P16INK4a expression and progression risk of low-grade intraepithelial neoplasia of the cervix uteri. Virchows Arch. 2004;445: 616–20.

[74] Volgareva G, Zavalishina L, Andreeva Y, Frank G, Krutikova E, Golovina D et al. Protein p16 as a marker of dysplastic and neoplastic alterations in cervical epithelial cells. BMC Cancer 2004;4: 58.

[75] Wang SS, Trunk M, Schiffman M, Herrero R, Sherman M, Burk R, et al. Validation of p16INK4a as a marker of oncogenic human papillomavirus infection in cervical biopsies from a population-based cohort in Costa Rica. Cancer Epidemiol Biomarkers Prev. 2004;13: 1355–60.

[76] Dray M, Russell P, Dalrymple C, Wallman N, Angus G, Leong A, et al. p16INK4a as a complementary marker of high-grade intraepithelial lesions of the uterine cervix. I: Experience with squamous lesions in 189 consecutive cervical biopsies. Pathology 2005;37(2): 112–24.

[77] Murphy N, Ring M, Hefron CC, King B, Killalea A, Hughes C, et al. p16INK4A, CDC6, and MCM5: predictive biomarkers in cervical preinvasive neoplasia and cervical cancer. J. Clin. Pathol. 2005;58: 525–34.

[78] Ishikawa M, Fujii T, Saito M, Nindl I, Ono A, Kubushiro K, et al. Overexpression of p16INK4a as an indicator for human papillomavirus oncogenic activity in cervical squamous neoplasia. Int. J. Gynecol. Cancer 2006;16 (1): 347–53.

[79] Focchi G, Silva I, Nogueira-de-Souza N, Dobo C, Oshima C, Stavale J. Immunohistochemical Expression of p16(INK4A) in Normal Uterine Cervix, Nonneoplastic Epithelial Lesions, and Low-grade Squamous Intraepithelial Lesions. J. Low Genit. Tract Dis. 2007;11: 98-104.

[80] Hariri J, Oster A. The Negative Predictive Value of p16INK4a to Assess the Outcome of Cervical Intraepithelial Neoplasia 1 in the Uterine Cervix. Int. J. Gynecol. Pathol. 2007;26: 223–28.

[81] Van Niekerk D, Guillaud M, Matisic J, Benedet J, Freeberg J, Follen M, et al. p16 and MIB1 improve the sensitivity and specificity of the diagnosis of high grade squamous intraepithelial lesions: Methodological issues in a report of 447 biopsies with consensus diagnosis and HPV HCII testing. Gynecol. Oncol. 2007;107: S233–40.

[82] Godoy A, Mandelli J, Oliveira F, Calegari S, Moura L and Serafini E. p16INK4 expression in precursor lesions of squamous cell cervical cancer related to the presence of HPV-DNA. Brazilian Journal of Medical and Biological Research 2008;41: 583-588.

[83] Dijkstra MG, Heideman DA, de Roy SC, Rozendaal L, Berkhof J, van Krimpen K, van Groningen K, Snijders PJ, Meijer CJ, van Kemenade FJ. p16(INK4a) immunostaining as an alternative to histology review for reliable grading of cervical intraepithelial lesions. J. Clin. Pathol. 2010 Nov;63(11): 972-7. Epub 2010 Oct 5

[84] Tan GC, Norlatiffah S, Sharifah NA, Razmin G, Shiran MS, Hatta AZ, Paul-Ng HO. Immunohistochemical study of p16 INK4A and survivin expressions in cervical squamous neoplasm. Indian J. Pathol. Microbiol. 2010;53: 1-6.

[85] Ozaki S, Zen Y, Inoue M. Biomarker expression in cervical intraepithelial neoplasia: potential progression predictive factors for low-grade lesions. Hum. Pathol. 2011 Jul; 42(7): 1007-12. Epub 2011 Feb 11.

[86] Kalof AN, Evans MF, Simmons-Arnold L, Beatty B, Kumarasen C. p16INK4A immunoexpression and HPV in situ hybridization signal patterns: potential markers of high-grade cervical intraepithelial neoplasia. Am. J. Surg. Pathol. 2005;29: 674–79.

[87] Horn L, Reichert A, Oster A, Arndal S, Trunk M, Ridder R, et al. Immunostaining for p16INK4a Used as a Conjunctive Tool Improves Interobserver Agreement of the Histologic Diagnosis of Cervical Intraepithelial Neoplasia. Am. J. Surg. Pathol. 2008;32: 502–12.

[88] Ordi J., Garcia S, del Pino M, Landol S, Alonso I, Quinto' L, and Torne' A. p16INK4a immunostaining identifies occult CIN lesions in HPV-positive women. Int. J. Gynecol. Pathol. 2008;28: 90–97.

[89] Kitahara S, Chan RC, Nichols WS, Silva EG. Deceiving high-grade cervical dysplasias identified as human papillomavirus non-16 and non-18 types by Invader human papillomavirus assays. Ann. Diagn. Pathol. 2012 Apr;16(2): 100-06. Epub 2011 Dec 23.

[90] van Bogaert LJ. P16(INK4a) immunocytochemistry/immunohistochemistry: need for scoring uniformization to be clinically useful in gynecological pathology. Ann. Diagn. Pathol. 2012 Oct;16(5): 422-6. Epub 2012 Apr 24.

[91] Negri G, Bellisano G, Zannoni GF, Rivasi F, Kasal A, Vittadello F, et al. P16ink4a and HPV L1 immunohistochemistry is helpful for estimating the behavior of low-grade dysplastic lesions of the cervix uterii. Am. J. Surg. Pathol. 2008; Epub Aug 30.

[92] Pei XF. The human papillomavirus E6/E7 genes induce discordant changes in the expression of cell growth regulatory proteins. Carcinogenesis. 1996;17: 1395–401.

[93] Southern S, McDicken I, Herrington CS. Evidence for keratinocyte immortalization in high-grade squamous intraepithelial lesions of the cervix infected with high-risk human papillomaviruses. Lab. Invest. 2000;80: 539–44.

[94] Bahnassy A, Zekri A, Saleh M, Lotayef M, Moneir M and Shawki O. The possible role of cell cycle regulators in multistep process of HPV-associated cervical carcinoma. BMC Clinical Pathology 2007;7: 4.

[95] Arafa M, Boniver J, Delvenne P. Detection of HPV-induced cervical (pre) neoplastic lesions: a tissue microarray (TMA) study. Appl. Immunohistochem. Mol. Morphol. 2008 Oct;16(5): 422-32.

[96] Carreras R, Alameda F, Mancebo G, García-Moreno P, Mariñoso ML, Costa C, Fusté P, Baró T, Serrano S. A study of Ki-67, c-erbB2 and cyclin D-1 expression in CIN-I, CIN-III and squamous cell carcinoma of the cervix. Histol. Histopathol. 2007 Jun; 22(6): 587-92.

[97] Mimica M, Tomić S, Kardum G, Hofman ID, Kaliterna V, Pejković L. Ki-67 quantitative evaluation as a marker of cervical intraepithelial neoplasia and human papillomavirus infection. Int. J. Gynecol. Cancer. 2010 Jan;20(1): 116-19.

[98] Pinto A, Schlecht N, Woo T, Crum CP, Cibas E. Biomarker (ProEx C, p16INK4A, and MiB-1) distinction of high-grade squamous intraepithelial lesion from its mimics. Modern Pathology 2008;21; 1067–74.

[99] Pinto AP, Crum CP, Hirsch MS. Molecular markers of early cervical neoplasia. Diagn. Histopathol. (Oxf). 2010;16(10): 445-54.

[100] Walts AE, Bose S. P16/Ki-67 Immunostaining is Useful in Stratification of Atypical Metaplastic Epithelium of the Cervix. Clin. Med. Pathol. 2008;1: 35-42.

[101] Samarawardana P, Singh M, Shroyer KR. Dual stain immunohistochemical localization of p16INK4A and ki-67: a synergistic approach to identify clinically significant cervical mucosal lesions. Appl. Immunohistochem. Mol. Morphol. 2011 Dec;19(6): 514-18.

[102] Badr RE, Walts AE, Chung F, et al. BD ProEx C: a sensitive and specific marker of HPV-associated squamous lesions of the cervix. Am. J. Surg. Pathol. 2008;32: 899-906.

[103] Shi J, Liu H, Wilkerson M, et al. Evaluation of p16INK4a, minichromosome maintenance protein 2, DNA topoisomerase IIalpha, ProEX C, and p16INK4a/ProEX C in cervical squamous intraepithelial lesions. Hum. Pathol. 2007;38: 1335-44.

[104] Sanati S, Huettner P, Ylagan LR. Role of ProExC: a novel immunoperoxidase marker in the evaluation of dysplastic squamous and glandular lesions in cervical specimens. Int. J. Gynecol. Pathol. 2010 Jan;29(1): 79-87.

[105] Guo M, Baruch AC, Silva EG, Jan YJ, Lin E, Sneige N, Deavers MT. Efficacy of p16 and ProExC immunostaining in the detection of high-grade cervical intraepithelial neoplasia and cervical carcinoma. Am. J. Clin. Pathol. 2011;135(2): 212-20.

[106] Walts AE, Bose S. p16, Ki-67, and BD ProExC immunostaining: a practical `approach for diagnosis of cervical intraepithelial neoplasia. Hum. Pathol. 2009;40(7): 957-64. Epub 2009 Mar 9.

[107] Galgano MT, Castle PE, Atkins KA, Brix WK, Nassau SR, Stoler MH. Using biomarkers as objective standards in the diagnosis of cervical biopsies. Am. J. Surg. Pathol. 2010;34(8): 1077-87.

[108] Gatta LB, Berenzi A, Balzarini P, Dessy E, Angiero F, Alessandri G, Gambino A, Grigolato P, Benetti A. Diagnostic implications of L1, p16, and Ki-67 proteins and HPV DNA in low-grade cervical intraepithelial neoplasia. Int. J. Gynecol. Pathol. 2011;30(6): 597-604.

[109] Cameron RI, Maxwell P, Jenkins D, McCluggage WG. Immunohistochemical staining with MIB1, bcl2 and p16 assists in the distinction of cervical glandular intraepithelial neoplasia from tubo-endometrial metaplasia, endometriosis and microglandular hyperplasia. Histopathology. 2002;41(4): 313-21.

[110] Negri G, Bellisano G, Carico E, Faa G, Kasal A, Antoniazzi S, Egarter-Vigl E, Piccin A, Dalla Palma P, Vittadello F. Usefulness of p16ink4a, ProEX C, and Ki-67 for the diagnosis of glandular dysplasia and adenocarcinoma of the cervix uteri. Int. J. Gynecol. Pathol. 2011;30(4): 407-13.

[111] Little L, Stewart CJ. Cyclin D1 immunoreactivity in normal endocervix and diagnostic value in reactive and neoplastic endocervical lesions. Mod. Pathol. 2010;23: 611-18.

[112] McCluggage WG, Maxwell P. Bcl-2 and p21 staining of cervical tuboendometrial metaplasia. Histopathology 2002;40: 107.

[113] Snijders PJ, Heideman DA, Meijer CJ. Methods for HPV detection in exfoliated cell and tissue specimens. APMIS. 2010;118(6-7): 520-28.

[114] Kelesidis T, Aish L, Steller MA, Aish IS, Shen J, Foukas P, Panayiotides J, Petrikkos G, Karakitsos P, Tsiodras S. Human Papillomavirus (HPV) Detection Using In Situ Hybridization in Histologic Samples: Correlations With Cytologic Changes and Polymerase Chain Reaction HPV Detection. Am. J. Clin. Pathol. 2011;136(1): 119-27.

[115] Montag M, Blankenstein T, Shabani N, Bruning A, Mylonas I. Evaluation of two commercialised in situ hybridisation assays for detecting HPV-DNA in formalin-fixed, paraffin-embedded Tissue. Arch. Gynecol. Obstet. 2011;284: 999–1005.

[116] Cooper K, Herrington CS, Stickland J, Evans M, and McGee J. Episomal and integrated human papillomavirus in cervical neoplasia shown by non-isotopic in situ hybridization. J. Clin. Pathol. 1991;44: 990–96.

[117] Evans MF, Mount S, Beatty B, and Cooper K. Biotinyltyramide-based in situ hybridization signal patterns distinguish human papillomavirus type and grade of cervical intraepithelial neoplasia. Mod. Pathol. 2002;15: 1339–47.

[118] Hopman AH, Kamps MA, Smedts F, Speel EJ, Herrington CS, and Ramaekers FC. HPV in situ hybridization: impact of different protocols on the detection of integrated HPV. Int. J. Cancer 2005;115: 419–28.

[119] Ho CM, Lee BH, Chang SF, Chien TY, Huang SH, Yan CC, Cheng WF. Clinical significance of signal pattern of high-risk human papillomavirus using a novel fluorescence in situ hybridization assay in cervical cytology. Clin. Microbiol. Infect. 2011;17(3): 386-94.

[120] Guo M, Gong Y, Deavers M, Silva EG, Jan YJ, Cogdell DE, Luthra R, Lin E, Lai HC, Zhang W, Sneige N. Evaluation of a commercialized in situ hybridization assay for detecting human papillomavirus DNA in tissue specimens from patients with cervical intraepithelial neoplasia and cervical carcinoma. J. Clin. Microbiol. 2008;46(1): 274-80. Epub 2007 Oct 31.

[121] Kong CS, Balzer BL, Troxell ML, Patterson BK, Longacre TA. p16INK4A immunohistochemistry is superior to HPV in situ hybridization for the detection of high-risk HPV in atypical squamous metaplasia. Am J Surg Pathol. 2007;31(1):33-43.

[122] Voss JS, Kipp BR, Campion MB, Sokolova IA, Henry MR, Halling KC, Clayton AC. Comparison of fluorescence in situ hybridization, hybrid capture 2 and polymerase chain reaction for the detection of high-risk human papillomavirus in cervical cytology specimens. Anal. Quant. Cytol. Histol. 2009;31(4): 208-16.

[123] Zheng L, Liu AL, Qi T, Wang Q, Cai Z, Su YJ, Hu YW, Liu GB, Wei LH. Human telomerase RNA gene amplification detection increases the specificity of cervical intraepithelial neoplasia screening. Int. J. Gynecol. Cancer. 2010;20(6): 912-17.

[124] Andersson S, Sowjanya P, Wangsa D, Hjerpe A, et al. Detection of Genomic Amplification of the Human Telomerase Gene TERC, a Potential Marker for Triage of Women with HPV-Positive, Abnormal Pap Smears. Am. J. Pathol. 2009;175: 1831–47.

[125] Wang F, Flanagan J, Su N, Wang L, Bui S, Nielson A, Wu X, Vo H, Ma X, Luo Y. RNAscope. A Novel in Situ RNA Analysis Platform for Formalin-Fixed, Paraffin-Embedded Tissues. J. Mol. Diagn. 2012;14: 22–29.

[126] Coupe V, González-Barreiro L, Gutiérrez-Berzal J, Melián-Bóveda A, López-Rodríguez O, Alba-Domínguez J, Alba-Losada J. Transcriptional analysis of human papillomavirus type 16 in histological sections of cervical dysplasia by in situ hybridization. J. Clin. Pathol. 2012;65: 164-70.

[127] Andersson E, Kärrberg C, Rådberg T, Blomqvist L, Zetterqvist BM, Ryd W, Lindh M, Horal P. Type-dependent E6/E7 mRNA expression of single and multiple high-risk

human papillomavirus infections in cervical neoplasia. J. Clin. Virol. 2012;54(1): 61-65. Epub 2012 Feb 10

[128] Nuovo GJ, MacConnell P, Forde A, Delvenne P. Detection of human papillomavirus DNA in formalin-fixed tissues by in situ hybridization after amplification by polymerase chain reaction. Am. J. Pathol. 1991 Oct;139(4): 847-54.

[129] Nuovo GJ. In situ detection of human papillomavirus DNA after PCR-amplification. Methods Mol. Biol. 2011;688: 35-46.

[130] Uleberg KE, Munk AC, Furlan C, van Diermen B, Gudlaugsson E, Janssen E, Malpica A, Hjelle A, Baak JP: A Protein Profile Study to Discriminate CIN Lesions from Normal Cervical Epithelium. Cellular Oncology 2011;34: 443-50.

[131] Uleberg KE, Munk AC, Brede C, Gudlaugsson E, van Diermen B, Skaland I, Malpica A, Janssen EA, Hjelle A, Baak JP. Discrimination of grade 2 and 3 cervical intraepithelial neoplasia by means of analysis of water soluble proteins recovered from cervical biopsies. Proteome Sci. 2011; 9:36. Epub 2011 Jun 28.

Chapter 5

HPV L1 Detection as a Prognostic Marker for Management of HPV High Risk Positive Abnormal Pap Smears

Ralf Hilfrich

Additional information is available at the end of the chapter

1. Introduction

1.1. Cervical cancer and HPV

Cervical cancer is still the 2nd most common cancer in women worldwide, and especially women in developing countries are suffering from the disease [1].

If detected at an early stage Cervical Cancer is preventable. In almost all places around the world the traditional Pap smear is used as primary screening tool and even from being far away to be a perfect test, the benefits of Papanicolaou based cervical cancer screening programs in reducing morbidity and mortality are well accepted.

About 50 years after Papanicolaou has started his initial work, Meisels & Fortin published in 1976 a report in which they showed that the "halo cell" in pap smears, was a koilocyte - the pathognomic cell of an HPV infection [2] and that low grade or mild dysplasia of the cervix had the histological features of a papillomavirus infection [3].

Shortly thereafter Lutz Gissmann in the zur Hausen laboratory in Erlangen cloned from genital warts 'condyloma acuminata', a novel HPV DNA classified as HPV6 [4].

The idea that Cervical Cancer and cancers at other sides could be caused by a viral infection developed afterwards step by step.

In the meantime both concepts are merged and it is accepted that a persisting infection caused by the sexual transmitted human papillomavirus (HPV), is almost always the trigger for the occurrence of cervical cancer and the main agent for cervical epithelial dysplasias.

Of the more than 120 HPV subtypes known today, the anogenital ones are further divided into low risk (LR-HPV) and currently at least 15 high risk types (HR-HPV; HPV 16, 18, 45, 31, 33, 52, 58 are most frequent). While the former are only in rare cases cancerogenic, HR-HPV are detected virtually regularly in high-grade intraepithelial neoplasias and invasive cervical cancers, of which more than 70% are HPV 16 and HPV 18 [5].

The negative predictive value of the highly sensitive DNA determination of HR-HPV in the cervical smear cell material is with more than 99% very high, i.e. women not infected with these HPV subtypes very probably have no high-grade intraepithelial lesion and no cervical cancer.

On the other hand the use as primary screening tool for cervical cancer is limited because the positive predictive value of a HPV DNA test is low.

The majority of HR-HPV infections remain morphologically undetected and even in mild dysplasias with persisting infections the probability for the development of high grade intraepithelial lesions is only about 20% focusing on young women.

Therefore even if thinking about the possibility to replace cytology as primary screening tool, the Pap-test will remain to verify a positive HPV DNA test, to confirm the presence of abnormal cells and most important to determine the severity or grade of disease, a unique feature of the morphological methods.

2. Cervical cancer screening

Since the early days of cervical cytology it is known that the morphologically identified lesions of different grades are mixtures of distinct biological stages resulting in different clinical outcomes, remission or progression [6].

Today with the knowledge that HPV is a necessary but not sufficient cause for the development of most cervical cancers, transient HPV infection and precancer are often used synonymous for these biologically different conditions.

Traditionally cervical cancer prevention programs rely on the repeated application of a 3-step strategy:

1. Screening by cervical cytology with the Pap - Test;

2. Follow up of the cytology positive women with HPV DNA testing colposcopic evaluation and directed biopsy of abnormal-looking cervical tissue for diagnosis; and if necessary

3. Excisional or ablative treatment of the cervical tissue in women diagnosed with CIN2+ or precancer.

For Pap smear diagnosis different reporting systems are in use worldwide. Besides the original WHO classification [7], The Bethesda System (TBS) [8] is internationally accepted, while the Munich Nomenclature II is being recommended in Germany [9].

Based on Ostors meta-analysis it's common sense that treatment isn't warranted for early dysplastic lesions as for atypical squamous cells of undetermined significance (ASCUS) and mild dysplasia (LSIL) since only 10% of the mild dysplastic lesions will progress to CIN3+ [10].

A cytological follow up with colposcopic evaluation is recommended for these women and if necessary directed biopsies of abnormal-looking cervical tissue for diagnosis are taken.

The cervical histopathologic diagnoses of these samples are graded according to the cervical intraepithelial neoplasia (CIN) system as normal, CIN1, CIN2, CIN3, and cervical cancer [11].

So far diagnosis of CIN2 or worse is the clinical threshold leading to ablative or excisional therapy in the United States and Europe.

In the meantime a discussion started if moderate dysplasias, the cytological CIN2 equivalent, should be called low grade or high grade lesion. Ostor reported that only 20% of the moderate dysplasitic lesions progressed to CIN3+, typically a threshhold that should not warrant invasive procedures.

As a consequence of the current situation conisations are being performed frequently, with potentially negative impact on reproductive outcomes for fertile women, including preterm delivery and low-birth-weight infants [12] with possible life long fatal disabilities.

Despite the conservative recommendation in the Munich Nomenclature II, not to treat CIN2, conisation was one of the most common surgical procedures performed in women of fertile age in Germany during 2010, accounting for more than 50.000 cases [13].

The dilemma is that neither cytological follow up, colposcopy nor HPV DNA testing could indicate whether a remission or progression of the precursor lesion to invasive cancer will occur. Therefore more specific tools like prognostic markers would be of great value, allowing an individualized management of cervical lesions depending on their risk profil.

3. HPV L1 detection as prognostic marker for early dysplastic lesions

Over the last couples of years cytological samples as well as colposcopically guided punch biospsies, have been used to determine if Cytoactiv HPV L1 detection is able to predict the clinical outcome of HPV high risk positive early dysplastic lesions.

Moderate dysplastic lesions, being part of HSIL, have been investigated as well since the Munich nomenclature II, in contrast to TBS, groups moderate dysplastic lesions, together with mild dysplasias, in the category IIID, with recommendation for cytological follow up and colposcopy.

This different risk assesement offered the unique possibility to follow up these women with moderate dysplasias as well.

4. The HPV L1 capsid protein and the viral life cycle

L1 or the major capsid protein is one of eight known HPV specific proteins (E1, E2, E4, E5, E6, E7, L1 and L2).

It is produced within the cytoplasm and translocated into the nucleus, clearly visible by strong nuclear immunochemical staining reaction in intermediate and superficial squamous epithelial cells.

The L1 protein forms an icosahedral capsid with a T=7 symmetry and a 50 nm diameter. The capsid is composed of 72 L1 pentamers, linked to each other by disulfide bonds, and associated with the minor capsid protein L2, which encapsulates the viral DNA to build new infectious viral particles that are released in the upper epithelial layer. [14]

At the same time, L1 is a ligand for a still not reliably identified surface receptor, a heparan sulfate proteoglycan, on the basal cell layer of the epithelium to provide initial virion attachment to target cells. As a general rule, the HPV gains access to the basal epithelial layers as a result of epithelial erosions or mucosal ulcerations in the transformation zone susceptible to inflammation at the cervical/endocervical junction.

Once attached, the virion enters the host cell via a L2 dependant, clathrin-mediated endocytosis, the capsid becomes decraded, the virus DNA is released and routed into the nucleus of the cell [15].

The virus genome then separately lies outside the chromosomal DNA of the host cell as a ring-shaped, episomal DNA molecule.

These initial steps are not associated with cellular changes that can be detected by morphological methods. This individually variably long so called latent or silent virus infection can only be detected with molecular biological methods.

The signals to leave the latent virus infection and to initiate the productive or permissive phase of the viral life cycle, leading to a L1 synthesis, are not identified yet. Once differentiation of the immature squamous epithelial host cells begins, the viral DNA starts to replicate to high copy numbers. In the further course and dependent on the host cell differentiation the late proteins are synthesized, and encapsidates the viral DNA. Thus, mature, infectious viruses emerge, which are released from the perishing superficial squamous epithelia [16].

Within the scope of this productive phase, morphological epithelial changes mostly occur after several weeks or months post infection, which allow the cytological diagnosis of dysplasia in the smear. The typical morphological changes like nuclear enlargement, multinucleosis, changes in the chromatin structure and cytoplasm composition as well as koilocytes or 'halo cells' have already been described by Papanicolaou.

Upon termination of the productive phase, the viral life cycle from primary infection to the release of the virus is completed without any malignant neoplasia having occurred (Figure 1). The L1 capsid protein is detectable at that stage of the life cycle, only.

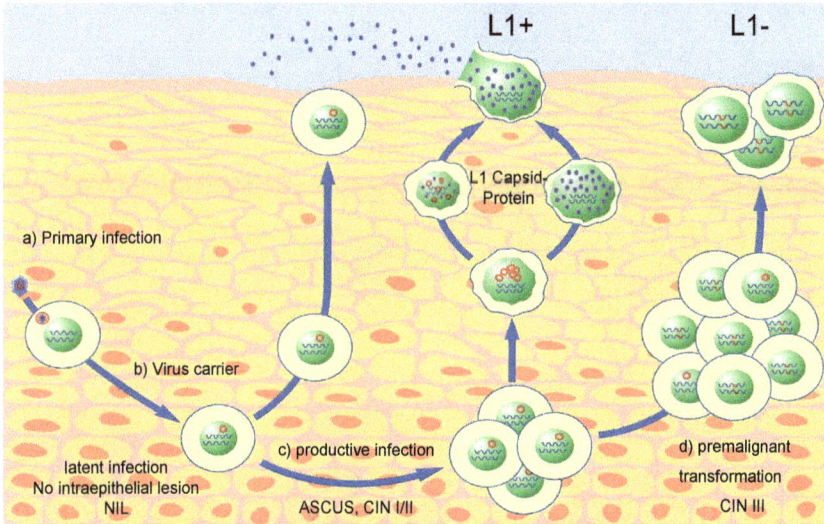

Figure 1. HPV life cycle, as described in the text.

5. Study results

A particular methodical advantage of the L1 capsid protein detection is that the protein is synthesized in the cells of the superficial layer of the epithelium that are easy to obtain by taking a smear (see Figure 2).

The typical L1 staining is a strong, homogenous nuclear stain (Figure 3-7), in contrast to other markers, leading to a very good interobserver reproducibility. Using histological sections Galgano et al. [17] reported for Cytoactiv a raw agreement and k of 96.9% and 0.88, respectively. With 98% raw agreement and 0.96 for kappa Mehlhorn et al. [26] reported similar results for the use of Cytoactiv in cytological samples.

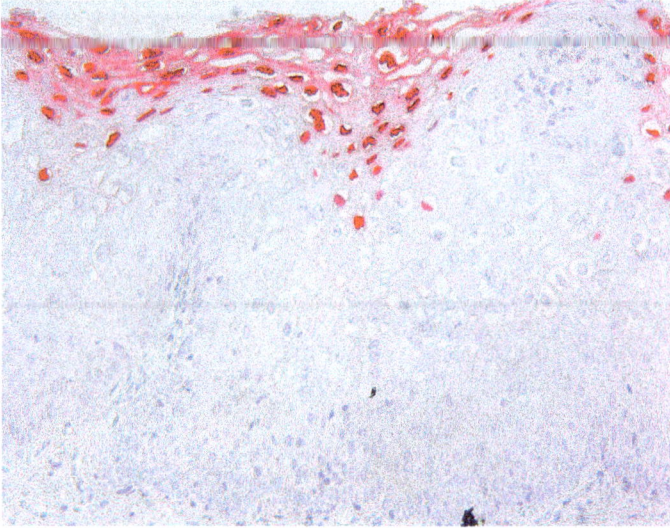

Figure 2. L1+ CIN1 -A particular methodical advantage of the L1 capsid protein detection is that the protein is synthesized in the cells of the superficial layer of the epithelium that are easy to obtain by taking a smear

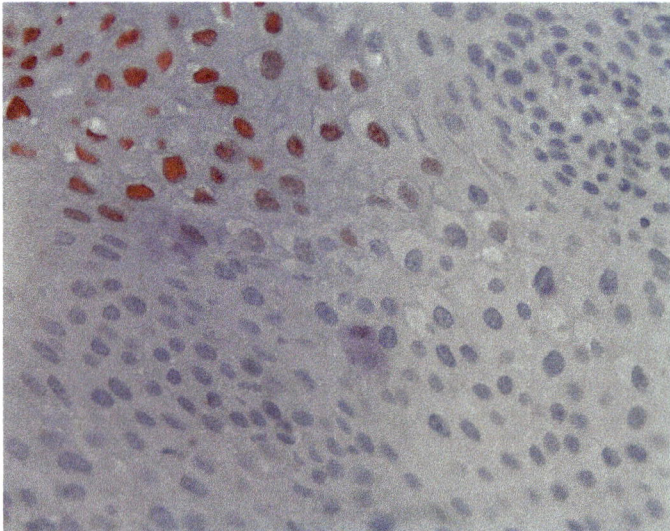

Figure 3. L1 staining intensity correlates with the amount of L1 capsid protein producedand it becomes more intense towards the surface of the epithelium

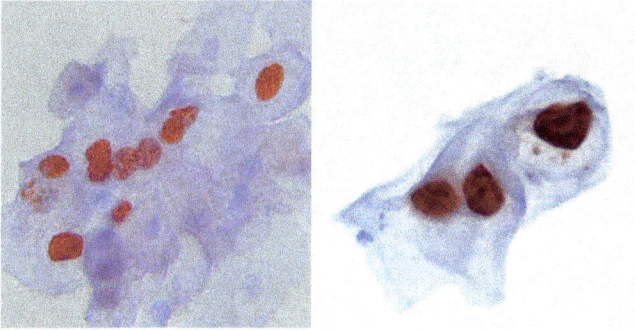

Figure 4. L1 positive LSIL

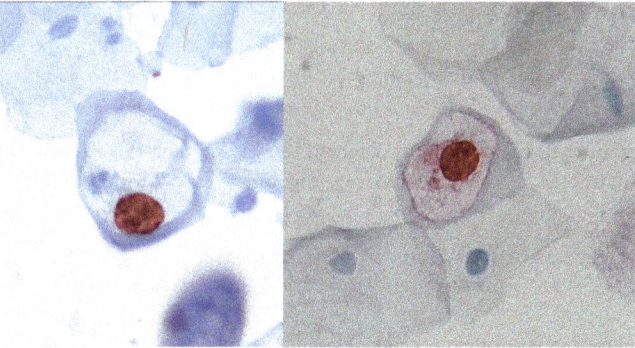

Figure 5. L1 + Koilocytes

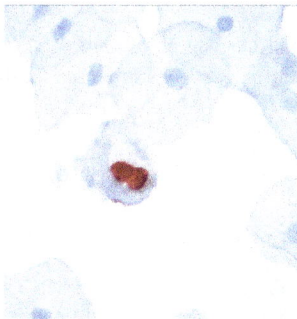

Figure 6. L1 + Koilocyte with 2 nuclei

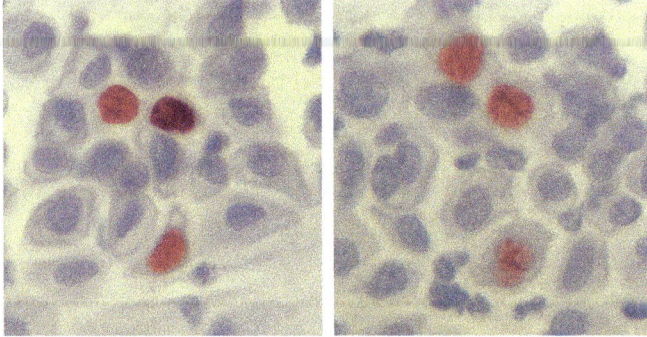

Figure 7. L1+ HSIL, Mehlhorn et al. [26]

Initial L1 studies faced the problem that the sensitivity of randomly choosen L1 antibodies was unacceptable low. One major problem was the well known high frequency of point mutations leading to a loss of the relevant epitopes, and false negative results as a viral strategy to escape immune recognition. This high variability is in clear contrast to the stability of epitopes recognized by antibodies detecting cellular proteins, like p16 or ki67.

During the product development of Cytoactiv it was possible to increase the sensitivity significantly by extensive selection processes generating an optimized antibody detecting a specific epitope.

Nevertheless there were a small number of cases where it was impossible to detect the L1 capsid protein. The reason for this finding was not clear in the beginning.

5.1. L1 and cytological samples

In 2003 Melsheimer et al. [18] have published that most of the HPV high risk associated LSIL expressed HPV L1 capsid protein, but in most of the HSIL cases the HPV L1 capsid protein was not synthesized (see Figure 3-6).

They suggested that a loss of viral L1 capsid protein, as a major target of the immune response in HPV infected SIL, could function as a prognostic marker for the development of CIN lesions.

Later on Griesser et al. [19] were able to confirm this suggestion in a retrospective study with 84 routinely performed conventional Pap smears. During a follow up time of 23 month they showed that the HPV high risk associated mild to moderate dysplastic squamous lesions without immunochemically detectable HPV L1 capsid protein progressed significantly more likely to CIN3+ (76,4%) than the L1 positive cases (23,6%).

Similar results were reported by Rauber et al. [20] in 2008 in a retrospective study of 279 HPV High risk positive conventional Pap smears with mild and moderate severe morphological changes. The progression rate to CIN3+ of L1 capsid protein positive cases was found to be only 12,3% (p-value <0,001).

In the same year Scheidemantel et al. [21] tested the Cytoactiv – Kit on 111 HPV High risk positive ThinPrep – slides. They reported that none of the L1 positive patients showed a progression towards cervical cancer and on the other hand all progredient cases were found to be L1 negative.

An additional advantage of choosing the ThinPrep system emerged in the meantime. The ThinPrep Imager allows the automated evaluation of the L1 stained slides, to speed up the reading process [22]. The benefit of computer based automatisation can be extended to conventional Pap smears and SurePath slides as well if choosing BD's focal point system.

The first prospective randomized study was published in 2009 by Griesser and colleagues [23]. The study included 211 HPV High risk-positive mild and moderate dysplasias (LSIL and HSIL) with a follow-up of the patients up to 48 months. The results of all former retrospective studies were confirmed and strengthened. Depending on patients age (<30 / >30) and the classification of the precancerous lesion (LSIL or HSIL) only 20 % of all L1 positive cases showed a progression to CIN3+. In contrast to this finding up to 97% of the L1 negative cases showed a progression.

In this study the mean duration from the initial L1 positively / negatively stained smears to the recognition of disease progression or remission were reported as well.

For L1 negative cases the time interval until progression was 6 months (range, 1-29) and 6.4 months (range 2-12) for clinical remission, whereas for the L1 positive cases it took 8.5 months (range, 1-13) until progression, and 7 months (range, 3-35) for clinical remission respectively.

	L1-	L1- LSIL	L1- HSIL	L1+	L1+ LSIL	L1+ HSIL
Remission	6.4 (2-12)	7.5 (3-12)	2	7 (3-35)	6.5 (3-18)	9 (3-35)
Progression	6 (1-29)	6 (1-29)	6 (1-20)	8.5 (1-13)	9 (6-13)	8 (1-13)

Table 1. Griesser et al., AJCP 2009: Time interval until clinical remission or progression to CIN3 in month (range)

Stemberger – Papic et al. [24] reported similar results for Croatian women and concluded that immunostaining for HPV L1 capsid protein could offer prognostic information about mild and moderate intraepithelial cervical squamous lesions.

In 2010 and 2011 two Korean studies reported that the prognostic significance of the L1 detection with Cytoactiv for the clinical outcome of early dysplastic lesions can be confirmed for East Asian women as well.

Lee et al [25] confirmed 2011 in a prospective trial of 318 women the benefit for Cytoactiv for the management of HPV high risk positive LSIL women. The positive predictive value of HPV L1-positive cases for no progression was 91.7%, and the negative predictive value of HPV L1-negative cases for progression to high-grade lesions was 27.7.

The results of the largest study so far, a prospective international multicenter study of 809 HPV High risk positive LSIL and HSIL was performed by Mehlhorn et al. [26].

During the follow up of 54 month 83,5% of the HPV-L1 negative progressed to CIN3+, as compared to only 19,8% of the HPV-L1 positive cases. The difference of the clinical outcome of HPV-L1 negative and HPV-L1 positive cases was statistically highly significant (p-value <0·0001) and independent of the classification as mild dysplasia (LSIL) and moderate dysplasia (HSIL).

The authors concluded that HPV-L1 detection allows identifying transient HPV infections and precancerous lesions within the group of HPV high-risk positive early dysplastic lesions.

The high progression rate of HPV-L1 negative mild and moderate dysplasia emphasizes the precancerous nature of these lesions.

As a clinical recommendation they suggested that a close follow-up with colposcopy and histological evaluation and removal of these lesions should be considered.

The low malignant potential of HPV-L1 positive cases, however, indicates transient HPV infection, justifying a watch and wait strategy with cytological follow-up thus preventing overtreatment especially for women in their reproductive age.

Author	classification	No.cases	L1 negative	L1 positive	Mean age	Follow up
Mehlhorn	LSIL	479	72,9	11,8	33,6	54 month
Griesser	LSIL	68	84	25	33,6	48 month
in total		547	75	13,1	33,6	

Table 2. Risk profil LSIL - Progression to CIN3+ for L1+ and L1- cases

Author	classification	No.cases	L1 negative	L1 positive	Mean age	Follow up
Mehlhorn	HSIL	322	92,7	37,4	33,6	54 month
Griesser	HSIL	119	96,9	33	33,6	48 month
in total		441	94,2	34,6	33,6	

Table 3. Risk profil HSIL - Progression to CIN3+ for L1+ and L1- cases

5.2. L1 and histological sections

As already mentioned earlier colposcopically guided punch biopsies are taken during the follow up of women with abnormal Pap smears as step 2 of the 3 step strategy of cervical cancer prevention.

Negri and colleagues [27] pointed out in their study that the possibility of predicting the behavior of low-grade cervical lesions could be of high value in clinical practice, potentially allowing an individualized management of cervical lesions depending on their progression risk.

Hilfrich and Hariri [28] have discribed first, the prognostic relevance of HPV L1 capsid protein detection on paraffin embedded histological sections, initially reported on routinely performed Papanicolaou stained cervical smears and on liquid based cytology (LBC) [18], [19] (see Figure 9).

In contrast to these cytology reports, the association of the cervical intraepithelial lesions with HPV high risk types was not confirmed by highly sophistic DNA methods like PCR [18] or Hybrid capture II [19], but the use of a second biomarker, p16, which together with L1, can be easily integrated in any histopathology lab.

Overall only 16.1% of the 87 L1 negative, p16 positive CIN lesions showed a remission of the lesion, compared to 72.4% of the double positive cases. None of the L1/p16 double negative CIN lesions progressed. Hariri found similar results for the combination of ProExC and Cytoactiv.

Negri and colleagues [27] included in their approach 38 conization specimens with coexisting cervical intraepithelial neoplasia grade 1 (CIN1) and 3 (CIN3) (group A) and 28 punch biopsies from women with CIN1 and proven spontaneous regression in the follow-up (group B). In group A, all CIN3 were p16 positive (p16+) and L1 negative (L1-). The CIN1 of this group were p16+ L1- and p16+ L1+ in 68.42% and 31.57%, respectively. No other expression pattern was found in this group. In group B, the p16+ L1-, p16+ L1+, p16- L1+, and p16- L1- patterns were found in 3.57%, 25%, 14.29%, and 57.14%, respectively. Overall, 96.29% p16+ L1- CIN1 were found in group A, whereas all the p16- L1+ and p16- L1- CIN1 were found in group B.

They found that no cases with both L1 and p16 negativity were found in group A, and proposed that this pattern might be classified as "low risk" or, unless the original section shows obvious dysplastic features, as "no evidence of CIN.'

The results of the study showed that p16 and L1 immunohistochemistry can be helpful for estimating the biologic potentiality of low-grade squamous cervical lesions. Particularly in cases in which the grade of the lesion is morphologically difficult to assess, the p16/L1 expression pattern could be useful for planning the clinical management of these women.

Staining pattern	Risk profile Negri et al.	Risk profile Hilfrich / Hariri
P16+ / L1 -	"high-risk", 3,6% remission	High risk 16.1% remission
P16+ / L1+	indeterminate" risk	72,4% remission not distinguished in p16+/-
P16- / L1+	"low-risk"	
P16- / L1-	"low risk", or "no evidence of CIN.'	No potential to progress

Table 4. Risk profils according to Negri et al./ Hilfrich, Hariri

Using 101 HPV High risk positive CIN1 Choi et al [29] published 2010 that the HPV L1 protein expression is closely related to spontaneous disease regression. Not using p16, but a type-specific HPV-DNA Chip, it was possible for the first time to correlate the HPV type with the regression of the L1 positive CIN1 lesions. 50% of the HPV16 positive CIN1, 72,7% of the HPV58, 76.9% of the HPV18, 77.8% of the HPV33, 83,3% of the HPV53 and 100% of the HPV31 positive cases regressed during the follow up period of 1 year (see Figure 8).

HPV 16	HPV 58	HPV 18	HPV 33	HPV 53	HPV 31
50%	72,7%	76,9%	77,8%	83,3%	100%

Table 5. Choi et al, Remission of Cytoactiv L1 positive cases within 1 year in relation to the HPV type

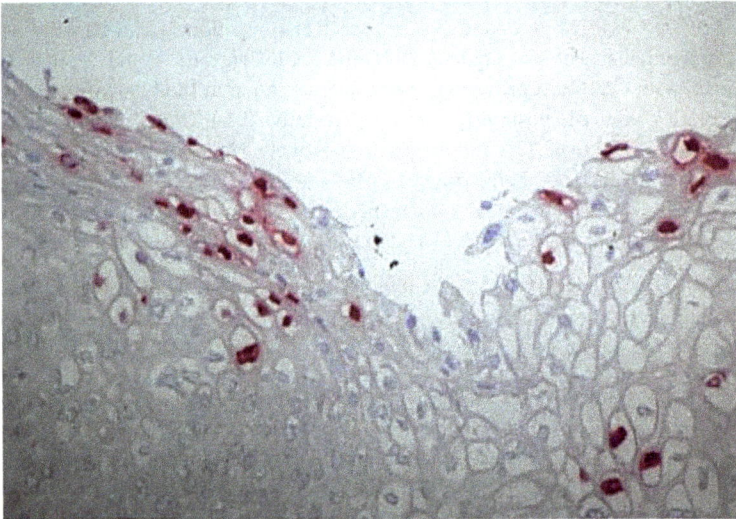

Figure 8. HPV16 / L1+CIN1 – according to Choi et al. regress in 50% of the cases within 12 month.

In contrast to all other studies Galgano et al. [17] asked if HPV L1 detection, as a stand alone marker, could be a useful diagnostic, but not prognostic, tool.

As HPV specific protein L1 is only detectable in HPV positive lesions. HPV negative CIN lesions have to be L1 negative, because the virus is absent.

According to Hilfrich/Hariri and Negri et al L1 negativ cases are mixtures of HPV associated and non HPV associated CIN lesions, especially analysing CIN1.

HPV positive (p16 positive) but L1 negative lesions are high risk lesions whereas on the other hand HPV negative (p16 negative) and L1 negative lesions are 'no risk' lesion or as Negri mentioned could be classified as 'no evidence of CIN'.

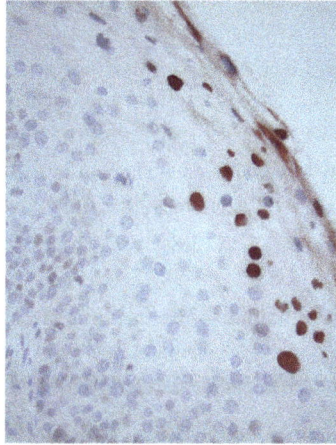

Figure 9. L1+ CIN2

Not surprisingly mixing and not differentiating the L1 negative 'high risk' and the L1 negative 'no risk' entities have to result in 'disappointing' results because remission and progression of the lesions are observed equally.

5.3. The combination of L1 / p16 in cytological samples

In the meantime the combination of L1 and p16 has been investigated on cytological samples by Ungureanu and colleagues [30] as well. As expressed in different phases of cervical carcinogenesis, the authors expected that p16 and L1 are potentially promising markers of progression risk of LSIL. The combination of p16 and L1 capsid protein immunostaining in LBC appears to be useful for an early diagnosis of precancerous lesions and for an appropriate clinical attitude.

Consistent with the previous data they found that expression of L1 capsid protein could be observed in 33.33% of ASC-US cases, 50% of LSILs, 18.51% of HSILs. No positive cases were found in the group of SCC, thus indicating that L1 capsid protein expression tends to decline with increasing severity of the lesions.

6. Discussion

6.1. L1 negative dysplastic lesions as proof of a non-productive, but deregulated life cycle

As already described a tight communication between the virus and the host cell is of critical importance for the viral life cycle. On the one hand it is strictly linked to the epithelial cell differentiation, on the other hand HPV need to modulate the proliferation / differentiation status of the host cells to allow replication in 'non dividing cells' and the maturation of new infectious virus particles.

As long as the L1 capsid protein can be detected within the nucleus of dysplastic cells the virus was successful in this 'walk on the edge'. Despite of all viral activities the cells are still in the condition to allow the normal, productive life cycle of the Human Papilloma Viruses.

L1 capsid protein negative dysplasias, however, are due to this virally induced cellular deregulation processes no longer capable to produce virions.

A shift from a productive HPV infection towards a non-productive or precancerous lesion has occurred.

The reasons for this event are multifarious since the differentiation dependent expression of L1 is controlled at multiple levels. A block at any of the following steps, such as transcription (integration and / or methylation of the DNA), post-transcriptional processing and translation, could be responsible for the loss of L1 capsid protein.

6.2. Transcriptional control

6.2.1. Loss of L1 due to integration of the HPV genome

Integration of the viral DNA is considered to be of critical importance for the progression from CIN to cancer, since the frequency of HPV-16 viral integration increase in parallel with the severity of cervical lesions.

During the integration process of the HPV genome into the host chromosome a linearization of the ring – shaped, episomal viral DNA is required. It's easy to imagine, that this non directed event is regularly associated with a deregulation of the strictly controlled episomal DNA. As a consequence of the integration process alterations of the control region and loss or disruption of HPV specific proteins like the early and late proteins can be observed [31].

Even if the L1 gene is not affected directly, the integration of the virus with loss of transcriptional control by E2 results in over expression of E6 and E7 leading to immortalization and transformation of the cells [32].

As a result, the epithelial host cell remains in the cell cycle and increasingly becomes genetically instable without being able to run its differentiating program.

L1 genes can functionally be inactivated afterwards too, as a result of mutation, gene deletion and insertion as well as DNA methylation so that no capsid protein will be produced anymore (discussed later).

A dysmaturational autonomous tumor emerges in the host epithelium; a 'point of no return' is crossed.

But for the background that many of the HPV-associated cancers do not even carry any integrated viral genome [31], [33] additional mechanisms have to exist to block L1 expression. In the meantime a discussion started if integration is the initial step towards cervical cancer, or maybe only the consequence of the E6/E7 induced genetic instability of the host cells.

6.2.2. Loss of L1 in precancerous lesions with an episomal HPV genome

Control of gene expression by epigenetic modification of distinct DNA sequences is a fundamental biological process, which affects for example embryonic development, cellular differentiation and others.

One important mechanism, affecting the chromatin conformation, is the methylation of DNA, specifically at cystidine-guanidine (CpG) dinucleotides. Methylated CpG dinucleotides bind repressors, which alter the conformation of nucleosomes through their interaction with histone deacetylases in a manner unfavourable to transcription [34].

In the meantime it's known that epigenetic mechanisms play a major role in the transcription of the HPV genome as well [35], [36].

Several reports showed that the HPV genome is differentially methylated during progression from simple infected to transformed cells.

Alterations were observed particularly in the control region, and the L1 and L2 gene in high grade precancer and invasive cancer. These observations lead to the suggestion that the lack of expression of these genes may be attributed at least in part to increasing methylation of the respective parts of the viral genomes.

Kalantari et al. for example reported that methylation exceeds 50% in the case of some CpG dinucleotides within the L1 gene [37].

In addition E2 expression seems to be strictly linked to the differentiation process from normal to malignant cells, indirectly affecting L1 expression as well. Vinokurova showed that E2 binding sites are highly methylated in undifferentiated cells, inhibiting E2-binding, and demethylation at the E2 binding sites occurs in association with the cell differentiation only [38].

That means different mechanisms are existing to prevent L1 mRNA transcription.

6.3. Post transcriptional control

Once the transcription of the late mRNA was successful, additional mechanisms have been reported that are able to control or block the L1 capsid protein expression.

6.3.1. Control of the stability of late mRNA

Mori et al. [39] showed that RNA instability elements are within the L1 and L2 coding mRNAs of HPV16, which function in undifferentiated cells. Although the mechanism for RNA destabilization are still subject of further investigations this mechanism could be important for L1 expression.

6.3.2. Nuclear export of late mRNAs,

Koffa et al. [40] reported that the L1 mRNA of HPV16 was retained in the nucleus in undifferentiated W12 epithelial cells, suggesting that the nuclear export of late mRNAs was inhibited in the dividing cells, thus preventing translation of the L1 protein in the cytoplasm. The factor(s) mediating the nuclear export of late mRNAs has not been identified yet [41].

6.4. Translational control of late mRNA

Last but not least the rare codon usages found in L1 and L2 might also contribute to the inhibition of late gene translation [42]. In terminally differentiated cells, the altered expression ratios of tRNA species could compensate for the inhibitory effect of the rare codon usages [43].

All these steps could be of critical importance for L1 capsid protein expression. As indicated a lot of questions are still remaining and need to be answered in the future. Most probably not only a single control mechanism is responsible for the oberserved loss of L1 capsid proteins.

7. Immune response against L1 capsid proteins

7.1. L1 positivity and clinical remission

The immune system developed special innate and adaptive immune mechanisms to recognize and fight against foreign agents that invade our body.

Sometimes these methods are ineffective especially when the agent uses mechanisms to evade the immune system, like HPV is doing.

Since the HPV infection remains located in the epithelium, mucosal ulceration is a prerequisite for antigen contact with the immune cells in the stroma and in addition to a sufficiently high antigen dose, an efficient immune response, against HPV, also requires supporting mediators.

However, HPV itself has own characteristics also due to its route of infection that protect it from access of the immune system.

The HPV infection does not cause a systemic spreading of the infection by means of a viraemia and the infected epithelia are not destroyed. Thus, any inflammatory tissue reaction support-ing the immune response is suppressed, and the virus material is only released on the epithelial surface which is poor in immune defence cells and distant from immune centers.

Finally, the virus itself express only very low levels of viral protein, suppresses the release of cytokines from epithelia and intraepithelial antigen-presenting Langerhans' cells and can suppress the expression of histocompatibility antigens required for the interaction of epithelial cells and immune cells. The E7 and E6 proteins are involved in this inhibition [44], [45].

Consequently, one could envision that in this setting an efficient transfer of antigen from HPV infected keratinocytes to the antigen presenting cells (APC) is not triggered.

Nevertheless a successful immune response to genital HPV infection is established in almost all cases. But the time required for clearance of high risk types, particulary HPV16, averages 8-14 month, which is considerably longer than 5-6 months needed for clearance of low risk types [44].

7.2. The role of the L1 capsid protein in immune recognition

The only fully accessible antigen sources in the earlier stage of virally induced SIL to promote an activation of the immune system are free viral particles consisting of 360 L1 capsid proteins.

Therefore it seems not to be surprising, that a clinical remission of the lesion is observed regularly if the L1 capsid protein is detectable in the dysplastic cells.

To generate an effective virus specific immune response the virus particles have to be detected by the antigen presenting cells (APC) of squamous epithelium, the Langerhans cells (LC) or Dendritic cells (DC), and armed effector cells, has to migrate back to the infected site, and destroy the infected keratinocytes leading to a spontaneous clinical remission of the lesion.

If such immunologic activation mechanisms are functional, they are quite effective since with about 20% the malignant potential for these L1-positive lesions, irrespective of the dysplasia being cytologically mild or moderate, is low.

On the other hand it is still not clear how L1 specific cytotoxic T-cells could be able to destroy the HPV reservoir in the basal cell layer to cause clinical remission, since the L1 capsid protein is only detectable in terminally differentiated cells.

In analogy to the basal cells it was shown for the L1 capsid protein negative C3 cell line, that these cells are sensitive to L1 specific cytotoxic T-cells [46]. The only explanation seems to be a L1 expression level in these cells (as well as the basal cells), lower than the detection limit used for analysis. As described earlier L1 mRNA is detectable in the nucleus of undifferentiated cells.

A second explanation for the clinical remission of L1 capsid protein positive dysplasias could be, that the viral capsids work as a kind of abjuvance, only triggering the cell mediated response to the early proteins, principally E2 and E6, which are thought to be important for lesion regression [47].

Nevertheless it was shown recently by Mehlhorn et al. [48] that the detection of antibodies against HPV16 L1 in the serum is always associated with clinical remission, if the L1 capsid protein is detectable in the smear of HPV high risk positive mild and moderate dysplasias. These L1 specific serum antibodies shouldn't be able to fight against the HPV infected cells, but it shows that a L1 specific activation of the immune system is of critical importance for the clearance of the HPV infection.

7.3. Progression of L1 capsid protein positive cases

An ineffective immune response maybe promoted by HLA incompatibilities, factors contributing to cervical cancer like tobacco smoking or the coexistence of dysplasias of different grade in the transformation zone, possibly reflecting a mixture of L1-positive and L1-negative lesions with different progressive potentials may be the reasons for a progression of some L1-positive intraepithelial lesions.

In addition Yang et al [49] identified several mutant HPV16 L1 isolates carrying genes encoding proteins that neither assemble nor activate VLP-dependent innate and adaptive immune responses. They concluded that this may represent an additional mechanism of the evasion of innate immune recognition during cervical carcinogenesis.

7.4. L1 negative dysplasias and progression to CIN3+

Absence of L1 capsid protein, as the only fully accessible antigen sources in the earlier stage of virally induced SIL, leads to the situation that the viral immune escape mechanisms are maintained and the dysplastic cells, unnoticed by the immune system, proceed in the process of malignant transformation.

With more than 80% in cytology and more than 90% for CIN1/2 the malignant potential of the L1-negative dysplasias is exceedingly high, similar to what is expected for a true precancerous lesion.

The differentiation dependent loss of the L1 stimulus may lead to a local 'lack of immunity' further supporting the virally induced alterations.

These may lead to additional disorders of cell cycle regulation at transcriptional, translational and genomic levels thus resulting in a progression of the early precursor lesions to CIN3+. [49]- [51].

7.5. L1 negative dysplasias and clinical remission

Reasons for the extremely rare cases of clinical remission of L1-negative cases (~5-10%) are most likely due to sampling errors with absence of L1 expressing cells in the sample or expression levels below the detection limit of the highly sensitive immunochemical assay, as reported for the C3 cell line [46].

8. Summary

To treat or not to treat that remains the last question, that has to be answered for women with abnormal Pap smears at the end of the cervical cancer prevention program.

As step 3 of the traditional programs it is common sense that excisional or ablative treatment of the cervical tissue is needed in women diagnosed with precancer.

A statement that is easy to agree on, but difficult to follow since mild, moderate and severe dysplasias or the histological equivalents CIN1, CIN2, CIN3 are mixtures of distinct biological stages resulting in different clinical outcomes and neither cytological follow up, colposcopy nor HPV DNA testing could indicate whether a remission or progression of the precursor lesion to invasive cancer will occur.

The good news is that the ratio of remission or transient HPV infection of the one hand, and progression or precancer on the other hand is moving to precancer with the severity of the lesion.

But even CIN3 is not uniform in being precancer. Ostor reported that 30% of these cases will show a spontaneous remission if untreated. Nevertheless we agree that a treatment is warranted.

Accepting CIN2 as the clinical threshold for treatment moves us towards a higher degree of overtreatment, increasing in parallel the potential harms on reproductive outcomes for fertile women, including preterm delivery and low-birth-weight infants with life long fatal disabilities.

As shown HPV L1 detection with Cytoactiv is an objective standard to optimize the clinical management of women with abnormal Pap smears.

The data published over the last decade shows uniform that HPV-L1 detection allows identifying transient HPV infections and precancerous lesions within the group of HPV high-risk positive early dysplastic lesions (mild and moderate dysplasia) see Figure 10.

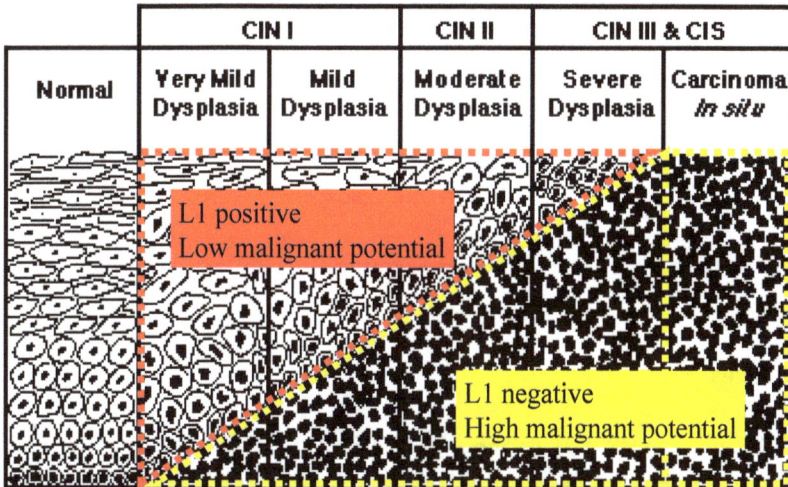

Figure 10. Histologically, CIN grading is based upon the proportion of the surface epithelium composed of undifferentiated cells characteristic of the basal layer. Increasing grade is associated with a progressive loss of epithelial maturation. L1 detection allows to identify the different progressive potentials of transient HPV infection (red) and precancer (yellow).

As summarized in Tables 2-4, 75% of the L1 negative LSIL and 94,2% of the L1 negative HSIL progressed to CIN3. Using CIN1 and CIN2 lesions with 83,9 – 96,4% the results are compareable.

These high progression rates of HPV-L1 negative mild and moderate dysplasia emphasizes the precancerous nature of these lesions. Only 5-25% of these lesions regress spontaneously a rate even better than what is accepted for treatment of CIN3, but years before the severe dysplasia arise.

As stated by different authors a close follow-up with colposcopy and histological evaluation is advisable and removal of these lesions should be considered.

On the other hand the low malignant potential of HPV-L1 positive cases indicates transient HPV infection, or true 'low grade lesions'.

Only 13,1% of the L1 positive LSIL, and 34,6% of the L1 positive HSIL progressed to CIN3, typically thresholds justifying 'a watch and wait strategy' with cytological follow-up.

Integrating the promising serological HPV L1 antibody rapid test into this procedure seems to be able to improve this data further, thus preventing overtreatment especially for women in their reproductive age.

Only in case of persistence of the L1 positive lesion a colposcopy should be performed.

At the end of the day a combination of cytology, colposcopy, HPV DNA determination and HPV L1 detection offers a unique possibility to increase the benfits of cervical cancer screening programs, by reducing the potentials harms.

Author details

Ralf Hilfrich

Cytoimmun Diagnostics GmbH Pirmasens, Germany

References

[1] Ferlay J, Shin HR, Bray F, Forman D, Mathers C and Parkin DM. GLOBOCAN 2008 v1.2, Cancer Incidence and Mortality Worldwide: IARC CancerBase No. 10.Lyon, France: International Agency for Research on Cancer; 2010. Available from: http://globocan.iarc.fr.

[2] Meisels A, Fortin R : Condylomatous lesions of the cervicx and vagina. I. Cytologic patterns. Acta Cytol 1976, 20 : 505-509

[3] Meisels A, Fortin R, Roy M : Condylomatous lesions of the cervic. II. Cytologic, colposcopic and histopathologic study. Acta Cytol 1977, 21 : 379-390

[4] Gissmann L, zur Hausen H : Partial characterization of viral DNA from human genital warts (Condylomata acuminata). Int J Cancer 1980, 25 : 605-609

[5] WHO/ICO information centre on Human Papilloma Virus (HPV) and Cervical Cancer, www.who.int/hpvcentre

[6] Papanicolaou GN; Traut HF. Diagnosis of uterine cancer by the vaginal smear. New York, Commonwealth Fund, 1943.

[7] Riotton G, Christopherson WM, Lunt R. Cytology of the Female Genital Tract. International Histological Classification of Tumours No. 8, World Health Organisation, Geneva, 1973.

[8] Solomon D, Davey D, Kurman R et al. The 2001 Bethesda System: terminology for reporting results of cervical cytology. JAMA 2002, 287 (16): 2114-9.

[9] Wagner D. Munich nomenclature II for gynaecologic cytodiagnosis. Acta Cytol 1990; 34: 900-901.

[10] Ostor A. Natural History of Cervical Intrepithelial Neoplasia: A critical review, Int J Gynecol Pathol 1993; 12(2): 186.

[11] Richart RM, Natural history of cervical intraepithelial neoplasia. Clin Obstet Gynecol 1967; 10 : 748-784

[12] Kyrgiou M, Koliopoulos G, Martin-Hirsch P, Arbyn M, Prendiville W, Paraskevaidis E. Obstetric outcomes after conservative treatment for intraepithelial or early invasive cervical lesions: systematic review and meta-analysis. Lancet 2006; 367:489-98.

[13] Soergel P, Makowski E, Makowski L, Schippert C, Hillemanns P. What are the costs of conisation when considering pregnancy – associated complications ? Geburtsh Frauenheilk 2011;71: 199-204).

[14] Zur Hausen H, Papillomaviruses and cancer: from basic studies to clinical application. Nat Rev Cancer. 2002; 2 : 342-350.

[15] Schiller JT, Day PM, Kines RC. Current understanding of the mechanism of HPV infection. Gynecol Oncol. 2010 Jun;118(1 Suppl):S12-7.

[16] Doorbar J. Papillomavirus life cycle organization and biomarker selection. Dis Markers 2007;23(4):297-313.

[17] Galgano MT, Castle PE, Atkins KA, Brix WK, Nassau SR, Stoler MH. Using biomarkers as objective standards in the diagnosis of cervical biopsies. Am J Surg Pathol, 2010 Aug; 34(8): 1077-1087.

[18] Melsheimer P, Kaul S, Dobeck S, Bastert G, Immunocytochemical detection of human papillomavirus high risk L1 capsid proteins in LSIL and HSIL as compared with detection of HPV L1 DNA. Acata Cytol. 2003; 47 : 124-128.

[19] Griesser H, Sander H, Hilfrich R, Moser B, Schenck U, Correlation of immunochemical detection of HPV L1 capsid protein in Pap smears with regression of high risk HPV DNA positive mild/moderate dysplasia. Anal Quant Cytol Histol, 2004;26; 241-245.

[20] Rauber D, Mehlhorn G, Fasching PA, Beckmann MW, Ackermann S. Prognostic significance of the detection of the human papillomavirus L1 protein in smears of mild

to moderate cervical intraepithelial lesions. Eur J Obstet Gynecol Reprod Biol 2008 Oct;140(2):258-62. Epub 2008 Jul 14

[21] Scheidemantel T, Simmerman K, Ji X, Dolar S, Brainard J, Tubbs R, Hilfrich R, Yang B. 2008. Expression pattern of HPV L1 capsid protein in PAP tests: a potential bio-marker in risk assessment for high grade SIL lesion. Abstract Ann. M. Am. Soc. of Cytopathology

[22] Hilfrich R, Weiss A, Griesser H, Use of the ThinPrep® Imager for evaluation of slides stained immunocytochemically with Cytoactiv®. Presentation ICC2010, Edinburgh.

[23] Griesser H, Sander H, Walczak C, Hilfrich R. HPV vaccine protein L1 predicts dis-ease outcome of high-risk HPV+ early dysplastic lesions. Am J Clin Pathol 2009 Dec; 132(6):840-5.

[24] Stemberger-Papic S, Vrdoljak-Mozetic D, Ostojic DV, Rubesa-Mihaljevic R, Manestar M, Evaluation of the HPV L1 capsid protein in prognosis of mild and moderate dys-plasia of the cervix uteri. Coll Antropol 2010, 34, 2 : 419-423.

[25] Lee SJ, Lee AW, Kim TJ et al. Correlation between immunocytochemistry of human papilloma virus L1 capsid protein and behavior of low-grade cervical cytology in Ko-rean women. Journal of Obstetrics and Gynaecology Research 2011 Sep;37(9):1222-8.

[26] Mehlhorn G, Obermann E, Negri G, Bubendorf L, Mian Chr, Koch M, Sander H, Simm B, Lütge M, Banrevi Zs, Weiss A, Gieri C, Hilfrich R, Beckmann M, Griesser H, HPV L1 detection discriminates cervical precancer from transient HPV infection – a prospective international multicenter study. Nature – Modern Pathology in press.

[27] Negri G, Bellisano G, Zannoni GF et al. p16 and HPV immunohistochemistry is help-ful for estimating the behaviour of low grade dysplastic lesions of the cervix uteri. Am J Surg Pathol 2008 Nov;32(11):1715-20.

[28] Hilfrich R, Hariri J. Prognostic relevance of HPV L1 capsid protein detection within mild to moderate dysplastic lesions of the cervix uteri in combination with a second biomarker p16. Anal Quant Cytol Histl 2008 Apr;30(2):78-82.

[29] Choi YS, Kang WD, Kim SM et al. Human Papillomavirus L1 Capsid Protein and Human Papillomavirus Type 16 as Prognostic Markers in Cervical Intraepithelial Ne-oplasia 1. Int J of Gynecological Cancer 2010 Feb;20(2):288-93.

[30] Ungureanu C, Socolov D, Anton G, Mihailovici MS, Teleman S, Immunocytochemi-cal expression of p16ink4a and HPV L1 capsid proteins as predictive markers of the cervical lesions progression risk. Rom J Morphol Embryol. 2010;51(3):497-503.

[31] Vinokurova S, Wentzensen N, Kraus I et al., Type-dependent integration frequency of human papillomavirus genomes in cervical lesions. Cancer Res 2008; 68: 307-313.

[32] Romanczuk H, Howley PM, Disruption of either the E1 and E2 regulatory gene of human papillomavirus type 16 increase viral immortalization capacity. Proc Natl Acad Sci USA, 89 : 3159-3163.

[33] Pett M, Coleman N, Integration of high-risk human papilloma virus a key event in cervical carcinogenesis?, J Pathol 212: 356-367.

[34] Goll MG, Bestor TH. Eukaryotic cytosine methyltransferases. Annu Rev Biochem. 2005;74:481-514.

[35] Kulis M, Esteller M, DNA methylation and cancer. Adv. Genet 2010, 70 : 27-56.

[36] Badal V, Chuang LS, Tan EH, Badal S, Villa LL et al., CpG methylation of human papillomavirus type 16 DNA in cervical cancer cell lines and in clinical specimen : Genomic hypomethylation correlates with carcinogenic progression. J Virol 77: 6227-6234.

[37] Kalantari M, Calleja-Macias IE, Tewari D, Hagmar B, Lie K, Barrera-Saldana HA, Wiley DJ, Bernard HU. Conserved methylation patterns of human papillomavirus type 16 DNA in asymptomatic infection and cervical neoplasia. J Virol. 2004 Dec;78(23): 12762-72.

[38] Vinokurova S , von Knebel Doeberitz M, Differential Methylation of the HPV 16 upstream regulatory region during epithelial differentiation and neoplastic transformation. PloS ONE 2011, 6 (9), 24451-24464.

[39] Mori S, Ozaki S, Yasugi T, Yoshikawa H, Taketani Y, Kanda T, Inhibitory cis-element-mediated decay of human papillomavirus type 16 L1-transcript in undifferentiated cells. Mol Cell Biochem 2006, 288, 47-57

[40] Koffa MD, Graham SV, Takagaki Y, Manley JL, Clements JB, The human papillomavirus type 16 negative regulatory RNA element interacts with three proteins that act at different posttranscriptional levels. Proc Natl Acad Sci USA, 2000, 97, 4677-4682.

[41] Zhao X, Rush M, Schwartz S, Identification of an hnRNA A1-dependent splicing silencer in the human papillomavirus type 16 L1 coding region that prevents premature expression of the late L1 gene. J Virol 2004, 78, 10888-10905.

[42] Gu W, Li M, Zhao WM, Fang NX, Bu S, Frazer IH, Zhao KN, tRNASer(CGA) differentially regulates expression of wildtype and codon-modified papillomavirus L1 genes. Nucl Acids Res 2004, 32, 4448-4461.

[43] Fang NX, Gu W, Ding J, Saunders NA, Frazer IH, Zhao KN, Calcium enhances keratinocyte differentiation in vitro to differentially regulate expression of papillomavirus authentic and codon modified L1 genes. Virology 2007, 365, 187-197.

[44] Stanley M, Immune responses to human papillomvirus. Vaccine 2006, 24 (Suppl.1): 16-22

[45] Scott M, Nakagawa M, Moscicki AB, Cell-mediated immune response to human pap-
      illomavirus infection. Clin Diagn Lab Immunol 2001, 8 : 209-220.

[46] Ohlschläger P, Osen W, Dell K, Faath S, Garcea RL, Jochmus I, Müller M, Pawlita M,
      Schäfer K, Sehr P, Staib C, Sutter G, Gissmann L. Human papillomavirus type 16 L1
      capsomeres induce L1-specific cytotoxic T lymphocytes and tumor regression in
      C57BL/6 mice. J Virol. 2003 Apr;77(8):4635-45.

[47] van Poelgeest MI, Nijhuis ER, Kwappenberg KM, Hamming IE, Wouter Drijfhout J,
      Fleuren GJ, van der Zee AG, Melief CJ, Kenter GG, Nijman HW, Offringa R, van der
      Burg SH. Distinct regulation and impact of type 1 T-cell immunity against HPV16 L1,
      E2 and E6 antigens during HPV16-induced cervical infection and neoplasia. Int J
      Cancer. 2006 Feb 1;118(3):675-83.

[48] Mehlhorn G, Koch M, Hilfrich R, Beckmann M, HPV16-L1-specific antibody rapidt-
      est improves the prognostic significance of Cytoactiv. HPV2011, Berlin.

[49] Yang R, Wheeler CM, Chen X et al. Papillomavirus capsid mutation to escape den-
      tritic cell dependent innate immunity in cervical cancer. J Virol 2005; 79 (11):
      6741-6750.

[50] Choo KB, Lee HH, Pan CC et al. Sequence duplication and internal deletion in the
      integrated human papillomavirus type 16 genome from cervical carcinoma. J Virol
      1998; 62: 1659-66.

[51] Icenogle JP, Clancy KA, Lin SY. Sequence variation in the capsid protein genes of hu-
      man papillomavirus type 16 and type 31. Virology 1995; 214: 664-669.

Chapter 6

Human Papillomavirus Prophylactic Vaccines and Alternative Strategies for Prevention

Lis Ribeiro-Müller, Hanna Seitz and Martin Müller

Additional information is available at the end of the chapter

1. Introduction

First evidence that transmissible agents are involved in the development of cervical cancer dates back to the mid 19th century and is based on investigations of the Italian physician Demonico Rigoni-Stern who recognized that cancer of the womb is found most frequently among women in their fourth and fifth decade and that factors such as age of sexual debut and promiscuity attribute to the risk of acquiring this type of cancer [1]. However, only with the advent of molecular biology in the early 1970s, and after ruling out Herpes Simplex Viruses, a link was established between cervical cancer and infections by certain types of human papillomaviruses (HPV). After isolation of HPV 6 from a condyloma and subsequently of HPV 11 from a laryngeal papilloma the genomic DNA of these two types allowed tracing of other, novel HPVs in biopsies of cervical tumors [2, 3]. The detection of HPV DNA in tumor cells, including the HeLa cell line, was initially met with much doubt and disbelief in the scientific community but could subsequently be confirmed. In fact, the initial observation by Dürst et al. [4] that 11 out of 18 cervical cancer biopsies from German patients were positive for HPV 16 is consistent with today's knowledge of HPV 16 being present in more than 50% of malignant tumors from the cervix. In the following years the findings by Harald zur Hausen and his colleagues were confirmed by numerous laboratories worldwide and a causative link between HPV infections and cervical cancer in humans was established due to the vast amount of epidemiological studies and an overwhelming body of data obtained in different *in vivo* and *in vitro* models. In 2008 Prof. Harald zur Hausen was awarded the Nobel Prize which recognizes his pioneering findings and fundamental role in HPV research.

2. HPV vaccines — Early studies in animal models

The first observations in respect to therapeutic or prophylactic vaccination against papillomaviruses (PV) were made using models of experimental induction of warts in rabbits and humans. In heroic and bold self-experimentation Findlay inoculated himself with wart extracts and noted that he became 'immune' to wart induction. Similarly, Grigg and Wilhelm noted patterns for the appearance of skin warts in school children and attributed their findings to a possible 'resistance' of some individuals [5]. In the first half of the last century a number of efforts were undertaken to treat skin and genital warts by the injection of autologous and heterologous wart extracts; some of these attempts were seemingly met with success [6].

A systematic development of prophylactic papillomavirus vaccines proved difficult without a virus that can be replicated in culture, suitable animal models, and markers for protection. Still, a number of prophylactic vaccine approaches were performed either by the use of formalin-fixed wart extracts or by inactivated purified viruses e.g. in dogs, rabbits, cattle and horses (for review see: [7]). By passive transfer Chambers et al. demonstrated that antibodies confer protection against induction of oral papillomas [8]. One of the first *in vitro* assays that allowed detection of virus-neutralizing antibodies, the so-called focus-formation assay, was based on transformation of mouse fibroblasts [9]. Initially, this assay was limited to the use of BPV but was later extended to HPV types, by encapsidating the BPV genome in an HPV capsid. Inhibition of virion induced agglutination (HI assay) of mouse erythrocytes by capsid-specific antibodies was employed as a simple surrogate assay before the development of functional reporter-based neutralization assays [10]. The HI assay has intrinsic limitations as it, first, only detects L1-specific antibodies that prevent binding of particles to the cell surface and, second, the nature of the interaction of PV virions with mouse erythrocytes is not well defined. On a different note, it should be mentioned that Kreider and colleagues were the first to develop a functional neutralization assay for HPV 11 by implanting human tissue under the renal capsule of nude mice and subsequently monitoring HPV induced lesions [11]. Because of the complex technique this assay was established only in very few laboratories.

In recent years, the so called pseudovirion-based neutralization assays (PBNAs) have been regarded as the gold standard for the detection of neutralizing antibodies against PVs [12]. These assays have in common that a plasmid encoding a reporter gene (such as secreted alkaline phosphatase, luciferases, fluorescent proteins) is encapsidated in mammalian cells by expression of codon-optimized L1 and L2 genes (Fig. 1). These pseudoviruses can be purified e.g. by gradient centrifugation and used to infect cells *in vitro* and *in vivo*. Presence of neutralizing antibodies will prevent infection and thus reporter gene expression. The assay is tedious and does not readily allow for screening of large serum sample collections e.g. for the monitoring of clinical vaccine trials. Recently, we have developed a modified, high-throughput PBNA that allows automated and reproducible detection of neutralizing antibodies (Sehr et al. in preparation).

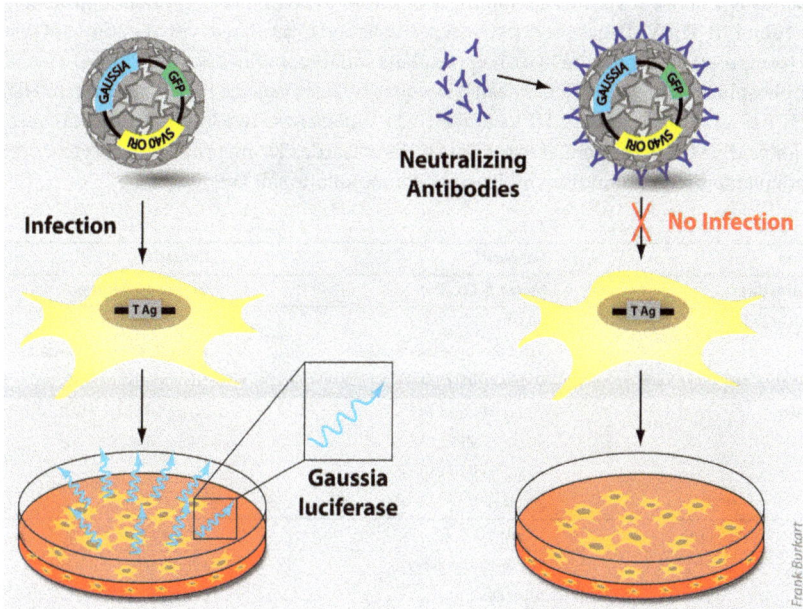

Figure 1. Pseudovirion-based neutralization assay (PBNA). Gaussia = Gaussia luciferase; GFP: green fluorescent protein; SV40 ORI = SV40 origin for replication. Pseudovirions (PSV) encapsidating a Gaussia luciferase reporter gene were produced in mammalian cells and used for infection of HeLa cells. The levels of secreted Gaussia (light blue arrows) can be quantified by a luminescence assay. The presence of neutralizing antibodies (dark blue) abrogates PSV infection and the subsequent secretion of Gaussia.

PV pseudovirions have also been used in a cervicovaginal mouse model for the detection of neutralizing antibodies. In this model, the female mouse genital epithelium is infected with pseudovirions carrying a firefly luciferase gene and luciferase activity is monitored by *in vivo* imaging. Compared to the *in vitro* PBNA, the mouse model shows increased sensitivity for the detection of L1 but moreover, of L2 antibodies [13].

3. Current HPV vaccines

3.1. The two commercial HPV vaccines — Similarities and differences

Many years of research showing that anti-L1 antibodies protect against HPV infection and L1 can assemble into particles called virus-like particles culminated and [14] triggered the development of the current HPV vaccines [15].

Two commercially available prophylactic HPV vaccines, Cervarix® (GSK) and Gardasil® (Merck) have been licensed in over 100 countries. Both are composed of the L1 major capsid protein assembled into non-infectious and highly immunogenic virus-like-particles (VLPs) [16].

Cervarix® is a bivalent vaccine containing VLPs from the two most prevalent high-risk HPV types 16 and 18. The VLPs are produced in insect cells and formulated with the adjuvant system AS04 (composed of aluminium hydroxyphosphate sulfate combined with MPL- 3-O-deacyl-4′-monophosphoryl lipid A) [17]. Gardasil® is a quadrivalent vaccine that in addition to HPV16 and HPV18 VLPs also contains HPV6 and HPV11 VLPs. These two low-risk types are responsible for nearly 90% of the genital warts. The VLPs in Gardasil® are produced in a yeast system and adjuvanted with aluminium hydroxiphosphate sulfate salt [18] (Table 1).

Vaccine	Gardasil®	Cervarix®
Manufacturer	Merck & Co., Inc.	GlaxoSmithKline
Producer cells	Yeast	Insect cells
	Saccharomyces cerevisiae	Spodoptera frugiperda Sf-9,
	CANADE 3C-5 (Stamm 1895)	Trichoplusia ni Hi-5
Antigen	20 µg HPV6 L1 VLP	20 µg HPV16 L1 VLP
	40 µg HPV11 L1 VLP	20 µg HPV 18 L1VLP
	40 µg HPV16 L1 VLP	
	20 µg HPV 18 L1VLP	
Vaccination schedule	Months 0, 2, 6	Months 0, 1, 6
Package	Ready-to-use syringe	Ampules
	Ampules	0.5 mL
	0.5 mL	
Vaccine recommendation	Vaccination of female at age 11 or 12 years	Vaccination of female aged 11
(ACIP)	(catch-up: 13-26 years old).	or 12 years old (can be started
	Vaccination of male aged 9 through 26	at 9 years).
	years.	

Modified from [19] and [20]

Table 1. Comparison of the two prophylactic HPV vaccines, Gardasil® and Cervarix®.

4. Safety

Since the main target groups for the HPV vaccines are children and young women that have not initiated sexual activity, safety was the highest priority for the two vaccine producers.

Over the past years many studies have been conducted to ensure safety and tolerability of Cervarix® and Gardasil® [21, 22]. Independent of age, sex or ethnicity, the HPV vaccines are highly safe and well tolerated with very little adverse effects and no significant differences between Gardasil® and Cervarix®. However, in a direct comparison study between the two vaccines, Cervarix® was associated with higher rates of local injection site reactions than Gardasil® [23] (Table 2). This effect might be associated with the differences in adjuvant formulation between the two vaccines.

The most common adverse effects for both vaccines are pain, reddening and swelling at the site of the injection as well as syncope, fatigue, nausea, dizziness and migraine. No severe side effects including auto-immune response abortion or abnormal pregnancy were observed with increased frequency after vaccination with Cervarix® or Gardasil® when compared to the control groups [24-26]

Symptom	Cervarix®	Gardasil®
Pain	92.9 [90.4, 95.0]	71.6 [67.5, 75.4]
Redness	44.3 [40.0, 48.6]	25.6 [21.9, 29.5]
Swelling	36.5 [32.3, 40.7]	21.8 [18.3, 25.5]
Fatigue	49.8 [45.5, 54.2]	39.8 [35.6, 44.1]
Headache	47.5 [43.2, 51.9]	41.9 [37.6, 46.3]
Fever ≥ 39.0 °C	0.4 [0.0, 1.4]	0.0 [0.0, 0.7]

Modified from [23]

Table 2. Percentage of women reporting symptoms at least once within seven days after any vaccine dose (total vaccinated cohort) – Einstein et al., 2009 study [23]

5. Immunity

5.1. Immunity of natural HPV infection

As HPV infection is limited to basal epithelial cells, the virus is normally "hiding" from circulating immune cells during initial stages of infection, limiting the host's immune responses. Additionally, to evade the host's immune system and achieve persistent infection, HPV has developed several mechanisms to down-regulate host immunity [27, 28]. The virus's success in evading the immune system is corroborated by the finding that of the women infected with HPV, only 50% develop anti-HPV antibodies (mainly anti-L1). Whether these antibodies can protect against re-incident infection remains unclear.

5.2. Vaccine induced immunity and duration of protection

The mechanisms of immunity induced by the HPV vaccines are not fully understood but it seems that humoral immunity (virus-specific neutralizing immunoglobulin G antibodies) plays an important role. Passive transfer of immune serum in pre-clinical animal models, for example, have demonstrated that L1 virus-specific antibodies are sufficient to prevent papillomavirus infection [14, 29, 30].

Cervarix® and Gardasil® induce production of high levels of anti-L1 antibodies that reach their peak seven months after the administration of the third dose. The level of antibodies gradually decreases over time but even after several years the titers remain higher than in naturally infected women.

Vaccine	Years (approximate) after vaccination	Cohort	Vaccine efficacy % (95% CI)				Reference
			HPV16 persistent* infection	HPV 18 persistent* infection	CIN2 lesions - HPV16/18	CIN3 lesions - HPV16/18	
Cervarix®	1.5	According -to -protocol	100%	N/A	–	–	[33]
	3	According -to -protocol	–	–	98.1%	100%	[34]
	4.5	According -to -protocol	100%	100%	100%	–	[35]
	5.5	According -to -protocol	100%	100%	100%	–	[36]
	7.3	According -to -protocol	100%	100%	100%	–	[37]
	8.4	According -to -protocol	100%	100%	100%	–	[38]
Gardasil®	3	Per protocol susceptible population	–	–	100%	97%	[39]
	3	Per protocol susceptible population	–	–	100%	100%	[40]
	5	Per protocol susceptible population	96.6%	90.6%	100%	100%	[41]

HPV = Human papillomavirus. According to protocol population = women HPV16 or HPV18 DNA negative during the vaccination schedule, that received 3 doses of the vaccine; Per protocol population = participants received 3 doses of vaccine or placebo within 12 months and were seronegative on PCR analysis for HPV6-, HPV-11, HPV-16, or HPV18 at day 1 through 1 month after the third dose.* Persistent infection correspond to infection detected for ≥6 months. N/A: not available.

Table 3. Cervarix® and Gardasil® efficacy

Both vaccines lead to seroconversion of nearly 100% of the immunized subjects. Cervarix® was shown to sustain relatively stable immunity against HPV16/18 for more than eight years [31]. Subjects immunized with Gardasil® were shown to be consistently seropositive for more than four years for HPV11, HPV6 and HPV16 but a decline in antibody titers was recorded for HPV18 (from 100% to approximately 47%) [32]. However, it cannot be excluded that this observed decline is a result of assay insensitivity. Nevertheless, the protection against HPV18 induced lesions did not decrease suggesting that low levels of anti-HPV18 antibodies are sufficient to confer protection. The Table 3 shows the efficacy of Cervarix® and Gardasil® for different clinical trials followed up for different periods of time.

6. Efficacy in clinical trials

Six major clinical trials enrolling around 44.000 females were conducted to evaluate the efficacy of Cervarix® (2 trials) and Gardasil® (4 trials). Most of the trials included subjects from the age of 15 to 26 years (except for Muñoz *et al*, 24-45 years) with a limited lifetime number of sexual partners (≤4-6, except for Muñoz *et al.*, with no restriction). The sole exclusion criteria were pregnancy and abnormal Pap smears [21, 42-46].

Since cervical cancer is an unethical endpoint for the HPV prophylactic vaccines efficacy evaluation, the clinical trials concentrated on prevention of pre-cancerous high-grade cervical intraepithelial neoplasias (CIN 2 and 3). Results from these trials have shown the high efficacy of the prophylactic vaccines in preventing persistent infection and CIN 2/3 lesions and genital warts for Gardasil® and Cervarix®.

6.1. Cervarix®

The double-blind randomized controlled PATRICIA (PApilloma TRIal against Cancer In young Adults) is the largest Cervarix® vaccine trial performed to date and it was conducted in more than 14 countries from Asia-Pacific, Europe, North America and Latin America. It included over 18.000 healthy women between 15 and 25 years of age with no more than six lifetime sexual partners; these women were enrolled irrespective of their HPV DNA status, HPV serostatus or cytology baseline.

Cervical cytologies and biopsies for 14 oncogenic HPV types were assessed by PCR. The primary endpoint for the vaccine efficacy was the development of CIN 2+ associated with HPV16 or HPV18 and as well non-vaccinated oncogenic HPV types (for cross-protection assessment) [34, 47].

Data from three different cohorts (ATP-E: according to protocol cohort for efficacy vaccinated: n=8093; control: n=8069; TVC: total vaccinated cohort = women receiving at least one dose of the Cervarix®: n=9319; control: n=9325; and TVC-naïve = no evidence of oncogenic HPV infection at baseline vaccinated: n=5822; control: n=5819) over a mean of 34.9 months was analyzed. The efficacy of the vaccine against CIN2/3 lesions associated with HPV16/18 was similarly high (around 98% for CIN2+ and 100% for CIN3+) in the ATP-E and TVC- naïve cohorts. For the TVC group the efficacy of the vaccine against CIN3+ lesions, irrespective of HPV DNA in lesions, was 30%.

6.2. Gardasil®

The randomized, double-blind, placebo-controlled trials FUTURE I and FUTURE II included 18.174 women between 16-26 years of age from 24 different countries from Asia-Pacific, North America, Latin America and Europe. The primary endpoints for the Gardasil® efficacy clinical trial were a) incidence of genital warts, vulvar or vaginal intraepithelial neoplasia or cancer and b) the incidence of cervical intraepithelial neoplasia CIN2/3 and adenocarcinoma *in situ* (AIS) lesions [48, 49]

For the FUTURE II study, which enrolled 12,167 women that were followed for an average of 3 years, Gardasil® efficacy for prevention of HPV-16/18 related CIN3 lesions was 97% in the per-protocol cohort (population negative for 14 HPV types and receiving all the three doses of the vaccine), 95% in the unrestricted susceptible population (population receiving one or more vaccination doses) and 45% in the intention-to-treat cohort (population with or without previous HPV infection). HPV16/11/16/18 related high grade vulvar and vaginal lesions could be prevented with 100% efficacy by vaccination with Gardasil® in the per-protocol, with 95% in the unrestricted susceptible, and with 73% in the intention-to-treat populations. Gardasil® efficacy for prevention of adenocarcinoma *in situ* was 100% in the per-protocol susceptible and unrestricted susceptible population and 28% in the intention-to-treat population. However, one subject in the per-protocol susceptible placebo population developed adenocarcinoma *in situ*, affecting the reliability of the vaccine efficacy in this group [50].

6.3. Cervarix® versus Gardasil®

After the data from several clinical trials ensuring safety, tolerability and efficacy of the HPV vaccines was published, discussions began about which vaccine should be implemented in public vaccination programs. To make this decision, the cost-effectiveness of the vaccines, potentially influenced by duration of protection, number of doses required for protection and the extend of cross-protection, needed to be evaluated.

It is a difficult and daunting task to directly compare results from the Cervarix® and Gardasil® clinical trials because of a) differences in the study population and cohorts for testing the vaccine efficacy, b) differences in the HPV typing and immunological assays and c) differences in the studies' endpoints.

For this reason, an observer-blind study was designed to directly compare the immunogenicity and safety of both vaccines [23]. In this study, a total of 1106 women aged 18 to 45 years were enrolled and vaccinated either with Gardasil® or Cervarix®. One month after the third vaccination, sera from all the subjects were collected and the presence of neutralizing anti-bodies was measured by pseudovirions-based neutralization assay (PBNA). The PBNA showed that all women in both vaccine groups were HPV16 and HPV18 seropositive with the exception of two HPV18 seronegative subjects in the Gardasil® group.

The titers of anti-HPV16 and HPV18 neutralizing antibodies from serum and cervicovaginal secretions induced by Cervarix® were significantly higher than those induced by Gardasil® in all the tested age strata. The frequency of antigen-specific (HPV16 and HPV18) and memory B-cells were also higher in the Cervarix® than in the Gardasil® group [23].

6.4. Dose

Although both vaccines were licensed as 3-dose administrations over six months, this regime has been questioned and re-evaluated either for cost-effectiveness or for difficulties with administering all the doses within the stipulated time frame.

Recently a comparative analysis between the Costa Rica Vaccine Trial cohort was published where it was suggested that two and maybe even one dose of Cervarix® might be as effective against persistent HPV16 and HPV18 infections as the three doses [51]. What remains unclear is the duration of protection for the vaccination with fewer doses.

6.5. Cross-protection

One surprising finding of the phase II and phase III clinical trials is that both vaccines induce cross-protection against non-vaccine HPV types.

A recent end-of-study analysis of the Cervarix® PATRICIA clinical trial, performed after 48 months of follow-up, evaluated the cross-protection against non-vaccine HPV types in persistent infection and high grade CIN2+ and CIN3+ lesions. In summary, this analysis reports consistent vaccine efficacy against HPV31, HPV33 and HPV45 for all the end-points [52]

The analysis of combined data from the Gardasil® FUTURE I and FUTURE II clinical trials reveals that vaccination reduced the rate of HPV-31/33/45/52/58 infection, CIN1-3 and AIS. However the reduction of HPV-31/33/45/52/58 related CIN2 lesions was not significant [53]

A meta-analysis study suggests that cross-protection efficacy against persistent HPV infection and CIN2 lesions is higher for Cervarix® than for Gardasil®. While Gardasil® can confer protection against the non-vaccine type HPV31, Cervarix® can efficiently protect against HPV 31, HPV 33 and HPV45. This study evaluated comparable populations in different clinical trials that used different methods to identify efficacy endpoints (e.g. genotyping of HPV to determine HPV persistent infection). The sensitivity of the methods used in clinical trials and population differences can influence the comparison between Cervarix® and Gardasil®[54].

A sub-analysis of an observer-blind study, performed to allow a direct comparison between Cervarix® and Gardasil®, evaluated cross-protection against non-vaccine HPV types for both vaccines. This study confirmed that both vaccines induce cross-reactive responses against HPV31 and HPV45 but that the responses were initially much lower for the Gardasil® vaccinated group. However, after 24 months the level of humoral responses for HPV31/45 was equally low for both vaccines. The only considerable difference between the vaccines shown in this study is the higher levels of T-cell response with the Cervarix® vaccine. Whether or not the T cell response is necessary for cross-protection remains unclear [55].

All the studies show lower levels of non-vaccine HPV antibody titers compared to the type-specific titers. One possibility to be considered is that the cross-protective responses will wane with time. There are on-going efforts in current phase IV surveillance studies addressing the degree and durability of cross-protective responses.

7. Age for HPV vaccination

7.1. Preadolescent girls and young women

Vaccination with Gardasil® or Cervarix® does not lead to clearance of pre-existing HPV infections [56]. Considering the decreasing age of sexual debut in many countries, both vaccines target preadolescent girls and young women. The Advisory Committee on Immunization Practices (ACIP) recommend vaccination of females aged 13 to 26 years for Cervarix® and vaccination of 9 to 26 year old males and females for Gardasil® [57, 58].

Most of the clinical trials performed to evaluate efficacy of the prophylactic vaccines included subjects older than the primary target population. This is explained by a) the need of a population where the HPV infection happens at higher frequency for efficacy proof-of-principle purposes and b) legal and ethical limitations regarding the evaluation of sexual activity in the preadolescent population.

A Cervarix® clinical trial, performed in Denmark, Estonia, Finland, Greece, Netherlands and Russia, with an extension study (4 years follow-up) conducted in Denmark, Estonia and Finland, was designed to evaluate safety and immunogenicity of the bivalent vaccine in two age groups (10-14 and 15-25 years). According to the follow-up study, Cervarix® induced higher systemic and mucosal immune responses, which sustained for more than four years, in the 10-14 years group compared to the 15-25 years group [59].

7.2. Older women

Women can acquire HPV infections at any age. However, epidemiological data report that the highest prevalence of HPV infections occur in sexually active women under 25 years of age and decline with age progression [60].

Recent meta-analysis studies have been showing a second peak of HPV prevalence in women over 44 years [61]. There are several hypotheses explaining this phenomenon but the most plausible one is associated with changes in sexual behavior of women and their partners at this age.

Humoral responses to HPV vaccines are known to decrease gradually with age progression but the antibody levels remain several fold higher for years in vaccinated (46-55 years) than in non-vaccinated subjects who developed natural immunity in response to infection [62]. A recent analysis of the FUTURE I and FUTURE II clinical trials evaluated the efficacy of Gardasil® in HPV DNA positive women who were treated for cervical, vulvar, or vaginal disease. This study showed that vaccination with Gardasil® decreases by more than 40% the incidence of subsequent HPV-related diseases including genital warts and CIN1/2 lesions, irrespective of the HPV type in the lesion [63]. This finding suggests that including women older than 26 years in the vaccination program might prevent HPV persistent infection in naïve women and reduce re-infection for those that were already infected.

7.3. Vaccination of males

HPV infection of males is associated with genital warts, anogenital cancer, oral cancer, and recurrent respiratory papillomatosis. The overall incidence of HPV infection is very similar for men and women, although, in contrast to the situation in women, HPV infection in males does not seem to be age related [64].

Currently, Gardasil® is the only HPV prophylactic vaccine licensed for use in males. Their target population is boys and men aged 9 to 26 years. Its high immunogenicity, safety and efficacy against anogenital warts and perianal/perineal intraephitelial neoplasia in males has been reported in several clinical trial studies [65, 66].

Even though several mathematical models suggest that the inclusion of males in vaccination programs will not be a cost-effective strategy [67], the potential reduction of the health burden associated with HPV infection in males (e.g.: anal cancer and anogenital warts) and the possibility to reduce the risk of HPV transmission to women argue in favor of extending HPV vaccination programs to males.

One of the arguments against the vaccination of males is that immunization of females might already lead to enhanced herd immunity and thereby reduce male lesions as well. One factor not considered with this argument is the scenario of men who have sex with men (MSM) who cannot benefit from female vaccination.

The MSM population is one of the most affected by HPV warts and anal cancer. It is clear that this population will not benefit from female vaccination. Recently, a clinical trial enrolling 602 healthy men who have sex with men (16 to 26 years of age) showed efficacy and safety of Gardasil® against high-grade anal intraepithelial neoplasia (AIN2/3) [68].

Based on data of Gardasil® safety, efficacy against AIN2/3, estimates of disease and cancer resulting from HPV and cost-effectiveness, the Advisory Committee on Immunization Practices (ACIP) recommended routine use of the quadrivalent HPV vaccine in males aged 11 or 12 years [58].

7.4. Vaccination of immunocompromised

Immunocompromised women and men are known to have higher incidences of HPV infection and HPV-related diseases including cervical and anal cancer. However, little is known about the efficacy and safety of the prophylactic vaccine in this population.

Few HPV clinical trials have been studying HIV positive populations. Among those, a clinical trial evaluated Gardasil® safety and immunogenicity in HIV infected children from 7 to 12 years, separated into three different groups according to their CD4+ T cells count. The vaccine was considered highly safe, with no CIN3 lesions being observed in the vaccinated group when compared to the control. Vaccination led to seroconversion of 99% of the immunized subjects; however, antibody titers for HPV16 and HPV18 were much lower (30-50%) than for the historical control (HIV uninfected children – Gardasil® vaccinated) [69], indicating a reduced response in this target population.

As levels of HPV16 and HPV18 antibodies were still comparable to HIV-uninfected women (16-26 years old) in whom the vaccine efficacy was confirmed, long-term studies with more subjects are necessary to determine vaccine efficacy in the HIV infected population.

8. Is there room and need for second generation vaccines?

As outlined above, the two commercial vaccines induce long lasting high titer, protective antibody responses against the HPV types included in the vaccines. The efficacy of preventing vaccine type induced lesions can reach up to 100%. This success is based on the exceptional immunogenicity of HPV virus-like-particles and the current vaccination programs will surely have significant impact on reducing the HPV associated cancer burden in the near future. Still, there are several shortcomings of the commercial vaccines which include costly production, need for invasive administration, low stability requiring intact cold chains in vaccine delivery and a narrow range of protection limited mainly to vaccine type papillomaviruses. Further, studies have shown that vaccination with the commercial vaccines has no impact on the progression of pre-existing lesions, i.e. neither Gardasil® nor Cervarix® seem to have a therapeutic effect [56]. Although basically all vaccines used in routine medicine are of pro-phylactic nature, this was not necessarily expected to be the case for the HPV VLP vaccines. In a number of preclinical studies it was demonstrated that vaccination of mice with VLPs induces strong cytotoxic T-cell responses against the L1 antigen and in case of L1-E7 chimeric particles also against the E7 portion [70-73]. The response had strong anti-tumorigenic properties in different tumor challenge models. Therefore, there was reason to hope for a vaccination benefit for humans already infected with the corresponding HPV type. Unfortu-nately, however, this benefit was not observed in clinical trials to date.

To overcome at least some of the limitations of the commercial vaccines a number of different approaches to develop a second generation PV vaccine are followed, some of which will be addressed in more detail below.

9. Second generation vaccines targeting L1

Both current commercial vaccines show excellent safety and efficacy profiles and there seems to be little room for improvement in either aspect when addressing the HPV type-specific protection. Some countries are considering or are in the process of implementing a two dose regiment, driven by the intention to minimize costs [74, 75]. Such deliberations would benefit from higher immunogenicity of the VLP vaccine, which could possibly be achieved by using stronger adjuvant systems. But naturally, it seems unlikely that Merck or GSK would find a sufficient economical motivation to move along this road. What's more, there is only a limited repertoire of adjuvants that can be used in prophylaxis for a young target population.

Both Merck and GSK are probably not highly motivated in developing second generation HPV vaccines that would compete with their blockbusters. An exception is the nonavalent HPV VLP vaccine that is currently evaluated by Merck in clinical trials. A number of pre-clinical studies focused on the development of L1-based vaccines that overcome one or more of the limitations discussed above. These second generation approaches addressed delivery (e.g. oral), production systems (plant, E. coli), stability (e.g. capsomeres) and extension to thera-peutic applications (chimeric L1 proteins) [76-78]. In light of the fact that the current VLP vaccines are inducing a limited degree of cross-protection, for which the nature is not yet known, one could envision modifying the L1 protein so as to extend the breadth of protection, but to our knowledge, this strategy is currently not pursued.

As indicated above, the protective range of Cervarix® and Gardasil® is mainly limited to the vaccine type papillomaviruses. In their clinical trial GSK could show that immunization with

Cervarix® induces cross-protection against additional types such as HPV 31, 33 and 45 and Gardasil® induces protection against HPV 31, albeit at lower efficacy. As a consequence, in 2010 the European Medicines Agency has approved the amendment of the license of Cervarix® in prevention of HPV 31, 33 and 45 induced lesions. The molecular mechanisms for the enhanced cross-protection of Cervarix® in comparison to Gardasil® is not fully understood. One explanation could be the fact that Cervarix® is inducing higher titers against HPV 16 and HPV 18, possibly due to the stronger adjuvants used in the formulation of Cervarix®. Another explanation could be structural differences of the VLPs contained in the two vaccines.

However, despite this extended cross-protection observed for Cervarix® about 20% of cervical cancer cases remain uncovered by the vaccine. To breach this gap, Merck MSD is currently evaluating a nonavalent HPV VLP vaccine in phase III clinical trials. In addition to the non-oncogenic HPVs 6 and 11, this vaccine includes VLPs of HPV types 16, 18, 31, 33, 45, 52 and 58 and theoretically would reach close to 88% efficacy. It remains to be determined whether this cocktail of nine different VLPs is able to induce prolonged protective responses against the corresponding HPV types or if due to interference this may not be possible. Further, because of increasing vaccine complexity this strategy will be limited due to rising costs in production. Also, it will be difficult to prove vaccine efficacy in preventing cervical dysplasia induced by rather rare HPV types, such as HPV 52 and HPV 58, if neutralizing antibodies or at least prevention of infection by these types are not accepted as surrogate markers by the licensing agencies.

10. Examples for second generation L1-based vaccines

10.1. Genetic vaccination

There are more than 200 different papillomaviruses infecting vertebrates. Among them are roughly 50 types for which there is a theoretical interest of implementing prophylaxis and these include oncogenic HPVs, skin type HPVs relevant in immune compromised patients, bovine PV infecting cattle [79] and horses and PV viruses infecting pets. It has been shown in a number of studies that genetic vaccination with codon-adapted L1 genes leads to the induction of high titer neutralizing antibodies. Vaccination has been performed by intramus-cular needle injection or by the use of a gene gun [80-90]. We observed particularly strong neutralizing antibody responses when administering codon-modified L1 genes using a tattooing device [84, 91]. In addition to delivering the expression constructs to muscle and/or antigen presenting cells, tattooing induces a certain degree of local tissue damage which might serve as a danger signal [92, 93]. The great advantage of immunization with naked DNA is the ease of constructing and producing the vaccine vectors for many different L1 antigens since standardized procedures can be applied. Also, DNA is a very stable molecule making the need for intact cold chains in vaccine distribution obsolete. In addition, it has been shown that cocktails of different L1 expression constructs can be applied to mount a broad range of protection, although some kind of interference between different L1s has been observed [94].

Currently, no clinical testing involving human subjects is being performed with naked DNA or with a genetic vector. For one, DNA immunization has not found its way to human immune prophylaxis to date. The main reason is the much lower efficacy of DNA vaccines in primates compared to the murine system. Further, there are concerns about the safety of DNA vaccines in general. Although these concerns are of theoretical nature only, they still pose a major hurdle for application in routine vaccine prophylaxis.

The ease of targeting multiple L1 antigens has also been a motivation to evaluate viral vector based genetic approaches. Different viral vectors have been used and these include vaccinia virus, vesicular stomatitis virus, and adenoviruses [95-98]. High titer neutralizing antibody responses were induced in vaccinated mice. Additionally, in some of the studies strong cellular immune responses against the L1 antigen could be demonstrated. Using the cottontail rabbit papillomavirus model, it was shown that single intranasal administration of recombinant vaccinia virus [99] or vesicular stomatitis virus (VSV) [96, 97] induces anti-L1 antibodies and protections against CRPV challenge, although the latter could also have been a consequence of the induction of cellular immune responses against L1.

Berg et al. ([98] [100] produced correctly folded canine oral PV VLPs using recombinant adenoviruses. Immunization of mice led to high titer neutralizing antibody responses, but the recombinant adenoviruses have not yet been tested in the COPV challenge model.

When considering administration, the use of complex virus systems including vaccinia virus, VSV and adenoviruses faces significant safety issues. Moreover, most vaccinations will likely be limited to single administration due to the strong responses against the vectors. In this light it might not be possible to generate responses against L1 proteins of multiple PVs.

Adeno-associated virus (AAV) vectors combine the simplicity of naked DNA with the efficacy of viral vector gene delivery. AAV vectors are extremely stable and can be lyophilized without compromising their transduction activity. Also, these viral vectors do not encode for viral gene products. We have used AAV vectors for intranasal and systemic delivery of the L1 gene. Single doses of AAV-L1 induce long lasting (>1 yr) neutralizing antibody responses in mice. The intranasal application also induced mucosal antibodies and cellular immunity. Non-adjuvanted intranasal application in macaques with recombinant AAV9 vectors also induced immunity against the encoded L1 antigen [101-104]. Liu and colleagues reported on the co-administration of AAV-L1 vectors together with a recombinant adenoviruses encoding for granulocyte macrophage colony-stimulating factor [105]. This strategy yielded higher neutralizing titers compared to VLP immunization but might prove difficult in translating into application in humans.

In addition to viral vectors, L1 has also been delivered by live prokaryotic vectors such as Salmonella enterica Typhii [106-109] and recombinant Bacille Calmette-Guerin (rBCG) [110, 111]. Nardelli-Haefliger was the first to demonstrate that live L1-recombinant bacteria (S. typhii) induced mucosal and systemic antibody responses in mice. In another study, Govan et al. showed that rabbits vaccinated with rBCG encoding the CRPV L1 protein are protected against viral challenge [110]. This protection might, however, in part be due to cellular immune responses against the L1 antigen, although the authors could demonstrate *in vitro* neutralization activity of the rabbit sera.

11. Alternative production systems

The current HPV vaccines are produced either in yeast (Gardasil®) or insect cells infected with recombinant baculoviruses (Cervarix®). It is not disclosed by the vaccine manufacturers what the production costs per dose really are, but insect cells present a rather complex platform and yeast cells provide challenges in the extraction procedures. In the early phases of HPV VLP technology, several labs worked on expressing L1 in *E. coli* but only recently has it been possible to produce properly folded L1 in this system. It was Chen et al. who showed in 2001 that N-terminally modified L1 protein of HPV 11 and 16 can be expressed in *E. coli* and purified in the form of native pentamers (capsomers) [112]. Yuan and colleagues reported that two doses of 400 ng of a GST-L1 fusion protein, assembled in capsomere-like structures protected dogs from a challenge with COPV. HPV 16 L1 pentamers share essential conformational epitopes with VLPs [113, 114]. L1 pentamers are less immunogenic compared to VLPs but use of appropriate adjuvant systems (e.g. ASO4) can largely compensate for this [113]. In addition to being produced cost-effectively in *E. coli*, L1 pentamers are also more stable than VLPs making an intact cold-chain in vaccine distribution obsolete. Although clinical trials are in preparation, efficacy of L1 pentamers has not yet been assessed in human subjects. However, Stahl-Hennig could show capsomeres adjuvanted with synthetic double stranded RNA, either poly ICLC or poly IC induced strong anti-L1 antibody and T-helper responses in rhesus macaques [115].

In a number of studies the production of L1 antigens in transgenic plants has been evaluated. Earlier studies showed that the surface antigen of hepatitis B virus can be expressed and assembled in transgenic plants [116]. Importantly, oral delivery of unprocessed plant material induced HBsAg specific immunity in mice and healthy volunteers [117]. This report ignited the idea that vaccine antigens can be produced with the aid of transgenic plant technology. The great advantage of plants is the simplicity by which vast quantities of biomass can be produced with all required technology already in place. Bypassing the requirement for antigen extraction and purification would allow to meet the worlds growing, yet unmet, demand for cheap vaccines. In this light, production of L1 in plants was initiated, [118-128], and immunogenicity after either oral or systemic delivery was confirmed. Yield of L1, which initially posed a major problem, improved significantly to more than 10% of the total soluble protein [125].

Today's consensus on antigen production in plants stresses standardized extraction and purification to ensure antigens with defined properties and limited inter-batch variability will be an essential criteria. Also, much of the L1 antigen in the plant tissue is incorrectly folded and hence has only little immunogenicity. Overall, there are strong resentments by regulatory agencies and vaccine manufacturers on introducing poorly standardize-able oral vaccines originating from partially processed plant material.

In summary, there are tremendous hurdles that novel second generation vaccines based on the L1 antigen must be overcome starting with facing and competing with the two existing commercial vaccines. The main challenge seems to be the need for demonstrating non-inferiority. Licensing of Gardasil® and Cervarix® has been a mammoth task, involving tens of thousands participants in clinical trials. It is very unlikely that such evaluation can be reproduced with a vaccine approach that presents only an incremental improvement in one of the other shortcomings of Gardasil® and Cervarix®. Other equally important issues are safety and simplicity of second generation vaccines, especially in light of the target population's young age. Lastly, intellectual property is an important factor in vaccine development. While the tight patent situation on L1 VLP technology might eventually be less stringent in the coming years, this will also leave novel developments without sufficient protection, making major investments for manufacturers less attractive.

12. L2: Candidate for a potential pan HPV vaccine?

At the time when PV VLP technology started to have its major impact on papillomavirus research and vaccine development, the group of Saveria Campo in Glasgow reported that vaccination of cattle with a bacterially produced minor capsid protein L2 induced protection against challenge with infectious BPV 4 virus [129]. The authors identified epitopes located in a region of L2 encompassing amino acids 131-151 of BPV 4. Although the report describes these epitopes as B-cell epitopes, no neutralization assay could be performed at the time and hence an involvement of cellular immunity could not be ruled out. Also, the antigens that were either GST-L2 fusion proteins or conjugated peptides were of rather poor immunogenicity. As the field was moving towards VLP vaccines that induce very strong protective effects, L2 was not given further thought as a vaccine antigen at the time.

Later, Richard Roden and his colleagues investigated in detail the suitability of L2 as a vaccine antigen. They observed that L2 antigens purified from E. coli induced cross-neutralizing antibodies as assessed by the focus formation assay developed by the investigators [130]. Subsequently, they mapped a cross-neutralizing epitope to a region spanning amino acids 1-88, which was later pin-pointed to amino acids 17-36 [131-133]. Interestingly, human sera from a therapeutic vaccine study using a L2-E6-E7 fusion protein produced in E. coli (TA-CIN; [134]) came back positive for neutralizing activity [132].

The presence of neutralizing and cross-neutralizing epitopes in the N-terminus of L2 was reported and confirmed by others. Kondo and colleagues mapped several regions in the L2 protein between amino acids 1-140 [135]. Some of the neutralizing epitopes were later confirmed by others, however it seems clear today that only one epitope, comprising amino acids 17-36, consistently elicited cross-protection [136-138].

After identifying the target region in the L2 protein, the major challenge in developing L2 as a vaccine antigen was posed by L2's low immunogenicity compared to L1. No or very little neutralizing activity is induced when fragments or peptides of L2 are used as antigens [129, 137]. Further, VLPs composed of L1 and L2 do not induce measurable anti-L2 responses. Because of this, a number of strategies were pursued with the goal of increasing immunogenicity of the L2 cross-neutralizing epitope.

Alphs et al. observed a strong increase in immunogenicity of the 17-36 epitope when conjugating the L2 peptide to a synthetic lipopeptide (TLR2 agonist) and a broadly acting T-helper epitope [139]. This antigen induced rather high neutralizing titers against HPV 16 while responses against other high-risk HPVs including HPV 18 or HPV 45 were 1-2 orders of magnitude lower. Still, this fully synthetic L2 vaccine provided an elegant basis for the development of a L2 vaccine. Jagu et al. reported that a concatenated L2 fusion protein, consisting of the amino acids 11-88 of five different HPV types induced strong neutralization and cross-neutralization and was superior compared to monotypic HPV 16 L2 antigen. This approach is expected to enter a clinical phase in 2013.

Displaying the 17-36 epitope on bacteriophage PP7 capsids was shown to be an attractive alternative approach in generating a functional L2-based vaccine [140, 141]. VLPs of bacteriophage PP7 can be produced in large quantities and are tolerant for the insertion of heterologous peptides. Immunization of mice leads to high titers of ELISA reactive L2-specific antibodies. Cross-protective neutralization of HPV pseudovirions was shown in an *in vivo* challenge model. The authors did not titrate the sera in an *in vitro* neutralization assay and thus it is not clear how robust the anti-L2 responses were.

A 'natural' scaffold for the presentation of L2 epitopes would be to insert the cross-neutralizing epitope into L1 loops located on the VLP surface. This would provide for a highly repetitive presentation of the L2 region. Schellenbacher et al. pursued this approach and tested various peptide insertions into the BPV1 and HPV 16 L1 protein [142]. Such insertions often interfere with proper assembly of the L1 into higher ordered structures but the authors were able to produce and purify a number of L1-L2 chimeric particles. They demonstrated that the CVLPs still induced L1-specific neutralization, indicating mostly correct conformation of the L1 protein. More importantly, chimeric particles carrying the 17-36 epitope of HPV 16 L2 induced neutralizing antibody responses in rabbits against HPV 5, 11, 16, 18, 45, 52, 58 pseudovirions with titers ranging from 1:100 to 1:10,000.

Recently, we have developed a strategy to boost the immunogenicity of the L2 cross-neutralizing epitope by using bacterial thioredoxin (*Trx*) as a carrier [137]. Due to its rigid structure, this small, 109 amino acid long protein can constrain rather large multi-peptide insertions of heterologous antigens without compromising carrier structure. Previously, presenting an amyloid-ß peptide in context of an *E. coli Trx* scaffold allowed induction of Aß immune responses in a mouse model for Alzheimer [143]. When we inserted the HPV 16 L2 cross-neutralizing epitope (aa 20-38 corresponding to 17-36 described by Roden et al.) we achieved a boost in immunogenicity by several orders of magnitude, compared to the peptide linked to keyhole limpet hemocyanin. Further, multimerization of the L2 epitope in the *Trx* led to further increase in induction of neutralizing antibodies. While we also confirmed the existence of other regions in the L2 N-terminus as targets for neutralizing antibodies, we only found cross-neutralization for the 20-38 epitope [136]. We also found that a subset of antibodies reactive against the different L2 epitopes fail to neutralize HPV pseudovirions *in vitro* and this might be due to steric hindrance of L2 epitope recognition in the context of virus capsids.

Ultimately, there is convincing evidence that the L2 protein of HPV contains a number of neutralizing epitopes and importantly one major cross-neutralizing epitope. It is also clear that due to the low immunogenicity of L2 an appropriate scaffold and/or adjuvant system is required. Still, there are several issues to be addressed. First, no systematic comparison of the different strategies of L2 epitope presentation has been carried out. No consensus has been reached as to which parameters for L2 vaccination would be an indicator for vaccine efficacy or would present a correlate for protection *in vivo*. Currently, there are a number of different assays to determine L2-directed humoral immune responses. Although anti-L2 antibodies can be readily measured by ELISA assays, this does not provide a meaningful result, as many antibodies recognizing the neutralizing epitopes seem to be non-functional. Typically, ELISA titers are orders of magnitude higher compared to titers obtained in functional neutralization assays.

13. Approaches to measure induction of neutralizing antibodies

A nowadays routine assay is the pseudovirion-based neutralization (PBNA) assay developed by Buck et al. that measures transduction efficiency of PV capsids encapsidating a reporter gene. In the presence of L1 or L2 neutralizing antibodies or compounds that interfere with virus infection such as carrageenan (see below), transduction of cells is inhibited. This assay is considered the gold-standard for *in vitro* assays and (theoretically) measures any antibody that prevents binding, uptake, uncoating and trafficking of viruses. Although the PBNA has been routinely used for the detection of L2-directed neutralization, recently, Day et al. described a modified *in vitro* neutralization assay with increased sensitivity for L2- (and L1-) specific neutralizing antibodies [144]. In this assay, the virus is treated with exogenous furin convertase after inducing a conformational change. Furin has been shown to be essential for PV infection and the L2 proteins have a conserved cleavage site at their N-terminus. Cleavage of L2 is a prerequisite for the binding of antibodies to the major cross-neutralizing epitope 17-36. Typically, the L2-specific titers in the L2-PBNA are at 10-100 fold higher compared to the standard PBNA.

As described above, early vaccination experiments have been carried out in rabbits and cows, followed by challenge with the corresponding virus, CRPV or BPV. Readout was induction of papillomas. The CPRV model was extended for the use of HPV by 'pseudotyping', i.e. encapsidating CRPV genomes into HPV 16 capsids. By this, rabbits can serve as an *in vivo* model for testing HPV vaccine antigens. Protection against oral papillomas in dogs infected with the canine oral papillomavirus was an essential milestone to demonstrate that VLPs can induce sterilizing immunity against PV infection. Also, by passive transfer it could be shown that antibodies are sufficient for protection.

However, despite the highly valuable contribution of BPV, CRPV, and COPV models, only a few laboratories around the world had the available means and resources to establish them for routine use.

The laboratory of John Schiller developed a mouse model for PV infection that can find widespread routine application more easily [13]. In this model, the genital mucosa is infected with pseudovirions encapsidating a luciferase reporter gene. Infection can be quantified by *in vivo* imaging. For efficient infection, microtraumata are induced into the mucosal epithelium, either mechanically or chemically. Vaccine antigens can be analyzed directly, i.e. by immunizing the mice before performing the challenge or indirectly by a passive transfer of antibodies from immunized animals or even humans. This model has later been translated to macaques. In one interesting study it was demonstrated that cytology specimen collection carried out in the macaques, as performed in routine pap screening in women, increases the likelihood of infection by papillomaviruses [145], which, in return, can be prevented by the use of carrageenan in the lubricant which is used in the pelvic exam.

Interestingly and similar to the L2-PBNA, the *in vivo* challenge model shows increased sensitivity compared to the standard PBNA. In fact, we have learned from these assays that extremely low amounts of L2-specific antibodies, which were not detected by the standard PBNA, are sufficient for protection *in vivo* in mice. It is not clear, whether this is due to the same mechanisms, e.g. better access of the L2 neutralizing epitopes. Further, it should be noted that it is not certain whether the increased sensitive of the L2-PBNA or the *in vivo* challenge model correlate with protection *in vivo* in humans.

The existing animal models are unlikely to make functional *in vitro* assays obsolete. First, they are not suited for analyzing large sets of samples and also, it is difficult to produce quantitative estimates of protection as they allow only very limited titration of sera.

14. Alternative strategies for HPV prevention

Concerns about the limitation of the HPV vaccines (e.g.: type specificity and costs) stimulate constant research on alternative strategies for HPV prevention.

Condoms, spermicides, microbicides, circumcision and contraceptives are included in the extensive list of preventive measures that have been shown to curb HPV infection and persistence.

Condoms are known to be protective against many sexual transmitted diseases such as HIV, gonorrhea, chlamydia and tricomoniasis. However, a cross- sectional analysis conducted in men (18-70 years old) from Brazil, Mexico and United States, showed that HPV infection can be reduced but not completely prevented by the use of condoms. Several factors can be attributed to the low efficacy of condoms in preventing HPV infection, including inappropriate usage leading to condom breakage and slippage and the fact that condoms cannot cover all the HPV infected genital areas [146].

Circumcision has been reported to play a role in preventing sexual transmission of HIV, herpes simplex and HPV [147-149]. A recent trial reported that circumcised males have a reduced prevalence of oncogenic HPV types by 32% to 35% and that this effect might be transferred to the partners of circumcised men [150]. Even though the positive effect of the circumcision against HPV persistence has been confirmed by several studies [151-153], ethical issues and complications make circumcision a procedure that most likely will not be routinely adopted.

Different microbicides have been studied for their properties to protect against sexual transmitted infections (STIs). Among those, the spermicide the nonoxynol-9 (N-9) was the most promising. This spermicide, largely available in the market during the 90s, has shown to be protective *in vitro* against several STDs as gonorrhea, candidiasis, herpes simplex and HIV [154-157] However, clinical trials showed that *in vivo* N-9 was not protective against HIV and HPV and could even promote higher infection ratio due to inflammatory and toxicity effects [13, 158].

Carrageenan is a sulfated polysaccharide compound routinely used as thickening ingredient in food products as well as in sexual lubricants and therefore has an excellent safety record. It is derived from seaweed and studies have shown that it confers protection against HIV and HPV *in vitro* [159, 160]. In a phase III clinical trial, carrageenan did not show any effect against HIV but it was tolerable and safe [161]. However, carrageenan was shown to confer HPV protection in a murine animal challenge model [162] and to minimize the increased susceptibility to HPV infection during or after cytology screening in rhesus monkeys [163].

Recently, a dendrimeric gel microbicide (VivaGel – SPL7013) was developed by Starpharma for prevention of infections by HIV and HSV-2. The efficacy and safety of the gel have been demonstrated *in vitro* and in *in vivo* in animal models [164]. Several clinical trials to evaluate the gel safety, tolerance and efficacy are ongoing. In 2008 Starpharma announced that their product can inhibit HPV infection in *in vitro* assays [165].

Acknowledgements

We would like to acknowledge Frank Burkart for designing figures.

Author details

Lis Ribeiro-Müller, Hanna Seitz and Martin Müller

German Cancer Research Center (DKFZ), Program Infections and Cancer, Heidelberg, Germany

References

[1] Rigoni S. Fatti statisici relativi alle malatie cancerose. G Serve Prog Pathol Terap. 1842;2:507-17.

[2] Gissmann L, Wolnik L, Ikenberg H, Koldovsky U, Schnurch HG, zur Hausen H. Human papillomavirus types 6 and 11 DNA sequences in genital and laryngeal papillomas and in some cervical cancers. Proceedings of the National Academy of Sciences of the United States of America. 1983 Jan;80(2):560-3.

[3] de Villiers EM, Gissmann L, zur Hausen H. Molecular cloning of viral DNA from human genital warts. Journal of virology. 1981 Dec;40(3):932-5.

[4] Dürst M, Gissmann L, Ikenberg H, zur Hausen H. A papillomavirus DNA from a cervical carcinoma and its prevalence in cancer biopsy samples from different geographic regions. Proceedings of the National Academy of Sciences of the United States of America. 1983 Jun;80(12):3812-5.

[5] Grigg WK, Wilhelm G. Epidemiological study of planter warts among school children. Public health reports. 1953 Oct;68(10):985-8.

[6] Biberstein. Immunization therapy of warts. Arch Dermatol Syphilol. 1943;50:12-22.

[7] Nicholls PK, Stanley MA. The immunology of animal papillomaviruses. Veterinary immunology and immunopathology. 2000 Feb 25;73(2):101-27.

[8] Chambers VC, Evans CA, Weiser RS. Canine oral papillomatosis. II. Immunologic aspects of the disease. Cancer research. 1960 Aug;20:1083-93.

[9] Roden RB, Greenstone HL, Kirnbauer R, Booy FP, Jessie J, Lowy DR, Schiller JT. In vitro generation and type-specific neutralization of a human papillomavirus type 16 virion pseudotype. Journal of virology. 1996 Sep;70(9):5875-83.

[10] Roden RB, Hubbert NL, Kirnbauer R, Breitburd F, Lowy DR, Schiller JT. Papillomavirus L1 capsids agglutinate mouse erythrocytes through a proteinaceous receptor. Journal of virology. 1995 Aug;69(8):5147-51.

[11] Howett MK, Kreider JW, Cockley KD. Human xenografts. A model system for human papillomavirus infection. Intervirology. 1990;31(2-4):109-15.

[12] Buck CB, Pastrana DV, Lowy DR, Schiller JT. Efficient intracellular assembly of papillomaviral vectors. Journal of virology. 2004 Jan;78(2):751-7.

[13] Roberts JN, Buck CB, Thompson CD, Kines R, Bernardo M, Choyke PL, Lowy DR, Schiller JT. Genital transmission of HPV in a mouse model is potentiated by nonoxynol-9 and inhibited by carrageenan. Nature medicine. 2007 Jul;13(7):857-61.

[14] Day PM, Kines RC, Thompson CD, Jagu S, Roden RB, Lowy DR, Schiller JT. In vivo mechanisms of vaccine-induced protection against HPV infection. Cell host & microbe. 2010 Sep 16;8(3):260-70.

[15] Inglis S, Shaw A, Koenig S. Chapter 11: HPV vaccines: commercial research & development. Vaccine. 2006 Aug 31;24 Suppl 3:S3/99-105.

[16] Schiller JT, Castellsague X, Villa LL, Hildesheim A. An update of prophylactic human papillomavirus L1 virus-like particle vaccine clinical trial results. Vaccine. 2008 Aug 19;26 Suppl 10:K53-61.

[17] Keam SJ, Harper DM. Human papillomavirus types 16 and 18 vaccine (recombinant, AS04 adjuvanted, adsorbed) [Cervarix]. Drugs. 2008;68(3):359-72.

[18] Siddiqui MA, Perry CM. Human papillomavirus quadrivalent (types 6, 11, 16, 18) recombinant vaccine (Gardasil). Drugs. 2006;66(9):1263-71; discussion 72-3.

[19] GlaxoSmithKline Inc. Product Monograph : CERVARIX® Human Papillomavirus vaccine Types 16 and 18 (Recombinant, AS04 adjuvanted). 2012; Available from: http://www.gsk.ca/english/docs-pdf/product-monographs/Cervarix.pdf.

[20] MERCK Canada Inc. Product monograph: GARDASIL® [Quadrivalent Human Papillomavirus (Types 6, 11, 16, 18) Recombinant Vaccine]. 2011 [cited 2012 October]; Available from: http://www.merck.ca/assets/en/pdf/products/GARDASIL-PM_E.pdf.

[21] Munoz N, Manalastas R, Jr., Pitisuttithum P, Tresukosol D, Monsonego J, Ault K, Clavel C, Luna J, Myers E, Hood S, Bautista O, Bryan J, Taddeo FJ, Esser MT, Vuocolo S, Haupt RM, Barr E, Saah A. Safety, immunogenicity, and efficacy of quadrivalent human papillomavirus (types 6, 11, 16, 18) recombinant vaccine in women aged 24-45 years: a randomised, double-blind trial. Lancet. 2009 Jun 6;373(9679):1949-57.

[22] Descamps D, Hardt K, Spiessens B, Izurieta P, Verstraeten T, Breuer T, Dubin G. Safety of human papillomavirus (HPV)-16/18 AS04-adjuvanted vaccine for cervical cancer prevention: a pooled analysis of 11 clinical trials. Hum Vaccin. 2009 May;5(5): 332-40.

[23] Einstein MH, Baron M, Levin MJ, Chatterjee A, Edwards RP, Zepp F, Carletti I, Dessy FJ, Trofa AF, Schuind A, Dubin G. Comparison of the immunogenicity and safety of Cervarix and Gardasil human papillomavirus (HPV) cervical cancer vaccines in healthy women aged 18-45 years. Human vaccines. 2009 Oct;5(10):705-19.

[24] Omer SB. Safety of quadrivalent human papillomavirus vaccine. J Intern Med. 2012 Feb;271(2):177-8.

[25] Wacholder S, Chen BE, Wilcox A, Macones G, Gonzalez P, Befano B, Hildesheim A, Rodriguez AC, Solomon D, Herrero R, Schiffman M. Risk of miscarriage with bivalent vaccine against human papillomavirus (HPV) types 16 and 18: pooled analysis of two randomised controlled trials. BMJ. 2010;340:c712.

[26] Forinash AB, Yancey AM, Pitlick JM, Myles TD. Safety of the HPV Bivalent and Quadrivalent Vaccines During Pregnancy (February). Ann Pharmacother. 2011 Feb 1.

[27] Lehtinen M, Nieminen P, Apter D, Namujju P, Natunen K, Rana M, Paavonen J. Immunogenicity, Efficacy, Effectiveness and Overall Impact of HPV Vaccines. In: Ridder FBaM, editor. HPV and Cervical Cancer: ; 2012. p. 257-72.

[28] Mariani L, Venuti A. HPV vaccine: an overview of immune response, clinical protection, and new approaches for the future. J Transl Med. 2010;8:105.

[29] Breitburd F, Kirnbauer R, Hubbert NL, Nonnenmacher B, Trindinhdesmarquet C, Orth G, Schiller JT, Lowy DR. Immunization with Virus-Like Particles from Cottontail Rabbit Papillomavirus (Crpv) Can Protect against Experimental Crpv Infection. Journal of Virology. 1995 Jun;69(6):3959-63.

[30] Ghim S, Newsome J, Bell J, Sundberg JP, Schlegel R, Jenson AB. Spontaneously re-gressing oral papillomas induce systemic antibodies that neutralize canine oral papil-lomavirus. Exp Mol Pathol. 2000 Jun;68(3):147-51.

[31] Rotelli-Martins CM, Naud P, De Borba P, Teixeira JC, De Carvalho NS, Zahaf T, San-chez N, Geeraerts B, Descamps D. Sustained immunogenicity and efficacy of the HPV-16/18 AS04-adjuvanted vaccine. Human vaccines & Immunotherapeutics. 2012;8(3).

[32] Castellsague X, Munoz N, Pitisuttithum P, Ferris D, Monsonego J, Ault K, Luna J, Myers E, Mallary S, Bautista OM, Bryan J, Vuocolo S, Haupt RM, Saah A. End-of-study safety, immunogenicity, and efficacy of quadrivalent HPV (types 6, 11, 16, 18) recombinant vaccine in adult women 24-45 years of age. Br J Cancer. 2011 Jun 28;105(1):28-37.

[33] Harper DM, Franco EL, Wheeler C, Ferris DG, Jenkins D, Schuind A, Zahaf T, Innis B, Naud P, De Carvalho NS, Roteli-Martins CM, Teixeira J, Blatter MM, Korn AP, Quint W, Dubin G. Efficacy of a bivalent L1 virus-like particle vaccine in prevention of infection with human papillomavirus types 16 and 18 in young women: a rando-mised controlled trial. Lancet. 2004 Nov 13-19;364(9447):1757-65.

[34] Paavonen J, Naud P, Salmeron J, Wheeler CM, Chow SN, Apter D, Kitchener H, Cas-tellsague X, Teixeira JC, Skinner SR, Hedrick J, Jaisamrarn U, Limson G, Garland S, Szarewski A, Romanowski B, Aoki FY, Schwarz TF, Poppe WA, Bosch FX, Jenkins D, Hardt K, Zahaf T, Descamps D, Struyf F, Lehtinen M, Dubin G. Efficacy of human papillomavirus (HPV)-16/18 AS04-adjuvanted vaccine against cervical infection and precancer caused by oncogenic HPV types (PATRICIA): final analysis of a double-blind, randomised study in young women. Lancet. 2009 Jul 25;374(9686):301-14.

[35] Harper DM, Franco EL, Wheeler CM, Moscicki AB, Romanowski B, Roteli-Martins CM, Jenkins D, Schuind A, Costa Clemens SA, Dubin G. Sustained efficacy up to 4.5 years of a bivalent L1 virus-like particle vaccine against human papillomavirus types 16 and 18: follow-up from a randomised control trial. Lancet. 2006 Apr 15;367(9518): 1247-55.

[36] Harper DM. Impact of vaccination with Cervarix (trade mark) on subsequent HPV-16/18 infection and cervical disease in women 15-25 years of age. Gynecol On-col. 2008 Sep;110(3 Suppl 1):S11-7.

[37] De Carvalho N, Teixeira J, Roteli-Martins CM, Naud P, De Borba P, Zahaf T, Sanchez N, Schuind A. Sustained efficacy and immunogenicity of the HPV-16/18 AS04-adju-vanted vaccine up to 7.3 years in young adult women. Vaccine. 2010 Aug 31;28(38): 6247-55.

[38] Roteli-Martins CM, Naud P, De Borba P, Teixeira JC, De Carvalho NS, Zahaf T, San-chez N, Geeraerts B, Descamps D. Sustained immunogenicity and efficacy of the

HPV-16/18 AS04-adjuvanted vaccine: up to 8.4 years of follow-up. Hum Vaccin Immunother. 2012 Mar;8(3):390-7.

[39] Quadrivalent vaccine against human papillomavirus to prevent high-grade cervical lesions. N Engl J Med. 2007 May 10;356(19):1915-27.

[40] Garland SM, Hernandez-Avila M, Wheeler CM, Perez G, Harper DM, Leodolter S, Tang GW, Ferris DG, Steben M, Bryan J, Taddeo FJ, Railkar R, Esser MT, Sings HL, Nelson M, Boslego J, Sattler C, Barr E, Koutsky LA. Quadrivalent vaccine against human papillomavirus to prevent anogenital diseases. N Engl J Med. 2007 May 10;356(19):1928-43.

[41] Villa LL, Costa RL, Petta CA, Andrade RP, Paavonen J, Iversen OE, Olsson SE, Hoye J, Steinwall M, Riis-Johannessen G, Andersson-Ellstrom A, Elfgren K, Krogh G, Lehtinen M, Malm C, Tamms GM, Giacoletti K, Lupinacci L, Railkar R, Taddeo FJ, Bryan J, Esser MT, Sings HL, Saah AJ, Barr E. High sustained efficacy of a prophylactic quadrivalent human papillomavirus types 6/11/16/18 L1 virus-like particle vaccine through 5 years of follow-up. Br J Cancer. 2006 Dec 4;95(11):1459-66.

[42] Harper DM, Franco EL, Wheeler C, Ferris DG, Jenkins D, Schuind A, Zahaf T, Innis B, Naud P, De Carvalho NS, Roteli-Martins CM, Teixeira J, Blatter MM, Korn AP, Quint W, Dubin G. Efficacy of a bivalent L1 virus-like particle vaccine in prevention of infection with human papillomavirus types 16 and 18 in young women: a randomised controlled trial. The Lancet. 2004;364(9447):1757-65.

[43] Villa LL, Costa RLR, Petta CA, Andrade RP, Ault KA, Giuliano AR, Wheeler CM, Koutsky LA, Malm C, Lehtinen M, Skjeldestad FE, Olsson S-E, Steinwall M, Brown DR, Kurman RJ, Ronnett BM, Stoler MH, Ferenczy A, Harper DM, Tamms GM, Yu J, Lupinacci L, Railkar R, Taddeo FJ, Jansen KU, Esser MT, Sings HL, Saah AJ, Barr E. Prophylactic quadrivalent human papillomavirus (types 6, 11, 16, and 18) L1 virus-like particle vaccine in young women: a randomised double-blind placebo-controlled multicentre phase II efficacy trial. The Lancet Oncology. 2005;6(5):271-8.

[44] Garland SM, Hernandez-Avila M, Wheeler CM, Perez G, Harper DM, Leodolter S, Tang GWK, Ferris DG, Steben M, Bryan J, Taddeo FJ, Railkar R, Esser MT, Sings HL, Nelson M, Boslego J, Sattler C, Barr E, Koutsky LA. Quadrivalent vaccine against human papillomavirus to prevent anogenital diseases. New England Journal of Medicine. 2007 May 10;356(19):1928-43.

[45] Villa LL, Perez G, Kjaer SK, Paavonen J, Lehtinen M, Munoz N, Sigurdsson K, Hernandez-Avila M, Skjeldestad FE, Thoresen S, Garcia P, Majewski S, Dillner J, Olsson SE, Tay EH, Bosch FX, Ault KA, et al.. Quadrivalent vaccine against human papillomavirus to prevent high-grade cervical lesions. New England Journal of Medicine. 2007 May 10;356(19):1915-27.

[46] Paavonen J, Jenkins D, Bosch FX, Naud P, Salmeron J, Wheeler CM, Chow SN, Apter DL, Kitchener HC, Castellsague X, de Carvalho NS, Skinner SR, Harper DM, Hedrick JA, Jaisamrarn U, Limson GAM, Dionne M, Quint W, Spiessens B, Peeters P, Struyf F,

Wieting SL, Lehtinen MO, Dubin G. Efficacy of a prophylactic adjuvanted bivalent L1 virus-like-particle vaccine against infection with human papillomavirus types 16 and 18 in young women: an interim analysis of a phase III double-blind, randomised controlled trial. Lancet. 2007 Jun 30;369(9580):2161-70.

[47] Paavonen J, Jenkins D, Bosch FX, Naud P, Salmeron J, Wheeler CM, Chow SN, Apter DL, Kitchener HC, Castellsague X, de Carvalho NS, Skinner SR, Harper DM, Hedrick JA, Jaisamrarn U, Limson GA, Dionne M, Quint W, Spiessens B, Peeters P, Struyf F, Wieting SL, Lehtinen MO, Dubin G. Efficacy of a prophylactic adjuvanted bivalent L1 virus-like-particle vaccine against infection with human papillomavirus types 16 and 18 in young women: an interim analysis of a phase III double-blind, randomised controlled trial. Lancet. 2007 Jun 30;369(9580):2161-70.

[48] Villa LL, Costa RLR, Petta CA, Andrade RP, Paavonen J, Iversen OE, Olsson SE, Hoye J, Steinwall M, Riis-Johannessen G, Andersson-Ellstrom A, Elfgren K, von Krogh G, Lehtinen M, Malm C, Tamms GM, Giacoletti K, Lupinacci L, Railkar R, Taddeo FJ, Bryan J, Esser MT, Sings HL, Saah AJ, Barr E. High sustained efficacy of a prophylactic quadrivalent human papillomavirus types 6/11/16/18 L1 virus-like particle vaccine through 5 years of follow-up. British Journal of Cancer. 2006 Dec 4;95(11):1459-66.

[49] Dillner J, Kjaer SK, Wheeler CM, Sigurdsson K, Iversen OE, Hernandez-Avila M, Perez G, Brown DR, Koutsky LA, Tay EH, Garcia P, Ault KA, Garland SM, Leodolter S, Olsson SE, Tang GWK, Ferris DG, Paavonen J, Lehtinen M, Steben M, Bosch FX, Joura EA, Majewski S, Munoz N, Myers ER, Villa LL, Taddeo FJ, Roberts C, Tadesse A, Bryan JT, Maansson R, Lu SA, Vuocolo S, Hesley TM, Barr E, Haupt R, Grp FIIS. Four year efficacy of prophylactic human papillomavirus quadrivalent vaccine against low grade cervical, vulvar, and vaginal intraepithelial neoplasia and anogenital warts: randomised controlled trial. British Medical Journal. 2010 Jul 20;341.

[50] FUTUREII. Quadrivalent vaccine against human papillomavirus to prevent high-grade cervical lesions. N Engl J Med. 2007 May 10;356(19):1915-27.

[51] Kreimer AR, González P, Katki HA, Porras C, Schiffman M, Rodriguez AC, Solomon D, Jiménez S, Schiller JT, Lowy DR, van Doorn L-J, Struijk L, Quint W, Chen S, Wacholder S, Hildesheim A, Herrero R. Efficacy of a bivalent HPV 16/18 vaccine against anal HPV 16/18 infection among young women: a nested analysis within the Costa Rica Vaccine Trial. The Lancet Oncology. 2011;12(9):862-70.

[52] Wheeler CM, Castellsague X, Garland SM, Szarewski A, Paavonen J, Naud P, Salmeron J, Chow SN, Apter D, Kitchener H, Teixeira JC, Skinner SR, Jaisamrarn U, Limson G, Romanowski B, Aoki FY, Schwarz TF, Poppe WA, Bosch FX, Harper DM, Huh W, Hardt K, Zahaf T, Descamps D, Struyf F, Dubin G, Lehtinen M, Group HPS. Cross-protective efficacy of HPV-16/18 AS04-adjuvanted vaccine against cervical infection and precancer caused by non-vaccine oncogenic HPV types: 4-year end-of-study

analysis of the randomised, double-blind PATRICIA trial. Lancet Oncol. 2012 Jan; 13(1):100-10.

[53] Paavonen J. Efficacy of human papillomavirus (HPV)-16/18AS04-adjuvanted vaccine against cervical infection and precancer caused by oncogenic HPV types (PATRI-CIA): final analysis of a double-blind, randomised study in young women (vol 374, pg 301, 2009). Lancet. 2010 Sep-Oct;376(9746):1054-.

[54] Malagón T, Drolet M, Boily M-C, Franco EL, Jit M, Brisson J, Brisson M. Cross-protective efficacy of two human papillomavirus vaccines: a systematic review and meta-analysis. The Lancet Infectious Diseases. 2012.

[55] Einstein MH, Baron M, Levin MJ, Chatterjee A, Fox B, Scholar S, Rosen J, Chakhtoura N, Lebacq M, van der Most R, Moris P, Giannini SL, Schuind A, Datta SK, Descamps D, Group HPVS. Comparison of the immunogenicity of the human papillomavirus (HPV)-16/18 vaccine and the HPV-6/11/16/18 vaccine for oncogenic non-vaccine types HPV-31 and HPV-45 in healthy women aged 18-45 years. Hum Vaccin. 2011 Dec;7(12):1359-73.

[56] Hildesheim A, Herrero R. Human papillomavirus vaccine should be given before sexual debut for maximum benefit. The Journal of infectious diseases. 2007 Nov 15;196(10):1431-2.

[57] CDC. Quadrivalent Human Papillomavirus Vaccine. 2007 [cited 2012 October]; Available from: http://www.cdc.gov/mmwr/preview/mmwrhtml/mm5920a4.htm.

[58] CDC. FDA Licensure of Quadrivalent Human Papillomavirus Vaccine (HPV4, Gardasil) for Use in Males and Guidance from the Advisory Committee on Immunization Practices (ACIP). 2010 [cited 2012 October]; Available from: http://www.cdc.gov/mmwr/preview/mmwrhtml/mm5920a5.htm.

[59] Petaja T, Pedersen C, Poder A, Strauss G, Catteau G, Thomas F, Lehtinen M, Descamps D. Long-term persistence of systemic and mucosal immune response to HPV-16/18 AS04-adjuvanted vaccine in preteen/adolescent girls and young women. Int J Cancer. 2011 Nov 1;129(9):2147-57.

[60] Woodman CB, Collins SI, Young LS. The natural history of cervical HPV infection: unresolved issues. Nat Rev Cancer. 2007 Jan;7(1):11-22.

[61] de Sanjosé S, Diaz M, Castellsagué X, Clifford G, Bruni L, Muñoz N, Bosch FX. Worldwide prevalence and genotype distribution of cervical human papillomavirus DNA in women with normal cytology: a meta-analysis. The Lancet Infectious Diseases. 2007;7(7):453-9.

[62] Schwarz TF, Spaczynski M, Schneider A, Wysocki J, Galaj A, Schulze K, Poncelet SM, Catteau G, Thomas F, Descamps D. Persistence of immune response to HPV-16/18 AS04-adjuvanted cervical cancer vaccine in women aged 15-55 years. Hum Vaccin. 2011 Sep;7(9):958-65.

[63] Joura EA, Garland SM, Paavonen J, Ferris DG, Perez G, Ault KA, Huh WK, Sings HL, James MK, Haupt RM. Effect of the human papillomavirus (HPV) quadrivalent vaccine in a subgroup of women with cervical and vulvar disease: retrospective pooled analysis of trial data. Bmj. 2012;344(mar27 3):e1401-e.

[64] Giuliano AR, Lu B, Nielson CM, Flores R, Papenfuss MR, Lee JH, Abrahamsen M, Harris RB. Age-specific prevalence, incidence, and duration of human papillomavirus infections in a cohort of 290 US men. J Infect Dis. 2008 Sep 15;198(6):827-35.

[65] Garnock-Jones KP, Giuliano AR. Quadrivalent human papillomavirus (HPV) types 6, 11, 16, 18 vaccine: for the prevention of genital warts in males. Drugs. 2011 Mar 26;71(5):591-602.

[66] Hillman RJ, Giuliano AR, Palefsky JM, Goldstone S, Moreira ED, Jr., Vardas E, Aranda C, Jessen H, Ferris DG, Coutlee F, Marshall JB, Vuocolo S, Haupt RM, Guris D, Garner EI. Immunogenicity of the quadrivalent human papillomavirus (type 6/11/16/18) vaccine in males 16 to 26 years old. Clin Vaccine Immunol. 2012 Feb;19(2): 261-7.

[67] Kim JJ, Goldie SJ. Cost effectiveness analysis of including boys in a human papillomavirus vaccination programme in the United States. Bmj. 2009;339(oct08 2):b3884-b.

[68] Palefsky JM, Giuliano AR, Goldstone S, Moreira ED, Aranda C, Jessen H, Hillman R, Ferris D, Coutlee F, Stoler MH, Marshall JB, Radley D, Vuocolo S, Haupt RM, Guris D, Garner EIO. HPV Vaccine against Anal HPV Infection and Anal Intraepithelial Neoplasia. New Engl J Med. 2011 Oct 27;365(17):1576-85.

[69] Levin MJ, Moscicki AB, Song LY, Fenton T, Meyer WA, 3rd, Read JS, Handelsman EL, Nowak B, Sattler CA, Saah A, Radley DR, Esser MT, Weinberg A, Team IPP. Safety and immunogenicity of a quadrivalent human papillomavirus (types 6, 11, 16, and 18) vaccine in HIV-infected children 7 to 12 years old. J Acquir Immune Defic Syndr. 2010 Oct;55(2):197-204.

[70] Jochmus I, Schäfer K, Faath S, Müller M, Gissmann L. Chimeric virus-like particles of the human papillomavirus type 16 (HPV 16) as a prophylactic and therapeutic vaccine. Archives of medical research. 1999 Jul-Aug;30(4):269-74.

[71] Schäfer K, Müller M, Faath S, Henn A, Osen W, Zentgraf H, Benner A, Gissmann L, Jochmus I. Immune response to human papillomavirus 16 L1E7 chimeric virus-like particles: induction of cytotoxic T cells and specific tumor protection. International journal of cancer Journal international du cancer. 1999 Jun 11;81(6):881-8.

[72] Nieland JD, Da Silva DM, Velders MP, de Visser KE, Schiller JT, Müller M, Kast WM. Chimeric papillomavirus virus-like particles induce a murine self-antigen-specific protective and therapeutic antitumor immune response. Journal of cellular biochemistry. 1999 May 1;73(2):145-52.

[73] Rudolf MP, Nieland JD, DaSilva DM, Velders MP, Müller M, Greenstone HL, Schiller JT, Kast WM. Induction of HPV16 capsid protein-specific human T cell responses by virus-like particles. Biological chemistry. 1999 Mar;380(3):335-40.

[74] Kreimer AR, Rodriguez AC, Hildesheim A, Herrero R, Porras C, Schiffman M, Gonzalez P, Solomon D, Jimenez S, Schiller JT, Lowy DR, Quint W, Sherman ME, Schussler J, Wacholder S. Proof-of-principle evaluation of the efficacy of fewer than three doses of a bivalent HPV16/18 vaccine. Journal of the National Cancer Institute. 2011 Oct 5;103(19):1444-51.

[75] CDC. Morbidity and Mortality Weekly Report: Progress Toward Implementation of Human Papillomavirus Vaccination - The Americas. http://wwwcdcgov/mmwr/preview/mmwrhtml/mm6040a2htm. 2011;60(40):1382-4.

[76] Müller M, Zhou J, Reed TD, RittMüller C, Burger A, Gabelsberger J, Braspenning J, Gissmann L. Chimeric papillomavirus-like particles. Virology. 1997 Jul 21;234(1): 93-111.

[77] Biemelt S, Sonnewald U, Galmbacher P, Willmitzer L, Müller M. Production of human papillomavirus type 16 virus-like particles in transgenic plants. J Virol. 2003 Sep;77(17):9211-20.

[78] Schädlich L, Senger T, Gerlach B, Mucke N, Klein C, Bravo IG, Müller M, Gissmann L. Analysis of modified human papillomavirus type 16 L1 capsomeres: the ability to assemble into larger particles correlates with higher immunogenicity. J Virol. 2009 Aug;83(15):7690-705.

[79] Schmitt M, Fiedler V, Müller M. Prevalence of BPV genotypes in a German cowshed determined by a novel multiplex BPV genotyping assay. J Virol Methods. 2010 Dec; 170(1-2):67-72.

[80] Cho HJ, Han SE, Im S, Lee Y, Kim YB, Chun T, Oh YK. Maltosylated polyethylenimine-based triple nanocomplexes of human papillomavirus 16L1 protein and DNA as a vaccine co-delivery system. Biomaterials. 2011 Jul;32(20):4621-9.

[81] Gupta SK, Singh A, Srivastava M, Akhoon BA. In silico DNA vaccine designing against human papillomavirus (HPV) causing cervical cancer. Vaccine. 2009 Dec 10;28(1):120-31.

[82] Lee HJ, Park N, Cho HJ, Yoon JK, Van ND, Oh YK, Kim YB. Development of a novel viral DNA vaccine against human papillomavirus: AcHERV-HP16L1. Vaccine. 2010 Feb 10;28(6):1613-9.

[83] Maeda H, Kubo K, Sugita Y, Miyamoto Y, Komatsu S, Takeuchi S, Umebayashi T, Morikawa S, Kawanishi K, Kameyama Y. DNA vaccine against hamster oral papillomavirus-associated oral cancer. J Int Med Res. 2005 Nov-Dec;33(6):647-53.

[84] Pokorna D, Rubio I, Müller M. DNA-vaccination via tattooing induces stronger humoral and cellular immune responses than intramuscular delivery supported by molecular adjuvants. Genet Vaccines Ther. 2008;6:4.

[85] Hu J, Cladel NM, Budgeon LR, Reed CA, Pickel MD, Christensen ND. Protective cell-mediated immunity by DNA vaccination against Papillomavirus L1 capsid protein in the Cottontail Rabbit Papillomavirus model. Viral Immunol. 2006 Summer;19(3): 492-507.

[86] Zheng J, Si L, Song J, Sun X, Yu J, Wang Y. Enhanced immune response to DNA-based HPV16L1 vaccination by costimulatory molecule B7-2. Antiviral Res. 2003 Jun; 59(1):61-5.

[87] Moore RA, Nicholls PK, Santos EB, Gough GW, Stanley MA. Absence of canine oral papillomavirus DNA following prophylactic L1 particle-mediated immunotherapeutic delivery vaccination. J Gen Virol. 2002 Sep;83(Pt 9):2299-301.

[88] Stanley MA, Moore RA, Nicholls PK, Santos EB, Thomsen L, Parry N, Walcott S, Gough G. Intra-epithelial vaccination with COPV L1 DNA by particle-mediated DNA delivery protects against mucosal challenge with infectious COPV in beagle dogs. Vaccine. 2001 Apr 6;19(20-22):2783-92.

[89] Matsumoto K, Kawana K, Yoshikawa H, Taketani Y, Yoshiike K, Kanda T. DNA vaccination of mice with plasmid expressing human papillomavirus 6 major capsid protein L1 elicits type-specific antibodies neutralizing pseudovirions constructed in vitro. J Med Virol. 2000 Feb;60(2):200-4.

[90] Schreckenberger C, Sethupathi P, Kanjanahaluethai A, Müller M, Zhou J, Gissmann L, Qiao L. Induction of an HPV 6bL1-specific mucosal IgA response by DNA immunization. Vaccine. 2000 Sep 15;19(2-3):227-33.

[91] Leder C, Kleinschmidt JA, Wiethe C, Müller M. Enhancement of capsid gene expression: preparing the human papillomavirus type 16 major structural gene L1 for DNA vaccination purposes. J Virol. 2001 Oct;75(19):9201-9.

[92] Bins AD, Jorritsma A, Wolkers MC, Hung CF, Wu TC, Schumacher TN, Haanen JB. A rapid and potent DNA vaccination strategy defined by in vivo monitoring of antigen expression. Nat Med. 2005 Aug;11(8):899-904.

[93] Gopee NV, Cui Y, Olson G, Warbritton AR, Miller BJ, Couch LH, Wamer WG, Howard PC. Response of mouse skin to tattooing: use of SKH-1 mice as a surrogate model for human tattooing. Toxicol Appl Pharmacol. 2005 Dec 1;209(2):145-58.

[94] Gasparic M, Rubio I, Thönes N, Gissmann L, Müller M. Prophylactic DNA immunization against multiple papillomavirus types. Vaccine. 2007 Jun 6;25(23):4540-53.

[95] Lin Z, Yemelyanova AV, Gambhira R, Jagu S, Meyers C, Kirnbauer R, Ronnett BM, Gravitt PE, Roden RB. Expression pattern and subcellular localization of human pap-

illomavirus minor capsid protein L2. The American journal of pathology. 2009 Jan; 174(1):136-43.

[96] Reuter JD, Vivas-Gonzalez BE, Gomez D, Wilson JH, Brandsma JL, Greenstone HL, Rose JK, Roberts A. Intranasal vaccination with a recombinant vesicular stomatitis virus expressing cottontail rabbit papillomavirus L1 protein provides complete protection against papillomavirus-induced disease. Journal of virology. 2002 Sep;76(17): 8900-9.

[97] Roberts A, Reuter JD, Wilson JH, Baldwin S, Rose JK. Complete protection from papillomavirus challenge after a single vaccination with a vesicular stomatitis virus vector expressing high levels of L1 protein. Journal of virology. 2004 Mar;78(6):3196-9.

[98] Berg M, Difatta J, Hoiczyk E, Schlegel R, Ketner G. Viable adenovirus vaccine prototypes: high-level production of a papillomavirus capsid antigen from the major late transcriptional unit. Proc Natl Acad Sci U S A. 2005 Mar 22;102(12):4590-5.

[99] Lin YL, Borenstein LA, Selvakumar R, Ahmed R, Wettstein FO. Effective vaccination against papilloma development by immunization with L1 or L2 structural protein of cottontail rabbit papillomavirus. Virology. 1992 Apr;187(2):612-9.

[100] Berg M, Gambhira R, Siracusa M, Hoiczyk E, Roden R, Ketner G. HPV16 L1 capsid protein expressed from viable adenovirus recombinants elicits neutralizing antibody in mice. Vaccine. 2007 Apr 30;25(17):3501-10.

[101] Nieto K, Stahl-Hennig C, Leuchs B, Müller M, Gissmann L, Kleinschmidt JA. Intranasal Vaccination with AAV5 and 9 Vectors Against Human Papillomavirus Type 16 in Rhesus Macaques. Hum Gene Ther. 2012 Jul;23(7):733-41.

[102] Nieto K, Kern A, Leuchs B, Gissmann L, Müller M, Kleinschmidt JA. Combined prophylactic and therapeutic intranasal vaccination against human papillomavirus type-16 using different adeno-associated virus serotype vectors. Antivir Ther. 2009;14(8):1125-37.

[103] Kuck D, Lau T, Leuchs B, Kern A, Müller M, Gissmann L, Kleinschmidt JA. Intranasal vaccination with recombinant adeno-associated virus type 5 against human papillomavirus type 16 L1. J Virol. 2006 Mar;80(6):2621-30.

[104] Kuck D, Leder C, Kern A, Müller M, Piuko K, Gissmann L, Kleinschmidt JA. Efficiency of HPV 16 L1/E7 DNA immunization: influence of cellular localization and capsid assembly. Vaccine. 2006 Apr 5;24(15):2952-65.

[105] Liu DW, Chang JL, Tsao YP, Huang CW, Kuo SW, Chen SL. Co-vaccination with adeno-associated virus vectors encoding human papillomavirus 16 L1 proteins and adenovirus encoding murine GM-CSF can elicit strong and prolonged neutralizing antibody. International journal of cancer Journal international du cancer. 2005 Jan 1;113(1):93-100.

[106] Echchannaoui H, Bianchi M, Baud D, Bobst M, Stehle JC, Nardelli-Haefliger D. Intravaginal immunization of mice with recombinant Salmonella enterica serovar Typhi-

murium expressing human papillomavirus type 16 antigens as a potential route of vaccination against cervical cancer. Infect Immun. 2008 May;76(5):1940-51.

[107] Baud D, Ponci F, Bobst M, De Grandi P, Nardelli-Haefliger D. Improved efficiency of a Salmonella-based vaccine against human papillomavirus type 16 virus-like particles achieved by using a codon-optimized version of L1. J Virol. 2004 Dec;78(23): 12901-9.

[108] Revaz V, Benyacoub J, Kast WM, Schiller JT, De Grandi P, Nardelli-Haefliger D. Mucosal vaccination with a recombinant Salmonella typhimurium expressing human papillomavirus type 16 (HPV16) L1 virus-like particles (VLPs) or HPV16 VLPs purified from insect cells inhibits the growth of HPV16-expressing tumor cells in mice. Virology. 2001 Jan 5;279(1):354-60.

[109] Nardelli-Haefliger D, Roden RB, Benyacoub J, Sahli R, Kraehenbuhl JP, Schiller JT, Lachat P, Potts A, De Grandi P. Human papillomavirus type 16 virus-like particles expressed in attenuated Salmonella typhimurium elicit mucosal and systemic neutralizing antibodies in mice. Infect Immun. 1997 Aug;65(8):3328-36.

[110] Govan VA, Christensen ND, Berkower C, Jacobs WR, Jr., Williamson AL. Immunisation with recombinant BCG expressing the cottontail rabbit papillomavirus (CRPV) L1 gene provides protection from CRPV challenge. Vaccine. 2006 Mar 15;24(12): 2087-93.

[111] Jabbar IA, Fernando GJ, Saunders N, Aldovini A, Young R, Malcolm K, Frazer IH. Immune responses induced by BCG recombinant for human papillomavirus L1 and E7 proteins. Vaccine. 2000 May 8;18(22):2444-53.

[112] Chen XS, Casini G, Harrison SC, Garcea RL. Papillomavirus capsid protein expression in Escherichia coli: purification and assembly of HPV11 and HPV16 L1. J Mol Biol. 2001 Mar 16;307(1):173-82.

[113] Thönes N, Herreiner A, Schädlich L, Piuko K, Müller M. A direct comparison of human papillomavirus type 16 L1 particles reveals a lower immunogenicity of capsomeres than viruslike particles with respect to the induced antibody response. J Virol. 2008 Jun;82(11):5472-85.

[114] Schädlich L, Senger T, Gerlach B, Mucke N, Klein C, Bravo IG, Müller M, Gissmann L. Analysis of modified human papillomavirus type 16 L1 capsomeres: the ability to assemble into larger particles correlates with higher immunogenicity. J Virol. 2009 Aug;83(15):7690-705.

[115] Stahl-Hennig C, Eisenblatter M, Jasny E, Rzehak T, Tenner-Racz K, Trumpfheller C, Salazar AM, Uberla K, Nieto K, Kleinschmidt J, Schulte R, Gissmann L, Müller M, Sacher A, Racz P, Steinman RM, Uguccioni M, Ignatius R. Synthetic double-stranded RNAs are adjuvants for the induction of T helper 1 and humoral immune responses to human papillomavirus in rhesus macaques. PLoS Pathog. 2009 Apr;5(4):e1000373.

[116]   Mason HS, Lam DM, Arntzen CJ. Expression of hepatitis B surface antigen in transgenic plants. Proc Natl Acad Sci U S A. 1992 Dec 15;89(24):11745-9.

[117]   Thanavala Y, Yang YF, Lyons P, Mason HS, Arntzen C. Immunogenicity of transgenic plant-derived hepatitis B surface antigen. Proc Natl Acad Sci U S A. 1995 Apr 11;92(8):3358-61.

[118]   Matic S, Masenga V, Poli A, Rinaldi R, Milne RG, Vecchiati M, Noris E. Comparative analysis of recombinant Human Papillomavirus 8 L1 production in plants by a variety of expression systems and purification methods. Plant Biotechnol J. 2012 May; 10(4):410-21.

[119]   Matic S, Rinaldi R, Masenga V, Noris E. Efficient production of chimeric human papillomavirus 16 L1 protein bearing the M2e influenza epitope in Nicotiana benthamiana plants. BMC Biotechnol. 2011;11:106.

[120]   Waheed MT, Thönes N, Müller M, Hassan SW, Gottschamel J, Lossl E, Kaul HP, Lossl AG. Plastid expression of a double-pentameric vaccine candidate containing human papillomavirus-16 L1 antigen fused with LTB as adjuvant: transplastomic plants show pleiotropic phenotypes. Plant Biotechnol J. 2011 Aug;9(6):651-60.

[121]   Paz De la Rosa G, Monroy-Garcia A, Mora-Garcia Mde L, Pena CG, Hernandez-Montes J, Weiss-Steider B, Gomez-Lim MA. An HPV 16 L1-based chimeric human papilloma virus-like particles containing a string of epitopes produced in plants is able to elicit humoral and cytotoxic T-cell activity in mice. Virol J. 2009;6:2.

[122]   Lenzi P, Scotti N, Alagna F, Tornesello ML, Pompa A, Vitale A, De Stradis A, Monti L, Grillo S, Buonaguro FM, Maliga P, Cardi T. Translational fusion of chloroplast-expressed human papillomavirus type 16 L1 capsid protein enhances antigen accumulation in transplastomic tobacco. Transgenic Res. 2008 Dec;17(6):1091-102.

[123]   Fernandez-San Millan A, Ortigosa SM, Hervas-Stubbs S, Corral-Martinez P, Segui-Simarro JM, Gaetan J, Coursaget P, Veramendi J. Human papillomavirus L1 protein expressed in tobacco chloroplasts self-assembles into virus-like particles that are highly immunogenic. Plant Biotechnol J. 2008 Jun;6(5):427-41.

[124]   Kohl TO, Hitzeroth, II, Christensen ND, Rybicki EP. Expression of HPV-11 L1 protein in transgenic Arabidopsis thaliana and Nicotiana tabacum. BMC Biotechnol. 2007;7:56.

[125]   Maclean J, Koekemoer M, Olivier AJ, Stewart D, Hitzeroth, II, Rademacher T, Fischer R, Williamson AL, Rybicki EP. Optimization of human papillomavirus type 16 (HPV-16) L1 expression in plants: comparison of the suitability of different HPV-16 L1 gene variants and different cell-compartment localization. J Gen Virol. 2007 May; 88(Pt 5):1460-9.

[126]   Kohl T, Hitzeroth, II, Stewart D, Varsani A, Govan VA, Christensen ND, Williamson AL, Rybicki EP. Plant-produced cottontail rabbit papillomavirus L1 protein protects

against tumor challenge: a proof-of-concept study. Clin Vaccine Immunol. 2006 Aug; 13(8):845-53.

[127] Varsani A, Williamson AL, Stewart D, Rybicki EP. Transient expression of Human papillomavirus type 16 L1 protein in Nicotiana benthamiana using an infectious to-bamovirus vector. Virus Res. 2006 Sep;120(1-2):91-6.

[128] Liu HL, Li WS, Lei T, Zheng J, Zhang Z, Yan XF, Wang ZZ, Wang YL, Si LS. Expression of human papillomavirus type 16 L1 protein in transgenic tobacco plants. Acta Biochim Biophys Sin (Shanghai). 2005 Mar;37(3):153-8.

[129] Campo MS, O'Neil BW, Grindlay GJ, Curtis F, Knowles G, Chandrachud L. A peptide encoding a B-cell epitope from the N-terminus of the capsid protein L2 of bovine papillomavirus-4 prevents disease. Virology. 1997 Aug 4;234(2):261-6.

[130] Roden RB, Yutzy WHt, Fallon R, Inglis S, Lowy DR, Schiller JT. Minor capsid protein of human genital papillomaviruses contains subdominant, cross-neutralizing epitopes. Virology. 2000 May 10;270(2):254-7.

[131] Pastrana DV, Gambhira R, Buck CB, Pang YY, Thompson CD, Culp TD, Christensen ND, Lowy DR, Schiller JT, Roden RB. Cross-neutralization of cutaneous and mucosal Papillomavirus types with anti-sera to the amino terminus of L2. Virology. 2005 Jul 5;337(2):365-72.

[132] Gambhira R, Karanam B, Jagu S, Roberts JN, Buck CB, Bossis I, Alphs H, Culp T, Christensen ND, Roden RB. A protective and broadly cross-neutralizing epitope of human papillomavirus L2. Journal of virology. 2007 Dec;81(24):13927-31.

[133] Gambhira R, Jagu S, Karanam B, Gravitt PE, Culp TD, Christensen ND, Roden RB. Protection of rabbits against challenge with rabbit papillomaviruses by immunization with the N terminus of human papillomavirus type 16 minor capsid antigen L2. Journal of virology. 2007 Nov;81(21):11585-92.

[134] Davidson EJ, Faulkner RL, Sehr P, Pawlita M, Smyth LJ, Burt DJ, Tomlinson AE, Hickling J, Kitchener HC, Stern PL. Effect of TA-CIN (HPV 16 L2E6E7) booster immunisation in vulval intraepithelial neoplasia patients previously vaccinated with TA-HPV (vaccinia virus encoding HPV 16/18 E6E7). Vaccine. 2004 Jul 29;22(21-22): 2722-9.

[135] Kondo K, Ishii Y, Ochi H, Matsumoto T, Yoshikawa H, Kanda T. Neutralization of HPV16, 18, 31, and 58 pseudovirions with antisera induced by immunizing rabbits with synthetic peptides representing segments of the HPV16 minor capsid protein L2 surface region. Virology. 2007 Feb 20;358(2):266-72.

[136] Rubio I, Seitz H, Canali E, Sehr P, Bolchi A, Tommasino M, Ottonello S, Müller M. The N-terminal region of the human papillomavirus L2 protein contains overlapping binding sites for neutralizing, cross-neutralizing and non-neutralizing antibodies. Virology. 2011 Jan 20;409(2):348-59.

[137] Rubio I, Bolchi A, Moretto N, Canali E, Gissmann L, Tommasino M, Müller M, Otto-
       nello S. Potent anti-HPV immune responses induced by tandem repeats of the
       HPV16 L2 (20 -- 38) peptide displayed on bacterial thioredoxin. Vaccine. 2009 Mar
       18;27(13):1949-56.

[138] Gambhira R, Karanam B, Jagu S, Roberts JN, Buck CB, Bossis I, Alphs H, Culp T,
       Christensen ND, Roden RB. A protective and broadly cross-neutralizing epitope of
       human papillomavirus L2. J Virol. 2007 Dec;81(24):13927-31.

[139] Alphs HH, Gambhira R, Karanam B, Roberts JN, Jagu S, Schiller JT, Zeng W, Jackson
       DC, Roden RB. Protection against heterologous human papillomavirus challenge by
       a synthetic lipopeptide vaccine containing a broadly cross-neutralizing epitope of L2.
       Proc Natl Acad Sci U S A. 2008 Apr 15;105(15):5850-5.

[140] Tumban E, Peabody J, Peabody DS, Chackerian B. A pan-HPV vaccine based on bac-
       teriophage PP7 VLPs displaying broadly cross-neutralizing epitopes from the HPV
       minor capsid protein, L2. PloS one. 2011;6(8):e23310.

[141] Caldeira Jdo C, Medford A, Kines RC, Lino CA, Schiller JT, Chackerian B, Peabody
       DS. Immunogenic display of diverse peptides, including a broadly cross-type neu-
       tralizing human papillomavirus L2 epitope, on virus-like particles of the RNA bac-
       teriophage PP7. Vaccine. 2010 Jun 17;28(27):4384-93.

[142] Schellenbacher C, Roden R, Kirnbauer R. Chimeric L1-L2 virus-like particles as po-
       tential broad-spectrum human papillomavirus vaccines. J Virol. 2009 Oct;83(19):
       10085-95.

[143] Moretto N, Bolchi A, Rivetti C, Imbimbo BP, Villetti G, Pietrini V, Polonelli L, Del Si-
       gnore S, Smith KM, Ferrante RJ, Ottonello S. Conformation-sensitive antibodies
       against alzheimer amyloid-beta by immunization with a thioredoxin-constrained B-
       cell epitope peptide. The Journal of biological chemistry. 2007 Apr 13;282(15):
       11436-45.

[144] Day PM, Pang YY, Kines RC, Thompson CD, Lowy DR, Schiller JT. A human papillo-
       mavirus (HPV) in vitro neutralization assay that recapitulates the in vitro process of
       infection provides a sensitive measure of HPV L2 infection-inhibiting antibodies.
       Clinical and vaccine immunology : CVI. 2012 Jul;19(7):1075-82.

[145] Roberts JN, Kines RC, Katki HA, Lowy DR, Schiller JT. Effect of Pap smear collection
       and carrageenan on cervicovaginal human papillomavirus-16 infection in a rhesus
       macaque model. Journal of the National Cancer Institute. 2011 May 4;103(9):737-43.

[146] Repp KK, Nielson CM, Fu R, Schäfer S, Lazcano-Ponce E, Salmeron J, Quiterio M,
       Villa LL, Giuliano AR, study HIM. Male human papillomavirus prevalence and asso-
       ciation with condom use in Brazil, Mexico, and the United States. J Infect Dis. 2012
       Apr 15;205(8):1287-93.

[147] Siegfried N, Müller M, Deeks JJ, Volmink J. Male circumcision for prevention of heterosexual acquisition of HIV in men. Cochrane Database Syst Rev. 2009(2):CD003362.

[148] Van Wagoner NJ, Geisler WM, Sizemore JM, Jr., Whitley R, Hook EW, 3rd. Herpes simplex virus in african american heterosexual males: the roles of age and male circumcision. Sex Transm Dis. 2010 Apr;37(4):217-22.

[149] Auvert B, Sobngwi-Tambekou J, Cutler E, Nieuwoudt M, Lissouba P, Puren A, Taljaard D. Effect of Male Circumcision on the Prevalence of High-Risk Human Papillomavirus in Young Men: Results of a Randomized Controlled Trial Conducted in Orange Farm, South Africa. Journal of Infectious Diseases. 2009 Jan 1;199(1):14-9.

[150] Gray RH, Serwadda D, Kong X, Makumbi F, Kigozi G, Gravitt PE, Watya S, Nalugoda F, Ssempijja V, Tobian AA, Kiwanuka N, Moulton LH, Sewankambo NK, Reynolds SJ, Quinn TC, Iga B, Laeyendecker O, Oliver AE, Wawer MJ. Male circumcision decreases acquisition and increases clearance of high-risk human papillomavirus in HIV-negative men: a randomized trial in Rakai, Uganda. J Infect Dis. 2010 May 15;201(10):1455-62.

[151] Castellsague X, Bosch FX, Munoz N, Meijer CJ, Shah KV, de Sanjose S, Eluf-Neto J, Ngelangel CA, Chichareon S, Smith JS, Herrero R, Moreno V, Franceschi S. Male circumcision, penile human papillomavirus infection, and cervical cancer in female partners. N Engl J Med. 2002 Apr 11;346(15):1105-12.

[152] Hernandez BY, Wilkens LR, Zhu X, McDuffie K, Thompson P, Shvetsov YB, Ning L, Goodman MT. Circumcision and human papillomavirus infection in men: a site-specific comparison. J Infect Dis. 2008 Mar 15;197(6):787-94.

[153] Giuliano AR, Lazcano E, Villa LL, Flores R, Salmeron J, Lee JH, Papenfuss M, Abrahamsen M, Baggio ML, Silva R, Quiterio M. Circumcision and sexual behavior: Factors independently associated with human papillomavirus detection among men in the HIM study. International Journal of Cancer. 2009 Mar 15;124(6):1251-7.

[154] Asculai SS, Weis MT, Rancourt MW, Kupferberg AB. Inactivation of herpes simplex viruses by nonionic surfactants. Antimicrob Agents Chemother. 1978 Apr;13(4): 686-90.

[155] Singh B, Utidjian HM, Cutler JC. Studies on Development of a Vaginal Preparation Providing Both Prophylaxis against Venereal Disease, Other Genital Infections and Contraception.3. In-Vitro Effect of Vaginal Contraceptive and Selected Vaginal Preparations of Candida-Albicans and Trichomonas-Vaginali. Contraception. 1972;5(5): 401-&.

[156] Singh B, Utidjian HM, Cutler JC. Studies on Development of a Vaginal Preparation Providing Both Prophylaxis against Venereal Disease and Other Genital Infections and Contraception.2. Effect in-Vitro of Vaginal Contraceptive and Non-Contraceptive Preparations on Treponema-Pallidum and Neisseria-Gonorrhoeae. British Journal of Venereal Diseases. 1972;48(1):57-&.

[157] Polsky B, Baron PA, Gold JW, Smith JL, Jensen RH, Armstrong D. In vitro inactiva-
       tion of HIV-1 by contraceptive sponge containing nonoxynol-9. Lancet. 1988 Jun
       25;1(8600):1456.

[158] Van Damme L, Ramjee G, Alary M, Vuylsteke B, Chandeying V, Rees H, Sirivon-
       grangson P, Mukenge-Tshibaka L, Ettiegne-Traore V, Uaheowitchai C, Karim SS,
       Masse B, Perriens J, Laga M. Effectiveness of COL-1492, a nonoxynol-9 vaginal gel,
       on HIV-1 transmission in female sex workers: a randomised controlled trial. Lancet.
       2002 Sep 28;360(9338):971-7.

[159] Schaeffer DJ, Krylov VS. Anti-HIV activity of extracts and compounds from algae
       and cyanobacteria. Ecotoxicol Environ Saf. 2000 Mar;45(3):208-27.

[160] Buck CB, Thompson CD, Roberts JN, Müller M, Lowy DR, Schiller JT. Carrageenan is
       a potent inhibitor of papillomavirus infection. PLoS pathogens. 2006 Jul;2(7):e69.

[161] Skoler-Karpoff S, Ramjee G, Ahmed K, Altini L, Plagianos MG, Friedland B, Govend-
       er S, De Kock A, Cassim N, Palanee T, Dozier G, Maguire R, Lahteenmaki P. Efficacy
       of Carraguard for prevention of HIV infection in women in South Africa: a rando-
       mised, double-blind, placebo-controlled trial. Lancet. 2008 Dec 6;372(9654):1977-87.

[162] Roberts JN, Buck CB, Thompson CD, Kines R, Bernardo M, Choyke PL, Lowy DR,
       Schiller JT. Genital transmission of HPV in a mouse model is potentiated by nonoxy-
       nol-9 and inhibited by carrageenan. Nat Med. 2007 Jul;13(7):857-61.

[163] Roberts JN, Kines RC, Katki HA, Lowy DR, Schiller JT. Effect of Pap Smear Collec-
       tion and Carrageenan on Cervicovaginal Human Papillomavirus-16 Infection in a
       Rhesus Macaque Model. Journal of the National Cancer Institute. 2011 May;103(9):
       737-43.

[164] Rupp R, Rosenthal SL, Stanberry LR. VivaGel (SPL7013 Gel): a candidate dendrim-
       er--microbicide for the prevention of HIV and HSV infection. Int J Nanomedicine.
       2007;2(4):561-6.

[165] Starpharma Holdings Limited. Shareholder Upadate: May 2008. Available from:
       http://asx.thebull.com.au/news-history?S=SPL&E=ASX&Year=2008.

Clinical Aspects of HPV-Infections

Chapter 7

Clinical Manifestations of the Human Papillomavirus

Miguel Ángel Arrabal-Polo,
María Sierra Girón-Prieto, Jacinto Orgaz-Molina,
Sergio Merino-Salas,
Fernando Lopez-Carmona Pintado,
Miguel Arrabal-Martin and Salvador Arias-Santiago

Additional information is available at the end of the chapter

1. Introduction

1.1. Skin injuries

1.1.1. Benign skin lesions

The global prevalence of papillomavirus in the 4- to 18-year-old population has been estimated to be 24% (12% for those aged 4 to 6 years and 24% for those aged 16 to 18 years) [1]. The prevalence is significantly reduced in adults (3.5%) [2]. There are no significant differences related to gender. There is, however, a higher prevalence in rural versus urban schools. While plantar and common warts generally number 1 or 2, flat warts frequently appear as multiple lesions [1].

HPV transmission requires the inoculation of the virus into the basal epithelia cells, which occurs on sites that are particularly predisposed to microtraumas. Therefore, it is not surprising to frequently find common warts on the hands and fingers (Figure 1). Lesion regression is frequently spontaneous, and the immune system plays an important role, as is reflected in practice by the increased HPV susceptibility of immunosuppressed patients. In these cases, the lesions are clinically more exuberant and recalcitrant to treatment [3]. It is important to highlight a particular collective group composed of butchers and slaughterhouse workers who, without immunosuppression, have a higher risk compared to the general population [4, 5]. This group has an increased incidence of the HPV7 subtype, and it is thought that some component of meat favors the replication of this viral subtype [6, 7].

1.1.1.1. Common warts

This infection is fundamentally produced by HPV subtypes 1, 2, 4, and 7 [8]. The lesions are usually asymptomatic, although they can be painful when located in pressure zones. Clinically, they are easily diagnosable; thus, the patient frequently brings up the presence of lesions during a consultation. Common warts can manifest as a single lesion; however, because of the virus's infectious nature, multiple lesions can be found in the same patient [1]. The lesions present progressive growth such that they are initially about the size of the head of a pin, and they are smooth and shiny. Over the course of weeks, they acquire their typical characteristics. On inspection, they present as papules with well-defined borders and with the same color as the skin. The surface is flattened; it may be whiter than the surrounding skin as an expression of hyperkeratosis of the lesion itself, and it may have a multilobulated aspect (Figures 1 and 2). The hyperkeratosis and multilobulate aspect confer a rough surface upon palpation. Occasionally, the exuberant development of hyperkeratosis can produce the formation of a cutaneous horn. Depending on the characteristics of the host and the anatomical location of the cutaneous horn, a histological study of the lesion may be necessary for a differential diagnosis with malignant lesions, such as epidermoid carcinoma. When the lesions are multiple, they can present as distinct isolated lesions, as close-by lesions and even as confluent lesions ("mosaic"). Lesions can be numerous in immunosuppressed patients (i.e., those who are transplanted or HIV-positive or have Hodgkin's lymphoma or leukemia) [3, 8-11]. Characteristically, lesions may be located on the nail fold. This location is particularly associated with the habit of nail biting [12]. Thus, breaking this habit can prevent new lesions in adjacent nails that have not yet been affected.

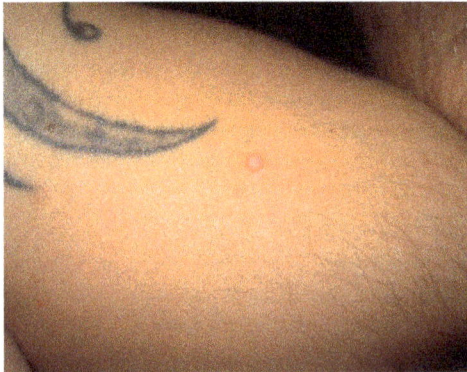

Figure 1. Erythematous hyperkeratotic papule on the arm: common wart.

Although the clinic is generally sufficient for diagnosis, dermatoscopy is a useful tool that provides complementary information for cases involving clinical doubts. Dermatoscopically, common warts are characterized by the presence of dense papillae, each centered around a

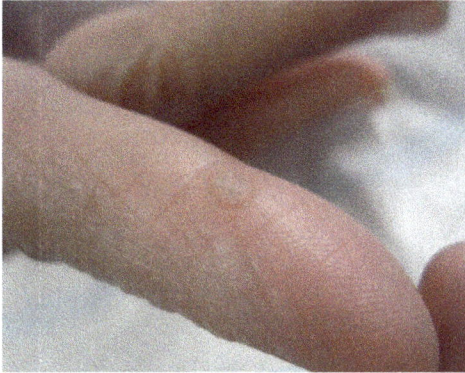

Figure 2. Papule with well-defined borders and with the same color as the skin on the finger compatible with common wart.

central red dot or a loop surrounded by a whitish halo. This combination of characteristics creates a "frog spawn" appearance [13].

Because of their frequency and similarity from a clinical point of view, the main differential diagnoses are nonpigmented seborrheic keratosis, fibrous papule of the nose (angiofibroma), intradermic nevus and warty epidermal nevus.

The histology is characterized by marked hyperkeratosis, acanthosis and papillomatosis. Nevertheless, these features are not specific to this type of lesion. As a characteristic sign of HPV's cytopathic effect, koilocytes (cells with a pyknotic nucleus surrounded by a clear halo) are observed [14].

1.1.1.2. Filiform warts

These are considered a special variant of common warts. They are predominantly localized in the palpebral and perioral regions and in the neck. Their distinctive characteristic is the special filiform or elongated morphology, with a narrow pedicle and pronounced digital projections on the surface (because of this, they are also called "digitiform papilloma") (Figure 3). The main differential diagnosis is with acrochordons, which can have a similar morphology but are differentiated by their smooth surface (they lack digital projections). The histological peculiarity of filiform warts is that the papillae are more elongated than those of common warts.

1.1.1.3. Plantar warts

HPV 1 frequently causes these lesions, and it occasionally causes Type 4 lesions [14]. They can manifest as single or multiple ("mosaic") lesions (Figure 4). Trauma plays an important role in the inoculation of the warts, as the most commonly affected sites are the heel and the heads of the metatarsi.

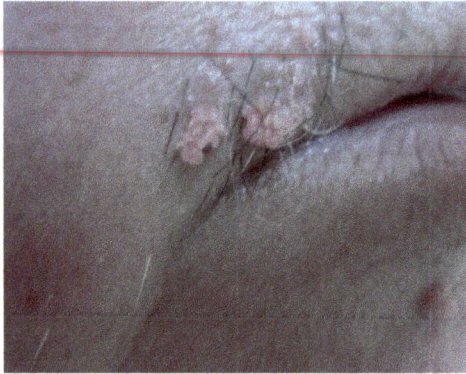

Figure 3. Filiform papule on the upper lip with pronounced digital projections on the surface compatible with filiform wart.

The main differential diagnosis between plantar warts and plantar callus is important because the two disorders are frequently confused in clinical practice. Although the most frequent locations for the emergence of warts are pressure zones, warts can also appear in areas that experience less pressure, such as the arch of the foot. This location, however, is not common for calluses, which are produced as a consequence of pressure on the skin. A clinical maneuver for distinguishing warts from calluses is tangential scraping: in calluses, the detachment of multiple hyperkeratosic layers with a clean central fundus is observed, whereas warts present a multilobulated aspect above the superficial hyperkeratosic layer, accompanied by multiple black dots that correspond to thrombosed capillaries. In contrast, warts are indicated by certain dermatoscopic signs, such as black to red dots, globules corresponding to dilated and thrombosed capillaries of the papillae and interrupted dermatoglyphics in the lesion. Calluses present a translucent central corn or a homogeneous opacity [15].

The use of the dermatoscope has been described as useful for monitoring the need for new treatment sessions for warts because dermatoscopes are more sensitive than the naked eye [15].

1.1.1.4. Flat warts

HPV 3 and 10 commonly produce this lesion. [14] This type of wart is typical in childhood. It is very rare in male adults and has been described in the context of HIV infection [16]. The most commonly affected area is the face, followed by the back of the hands and the shins. [14] The aspect is that of a papule or slightly elevated flat plaques (2-3 mm) and low desquamation (smooth surface). Coloration ranges from light brown to the color of the individual's skin, thus making flat warts hard to detect with simple inspection. Histologically, flat warts are characterized by less acanthosis than common or plantar warts, and papillomatosis is minimal or absent.

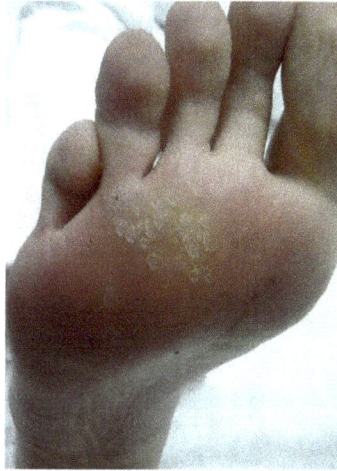

Figure 4. Plantar wart: Multiple hyperkeratotic lesion on the sole of the foot with thrombosed capillaries (black dots).

For differential diagnosis in the face, the syringomas, seborrheic keratosis, and papulosis nigra standout. Warty epidermal nevus, present from early childhood and following the Blaschko lines, is another diagnosis to consider.

1.1.1.5. Pigmented warts

Subtypes 65, 4 and 60 are the main causes of pigmented warts [17]. Egawa was the first to describe these subtypes in 1988 [18]. Although common warts and molluscum contagiosum can transform to a black color [19, 20] in their involutionary phases, pigmented warts are pigmented from the initial phases. They are fundamentally located on the hands and feet. The lesions are morphologically similar to common warts when they are located in the lateral side of the hands and feet and on the fingers and toes (Figure 5); when they are located on the sole, they can have the aspect of flat, pigmented warts with light hyperkeratosis on the surface [17], but with the particularity of their brown-black coloration. Although the clinical diagnosis is not difficult, lesions on the sole can be proposed for a differential diagnosis with acral melanoma. Surface hyperkeratosis usually guides diagnosis. However, when in doubt, histological analysis can be used for diagnosis.

One histological peculiarity of pigmented warts is the presence of intracytoplasmic inclusion bodies consisting of a homogeneous eosinophilic substance together with swollen nuclei, very similar to cases associated with Types 65 and 4. In the case of HPV 60, the inclusion bodies are similar but have a much rounder shape and no edema in the nucleus [17]. In contrast, not all of the other HPV subtypes are associated with inclusion bodies; when present, inclusion bodies are characterized by eosinophilic bodies and not by a homogeneous substance [21].

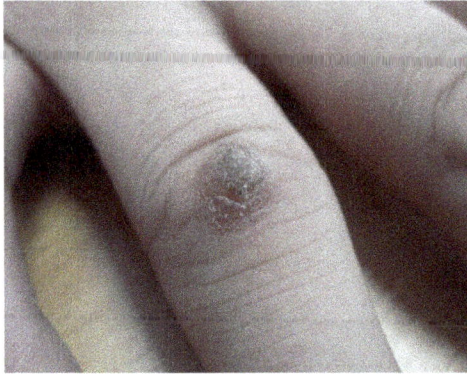

Figure 5. Pigmented hyperkeratotic papule on the finger: pigmented wart

1.1.1.6. Epidermodysplasia verruciformis

This is a rare genodermatosis that is generally autosomal recessive hereditary, although X-associated heritage has also been described. It has been classified as a primary immunodeficiency [22] in which there is a curious and particular susceptibility to infection by HPV-β subtypes [23]. The types most frequently implicated are HPV 5 and 8, although many others have also been associated. Most of the cases are associated with mutations in one of the genes located in the long arm of chromosome 17 (EVER1 or TMC6, and EVER2 or TMC8) [24]. These genes code for transmembrane proteins that are fundamentally found in the endoplasmic reticulum and interact with the zinc transporter (ZT1) [23]. It is believed that a selective inhibition of T lymphocyte immune responses against HPV exists, most likely because of defective viral antigen presentation on keratinocyte surfaces [25].

Clinically, this infection is characterized by the appearance at an early age of multiple flat warts, pityriasis versicolor-type lesions, and other lesions similar to seborrheic keratosis (Figure 6) [14]. However, the major interest is in the high risk of developing squamous cell carcinoma, especially in photoexposed zones (30 to 50% of patients) between the third and fourth decades of life [14, 23]. Based on the risk of developing malignant lesions, two phenotypes have been distinguished. One phenotype is indicated by more benign lesions that are flat, desquamous and hypo- or hyperpigmented in a manner similar to that of tinea versicolor; these lesions are distributed on the neck, torso and extremities. The other phenotype is characterized by seborrheic keratosis-type warty lesions that have a higher malignant potential. These lesions are distributed primarily on photoexposed zones, such as the face and hands, and on the feet. The development of these malignant lesions is usually associated with Types 5 and 8. However, unlike the pathogenesis of other oncogenic HPV, these types do not seem to require integration into the host genome [23].

Recently, epidermodysplasia verruciformis (EV)-like clinical appearances have been described in immunosuppressed patients, such as HIV and transplantation patients [26, 27] This phenomenon has been called "acquired EV form" [26]. It has been hypothesized that these forms can create minor defects in patients with predisposing genes, and these defects manifest clinically upon immunosuppression [24].

From a histology perspective, EV is characterized by the presentation of hyperkeratosis, hypergranulosis, and acanthosis. However, the characteristic feature is the presence of large keratinocytes with a blue-grey granular cytoplasm in the superior portions of the squamous stratum and in the granulose. As has been noted, the lesions can present a progressive atypia until the development of invasive squamous cell carcinoma [14].

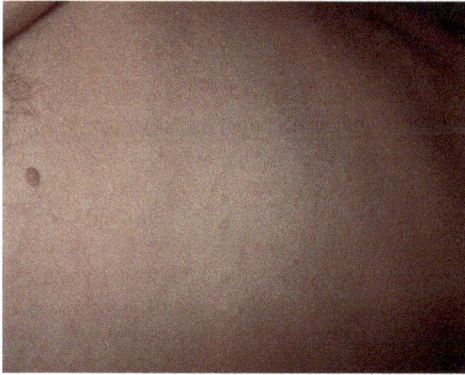

Figure 6. Multiple flat warts and pityriasis versicolor-type lesions in a patient with epidermodysplasia verruciformis

1.2. Malignant skin lesions

1.2.1. Squamous cell carcinoma of the skin

Squamous cell carcinoma (SCC) is the second commonest malignant skin tumor (the first one is basal cell carcinoma). Ultraviolet (UV) radiation is the main risk factor for skin cancer and this tumor usually appears in sun-exposed areas specially the face, neck, arms and hands. Changes in lifestyle over recent decades have led to greater exposure to ultraviolet radiation; this phenomenon increases the risk of developing skin cancer. In the last 25 years there have been an increased in the incidence of this tumor due to sun exposure and increased life expectancy [28]. SCC can complicate other lesions as burn scar, lichen planus, discoid lupus, epidermoid cyst or venous ulcers. Other risk factors include older age, fair skin and immuno-supression. Emerging evidence suggests that cutaneous human papillomavirus (HPV) infection may also be a risk factor for SCC.

Despite the role of HPV in sunlight induced malignancies is uncertain as in squamous cell carcinoma there have been some evidence of the association between some subtypes of HPV and squamous cell carcinoma of the genital area. HPV 16 has been detected in squamous cell carcinoma of the vulva, penis and perianal region. [29] The inactivation of tumor suppressor genes by HPV has been implicated in the development of SCC. In HPV infection, the oncoprotein E7 inactivates the tumor suppressor Rb, leading to p16 upregulation. Recently new studies have shown that Genus-beta HPV (seropositivity) infections were associated with SCC in any locations [30]. Patients with HPV related squamous cell carcinoma are characterized by a higher rate of recurrences but not more metastases compared to ordinary SCC and also many patients present genital lesions containing the same HPV type [31]. Moreover patients with SCC of penis, scrotum an anus are associated with higher risk of metastases. Also immuno-suppressed patients for renal transplantation or with epidermodysplasia verruciformis (HPV 5) develop SCC associated with VPH. UV radiation and HPV may play a synergic role in the development of squamous cell carcinoma and a recent study has shown that seropositivity for HPV types in genera alpha or beta increased the risk of SCC associated with poor tanning ability [32].

Clinically SCC presents as shallow ulcers, papules or plaques often with keratinous crust and elevated surrounds commonly in photo-exposed areas (Figure 7). It is not uncommon to find an in situ SCC under a cutaneous horn. Patients rarely complain about pain or pruritus. SCC usually bleeds with minor trauma. The adjacent skin usually shows features of actinic damage (actinic keratosis). Pigmented variants are rare. SCC should be suspected in patients with permanent or bleeding recurrent ulcer. Prognosis depends on the risk of recurrence and metastasis. The overall recurrence rate varies from 3 to 11% and the overall metastatasis rate is around 5%. Tumor thickness and desmoplasia are multivariate factors associated with local recurrence and tumor thickness, immunosuppression, ear location and tumor diameter with the risk of metastasis.

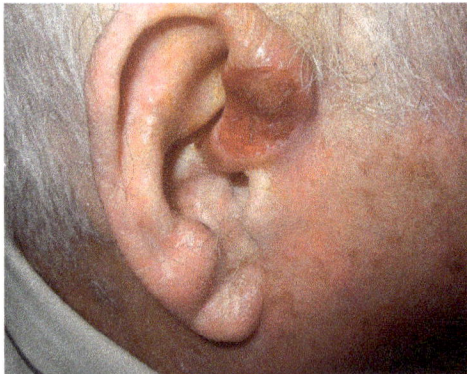

Figure 7. Infiltrated and erosive tumor of the helix compatible with squamous cell carcinoma of the skin

Actinic keratosis is a well-established precancerous skin lesion that has the potential to progress to squamous cell carcinoma. Clinically it is presented as a circumscribed scaly erythematous lesions, usually less than 1cm in diameter on the sun-exposed (face, ears, scalp, hands) skin of older individuals. They may remit or remain unchanged for a long time but between 8-20% gradually transform into a SCC. Several clinical variant of actinic keratosis has been described: hypertrophic, acantholytic, pigmented and lichenoid. Intermittent sun exposure and sunburns during the childhood are strongly associated with the prevalence of actinic keratosis. Recently HPV infection has been associated also with the risk of developing these lesions [33].

A clinical well-differentiated variant of SCC is verrucous SCC which is named different according to the localization, in oral mucosa florid oral papillomatosis, in the genital area giant condyloma of Buschke-Lowenstein and in the soles caniculatum carcinoma. Differential diagnosis includes verrucous hyperplasia, pseudoepitheliomatous hyperplasia and giant condylomas. These tumors present a low rate of metastases but tend to infiltrate easily. Radiotherapy is not indicated as usually recur in a more aggressive manner. The role of human papillomavirus infections in the development of verrucous carcinoma is controversial in the literature, and although some clinical cases have shown and HPV positivity (type 6, 11, 16, 18) a recent study do not support a causal role of HPV in the development of verrucous carcinoma. [34]

SCC of the oral or anogenital mucosa tends to metastasize and be more aggressive than the one originated in sun-exposed skin. Oral carcinoma usually affects lower lips but also in the tongue and inside the oral cavity (palate). Special risk factors for this location are smoking and alcoholism. SCC in oral mucosa begins as an eritroplasia plaque that evolves into a nodular and granulomatous plaque. A recent study which included 172 patients with advanced oral cavity squamous cell carcinoma detected a prevalence of HPV infection in 22% of the tumors [HPV-16 (9%) and HPV-18 (7%)]. A comparison with the group of patients with HPV-16 negative infection revealed that those with a single HPV-16 infection are at higher risk of distant metastases and poor survival despite undergoing radiation-based adjuvant therapy and require a more aggressive adjuvant treatment and a more thorough follow-up whereas HPV-18 infection had no impact on 5-year prognosis [35].

Keratoacanthoma is a rapidly growing skin tumor arising predominantly on the exposed surfaces of the body that should be considered as a variant of SCC rather than a benign or pseudomalignant neoplasm. Clinically they present as a smooth, hemispherical papule that rapidly enlarges over the course of a few weeks with a central keratin-filled crater. Usually involution occurs with tumor resorption and loss of the keratin plug. The role of HPV in keratoacanthoma remains thus elusive but a study showed that 51% of keratoacanthoma presented DNA of HPV. [36]

1.2.2. Bowen´S disease

Bowen's disease (BD) is considered a squamous cell carcinoma in situ that predominantly affects sun-exposed areas in middle-aged or elderly patients. It presents as an asymptomatic well-defined erythematous scaly plaque which grows centrifugally resembling psoriasis or dermatitis (Figure 8). It is not uncommon the presentation of Bowen's disease as non-steroid-responsive dermatitis. The clinical differential diagnosis of Bowen's disease includes psoriasis, eczema, superficial basal cell carcinoma or cutaneous Paget's disease. It may affect any part of the integument, mucous membranes or nail bed, but it commonly presents on the trunk, head, extremities or genitalia. Some clinical variants of Bowen's disease include a verrucous, nodular, eroded or pigmented variant that may be confused with melanoma. Invasive carcinoma develops in nearly 5-10% of untreated cases with a metastatic potential of 13-30% of cases. This complication should be suspected when a rapidly growing tumor is present in a previous scaly lesion. Complete or partial regression has been described in Bowen's disease [37] but this is not a common phenomenon. Some authors proposed that Bowen's disease was considered a marker of an internal malignancy; however a later meta-analysis showed that this association was inconsistent [38].

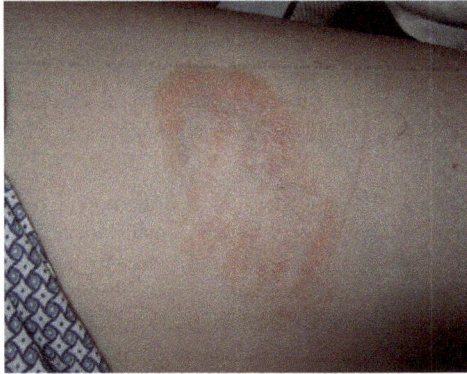

Figure 8. Well-defined erythematous scaly plaque on the limb clinically and histopathologically compatible with Bowen´s disease.

Bowen's disease of the penis is regarded as erythroplasia of Queyrat and this disease is characterized by slightly, erythematous, velvety, bleeding macules or plaques. Perianal lesions present the same clinical characteristics, but they are more common in females than males.

The etiology of Bowen's disease is mainly multifactorial and different factors have been associated as UV light or arsenic. Also HPV have been associated with Bowen's disease, initially periungueal and anogenital lesions, but later studies have shown an association in other locations. Many types of HPV have been associated with BD: HPV 2,16,18,27,31,33,34,39,52,56,58,59,67,76,82… and the implication in the prognosis of the disease remains elusive.[39]

1.2.3. Basal cell carcinoma of the skin

Basal cell carcinoma (BCC) is the most common malignant cutaneous neoplasm and the incidence is rising in the last decades [28]. They usually arise from the lowermost layer of the epidermis, although a small percentage may originate from the outer root sheath of the pilosebaceous unit. It is slightly more common in men than in women and although these tumors metastasize exceptionally rarely they have a tissue destruction potential particularly lesions on the face. This tumor is mainly found on areas of skin exposed to the sun. Up to 70% of all lesions are found on the head and neck and 30% on the shoulders, back, chest and lower extremities. This tumor has been described in nearly every location of the body, but lesions on the scrotum are of particular importance because of a high rate of metastasis associated. The most common sites of metastasis (less than 0.5% of the cases) include lymph nodes, lung, bone and skin. In sunny climates the clinical presentation is in much younger patients but in less sunny climates it usually happens during the sixth decade [40].

Basal cell carcinoma may develop in some benign lesion as organoid nevi, pore of Winer, rhinophyma, epidermal nevi, "port wine" stain, epidermal cysts, multiple trichoepiteliomas, solar lentigos… The presence of multiples BCC in young people is associated with different syndromes as Gorlin syndrome, Bazex syndrome, cartilage hair hypoplasia syndrome or ROMBO syndrome that should be discarded.

BCC is characterized by a papulonodular lesion with pearly translucent edge and it is usually ulcerated (Figure 9). The lesion is usually indurated and telangiectasias on the surface of the lesion are easily visible. Five main clinical variants have been described: nodular/ulcerative, superficial, pigmented, infiltrative or morpheaform and fibroepithelioma of Pinkus. Nodular variant resembles a cutaneous cyst with telangiectasias on the surface, the sizes varies from 1 to various centimeters. The ulcerative variant usually starts as a small translucent papule with a pearly appearance with a central erosion or ulceration with a rolled margin (*ulcus rodens*). The superficial variant is usually located on the trunk as a slowly enlarging, scaly red patch for a long time. Lesions may be confused with psoriasis, dermatits or eczema.. These lesions are usually treated with topical corticosteroids but a careful examination of the edges of the lesions shows a rolled translucent border and dermatoscopy may be useful for the diagnosis of these tumors. Infiltrative or morpheaform BCC presents a poorly demarcated and cicatricial lesion which enlarges over several years. BCC may contain pigment on it and in some cases it is necessary to differentiate from melanocytic lesions. BCC tends to enlarge progressively and to be destructive, also atypical forms simulating cervical adenopathies have been described [41-42]. Fibroepithelioma of Pinkus is an uncommon erythematous tumor usually located on the trunk or extremities with typical histopathologic features.

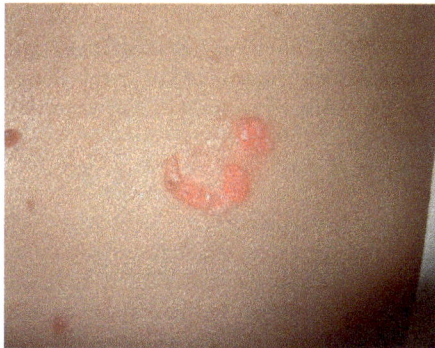

Figure 9. Basal cell carcinoma: papulonodular lesion with pearly translucent edge on the upper back.

UV radiation and sunburns correlates properly with BCC of the head and neck. The history of sunburns during the childhood and recreational exposure during the first two decades of live are associated with higher risk of this tumor. Low phototype is also a risk factor (fair skin and red hair). Primary prevention is very important and recently a study has demonstrated that a programme entirely conducted via Internet significantly reduces by half self-reported sunburn risk (main risk factor of melanoma and BCC) in an adolescent population achieving very high satisfaction rates [43]. BCC can be a complication of PUVA therapy, irradiation, burns, immunosuppression, renal transplant recipients, HIV infection, or leukemia. Mutation in PTCH1 has been found in sporadic and syndromes associated wih BCC. The pathogenic role of beta-HPVs in non melanoma skin cancer (NMSC), is not still completely understood, and literature data indicate that they might be at least cofactors in the development of certain cutaneous squamous cell carcinomas. However, only few reports contain data on basal cell carcinoma (BCC). Some studies have shown an overexpression of some protein associated with beta-HPV species [44] but other authors conclude that HPV does not seem to play a funda-mental role in the aetiopathogenesis of either nodular or superficial BCC. The presence of HPV appears to be more related to actinic damage and possibly to an alteration of the barrier function associated with ageing [45].

2. Mucosal lesions

2.1. Benign mucosal lesions

Human papillomavirus (HPV) produces a wide variety of lesions in all the mucosae that are in contact with the environment outside the organism. In addition to genitourinary lesions, benign lesions associated with HPV have been described in the oral cavity, nasal mucosa, and ocular conjunctiva [46]. Some serotypes are frequently associated with specific lesions: focal epithelial hyperplasia (13, 32), buccal papilloma (2, 6, 11, 57), condyloma acuminata (6, 11), laryngeal papilloma (11), squamous conjunctival papilloma (6, 11, 16) and nasosinal papilloma (6, 11).

The diagnosis can be made clinically, but some cases require the use of DNA techniques or microscopy techniques to establish the presence of koilocytes (elongated cells with eccentric and pyknotic nuclei that are frequently surrounded by a perinuclear halo).

2.1.1. Focal epithelial hyperplasia or Heck's disease

Although several etiopathogenic factors have been considered, this disease is associated with HPV, particularly Types 13 and 32. However, other factors play a role, as the zones where the disease is most frequently observed (the oral mucosa) are contact areas with dental prostheses [47]. There are also family and ethnic associations (the disease was first described in Inuits and is not common in Caucasians), thus supporting a possible genetic component associated with HLA-DR4 [48]. Sexual transmission is not considered common, as the disease is most common in patients before the second decade of life.

The basic lesion consists of a rounded or oval papule with a soft consistency that is usually multiple (figure 10). Its surface is smooth, not keratinized, and the same color as the mucosa or slightly lighter. Its maximum diameter is usually 5 mm, although it can be confluent; therefore, the sizes reported in the literature vary between 1 and 10 mm, and the lesion may even have a cobbled aspect. It is asymptomatic [47, 48]

Heck's disease lesions have been described almost exclusively in the oral mucosa. The most common location is the lower lip, followed by the jugal mucosa, the upper lip and the tongue. Lesions are also associated with contact zones. Much more rarely, lesions occur on the palate, the floor of the mouth, or the oropharynx.

Histologically, epithelial hyperplasia is observed with elongation and horizontal anastamosis between the interpapillary crests. Also described are hyperkeratosis, parakeratosis, focal acanthosis, koilocytosis and mitosoid figures (cells that present degenerative nuclear changes that simulate mitosis) in superficial keratinocytes [3,4]. When HPV DNA is detected, either by PCR or in situ hybridization, Genotypes 12 and 32 are appreciated in more than 90% of cases and in Types 1 and 11. To date, no malignant potential has been demonstrated [49].

Differential diagnosis is made against other benign lesions produced by HPV, such as the common wart, squamous papilloma and condyloma acuminata, all of which are associated with sexual transmission and with possible abuse, in the case of a minor. It is necessary to differentiate against fibroma and bite papilloma, as lesions occur in a friction zone. Mucosal neuroma, white sponge nevus, florid oral papillomatosis and diffuse epithelial hyperplasia in tobacco chewers are considered in the differential diagnosis. Neurofibromas on the mucosal affectation of the neurofibromatosis and the papule or labial papillomas of Cowden's syndrome are usually located in similar zones, thus indicating these systemic diseases [47, 48].

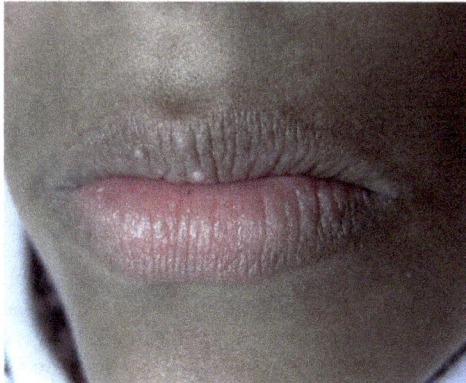

Figure 10. Heck´s disease: rounded papule with a soft consistency on the upper lip.

Treatment deserves a brief mention. Because the lesions usually remit spontaneously in months or years, no specific treatment is suggested. However, if treatment is needed in the absence of remission or because of aesthetics or friction-related nuisance, surgery (cryosurgery, electrosurgery, CO_2 laser) or pharmacological therapy similar to any other HPV lesion can be considered (imiquimod, salicylic acid, podophyllin or trichloroacetic acid)

2.1.2. Condyloma acuminata

The prevalence of this entity, which is associated with human papillomavirus, has progressively increased in the developed world, affecting an estimated 6% of the population with an incidence close to 2% [50]. The most common viral types are 6 and 11. These types have a low carcinogenic potential, although others types with a higher carcinogenic potential are also associated with these lesions.

The most frequent mode of transmission is sexual contact, although it is not exclusive. The disease can also be transmitted vertically in the birth canal or by direct contact via the hands. Consequently, its presence in children does not necessarily imply sexual abuse.

In addition to infection by papilloma viruses Types 6 and 11 (HR of 12.42), the risk factors associated with condyloma age (HR of 0.43; if we compare 45-70 years against 18-30 years), high number of female sexual partners (HR of 5.69) and number of male partners (HR 4.53) [51]. Classically, it has been considered that there is an inverse association between circumcision and HPV prevalence in men, although meta-analyses are inconclusive [52].

The incubation period is variable, lasting from 3 weeks to 8 months (2 to 3 months on average) [50]. In addition, the infection can be present and contagious in the absence of lesions (subclinical infection). Consequently establishing the source of infection is practically impossible, and it should be assumed that both members of a couple are infected at the time of diagnosis.

In the beginning, the lesion is asymptomatic because it initially affects the basal epidermal cells. With time, a papule lesion appears, and new lesions develop from there. The evolution of the disease depends on viral (type, virulence), host (e.g., age, sex, promiscuity, immune system, toxic abuse) and other factors (location, friction). After infection, evident lesions may appear, or the lesions may be difficult to appreciate, even with the help of 3 to 5% acetic acid (inapparent subclinical forms). In other cases, it is impossible to diagnose the lesion even after histopathological study, and only in situ hybridization (latent forms) can provide a diagnosis. The evolution of the disease allows the coexistence of the three types of lesions.

Clinically, several forms have been described:

- Classical form: These lesions are defined as a fleshy mass, exophytic and vegetating, pedunculated, with digitations, classically described as having the shape of a cauliflower (Figure 11). They are keratinized, and the color is variable but generally clear. They are located in humid areas exposed to friction, such as the balanopreputial sulcus, the frenulum and the introitus or meatus of the genitals. When they are located in the oral cavity, the nodules and digitations are frequently softer, but the cauliflower shape is more pronounced [53]. Their most frequent location is on the superior lip, the lingual frenulum, the back of the tongue, the inferior lip and the corner of the mouth. The size is also variable, from 1-2 cm to 15 or 20 cm.

- Spicule form: These lesions are more hyperkeratosic, rough and digitiform than the classical form. They are usually isolated on the preputial mucosa or plate-clustered in the perianal zone.

- Papule form: These lesions are 1-mm papules that are well delimited, non-confluent, cupuliform and disseminated. When located in the penis, they require differential diagnosis from hypertrophic sebaceous glands; heterotypic, pearly papules or hirsutoid papillomas; and Tyson's glands.

- Flat condyloma or leukoplakia: These lesions present a confluence of viral papules. They react poorly to acetic acid and do not respond to treatment.

- Macular form: These lesions take the form of erythematous spots with a vascular or granulomatous aspect, with or without a hypopigmented halo. They have a moist surface with a velvety aspect. They must be differentiated from bacterial or candida chronic balanoposthitis in immunosuppressed patients and from with Queyrat's erythroplasia.

- Micropapillar form: These lesions are small fibroepithelial projection with central capillaries.

- Inverse punctuated form: These lesions present as erythematous spots.

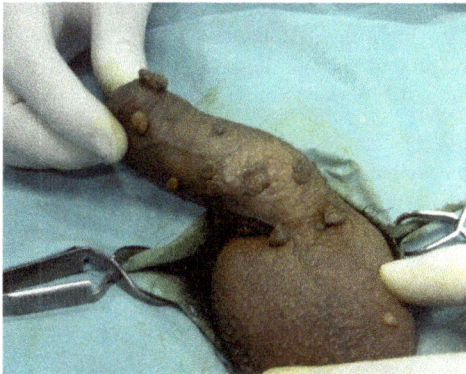

Figure 11. Multiple condyloma acuminata in penis in an HIV patient

All of these forms are usually asymptomatic, although they can produce pruritus, stinging or discrete hemorrhages from trauma. If they are large, they can produce a bad odor or pain. Dysuria, pollakiuria or hematuria can appear if the location is intraurethral, and a ureteroscopy will be necessary. If the lesions are located in the anus, they can produce constipation and dyschezia. An anuscopy with exfoliative cytology is recommended, particularly in passive homosexuals with lesions, as the risk of affecting the rectum is near 50%.

Other forms are much more striking and have benign tumor characteristics but are locally aggressive. These forms are the giant penile condyloma (Buschke-Lowenstein tumor) and the florid oral papillomatosis.

The diagnosis of acuminate condylomas is clinical, requiring a biopsy for confirmation because of atypical lesions, a malignant aspect, no improvement with therapy or immunological problems.

In addition to typical koilocytes, the histopathological study of the epidermis will show strong acanthosis with diverse degrees of papillomatosis, hyperkeratosis and parakeratosis and a total obliteration of the granule cell layer. The crests tend to be elongated and point towards the center of the lesion, and the dermis presents increased vascularization with the presence of capillary thrombosis. In unclear lesions, immunohistochemical staining with peroxidase-antiperoxidase or MIB1 antibody (against the protein Ki-67) allows the direct visualization of a viral presence [50].

Treatment will depend on the size and location of the lesion, and surgery is preferable when lesions are large or are located in the urethral meatus.

2.1.3. Bowenoid papulosis

This disease is fundamentally associated with HPV Type 16, although it is also related to Types 18 and 33 (along with Type 16, these are the most oncogenic types), 32 (in oral mucosa lesions) and, in a small percentage of cases, to Types 31, 34, 35, 39, 42, 48, 51 and 54 [54]. Bowenoid papulosis is most frequent in the second and third decades of life (earlier than for Bowen's disease). It is located in the prepuce and less frequently in the glans. In women, it appears in the labia majora and minora, the clitoris, the groin and around the anus. It is less common in the oral area and is generally associated with HIV, thus possibly posing a differential diagnosis problem [55].

The lesions are defined as macular lesions (less frequent), papular or multiple verruciform. They are less than 1 cm in size and are usually confluent. They are usually hyperpigmented, pink to red-violet or brown (Figure 12). The surface is regular with scales or velvety with a soft consistency. The disease is asymptomatic, and the lesions rarely ulcerate or bleed (unlike in Bowen's disease).

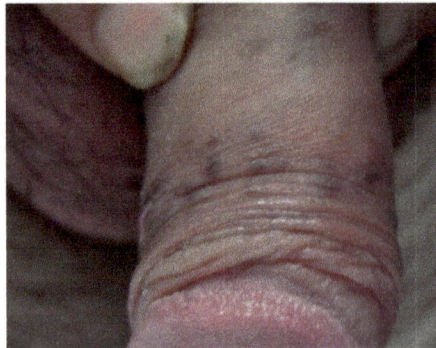

Figure 12. Violaceous papular lesions on the back of foreskin support Bowenoid papulosis

The pathological anatomy has similar characteristics to Bowen's disease and few differences from in situ squamous cell carcinoma. At times, Bowenoid papulosis is considered a low-degree in situ carcinoma [54, 56]. We find hyperkeratosis with parakeratosis foci and hyper-granulosis, irregular acanthosis, occasional papillomatosis and vacuolated keratinocytes with mitosis in the same phase. Such findings distinguish these lesions from those of Bowen's disease, in which maturation is disorderly and appears as dysplasia. The basement membrane is intact [9]. However, nuclear alterations can also appear, along with dyskeratosis, atypical mitosis and multinucleated keratinocytes [11]. In fact, some authors propose that there is a risk of neoplastic transformation in 2.6% of the cases, and the frequency is higher if there is some type of immunodeficiency [57].

The main differential diagnosis is made with Bowen's disease but may also involve condyloma acuminata, Queyrat's erythroplasia, lichen planus, psoriasis, seborrheic keratosis, anular granuloma and molluscum contagiousum [54, 57].

Treatment should be conservative because of the high percentage of spontaneous regression, although the terms are variable and the lesions can persist for 2-3 weeks to 2-3 years or longer. Simple partial or total excision has been used, as have ablative treatments and local or systemic pharmacological approaches [54, 56]. A wait-and-see approach with clinical management and/ or repeated biopsies is also a good option [54].

2.2. Malignant mucosal lesions

2.2.1. Queyrat's erythroplasia

Queyrat's erythroplasia is an in situ squamous carcinoma (intraepidermic) that can evolve into invasive squamous carcinoma in 3 to 5% of cases. Aside from human papillomavirus (princi-pally Serotypes 16 and 18), the risk factors that influence the development of erythroplasia include sun exposure, light skin, radiation, PUVA therapy, immunosuppression, smegma and poor hygiene [58].

Clinically, Queyrat's erythroplasia presents as an erythematous-squamous plate of slow growth and irregular borders (Figure 13), with a smooth surface, hyperkeratosic or warty appearance and pigmentation in less than 2% of the cases. It is usually present in the multiple form, although it can also appear as a single lesion. It is frequently located in the penis, although it can also be found in the urethra, vulva, oral mucosa, tongue and conjunctiva. The diagnosis must be made by a biopsy or the exeresis of the lesion, and cellular atypia with an intact basal membrane is typically observed. Differential diagnosis is required against psoriasis, seborrheic dermatosis, actinic keratosis, invasive squamous cell carcinoma, surface basocellular carcino-ma and Paget's disease [59].

2.2.2. Vulvar cancer

The vulva is the only visible and external part of the female genital system, and its pathology should be well-known and quickly diagnosed. However, vulvar pathology has been under-valued because it is not very symptomatic or very frequent. Vulvar cancer has a biological and

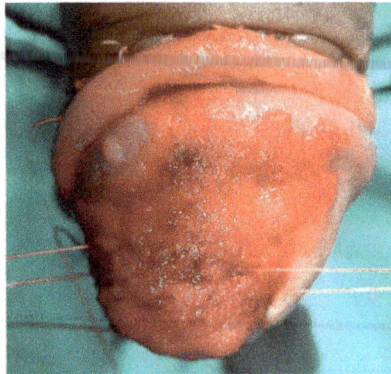

Figure 13. Slightly raised erythematous lesion occupying the glans. Queyrat's erythroplasia

social impact and requires early diagnosis. It represents 3 to 4% of gynecologic cancers; epidermoid carcinoma is the most frequent, representing 90% of malignant vulvar tumors.

Vulvar exploration must be meticulous and exhaustive, especially in women with referred symptomatology. Subclinical lesions frequently require special detection techniques. The study must be performed via simple vulvoscopy and expanded with a complete biopsy of the suspicious lesion. An adequate anamnesis, in which personal background is documented (sexually transmitted diseases, toxic habits, hygienic habits and immunosuppression status) is important. In addition, visual inspection and inspection with panoramic light must be performed to observe coloration, trophism and macroscopic lesions, and the other female genitalia must be examined [60]. The vulvoscopic exam should be undertaken with frequent applications of 5% acetic acid to corroborate the white color reaction. Another applicable study is the Collins test, which involves the application of 1% toluidine blue, followed by washing with 3% acetic acid. However, the most definitive test for diagnosis is a vulvar biopsy with a rongeur, punch, scalpel or scissors.

It has been observed that one of the etiological agents implicated in the development of vulvar cancer is the human papillomavirus, specifically Serotype 16, although other serotypes that influence molecular mechanisms associated with cancer development, such as inactivation of the p53 gene, have also been implicated.

Although epidermoid vulvar cancer is the most common type, other types include warty carcinoma, Paget's disease of the vulva, adenocarcinoma, basocellular carcinoma, Bartholin gland carcinoma and vulvar sarcoma.

Our primary focus will be the clinical description of squamous or epidermoid vulvar carcinoma, which is the type most directly related to human papillomavirus. Squamous or epidermoid carcinoma is characterized by the presence of long-evolution pruritus (between 40 and 50%); flux or vulvar exudate, sometimes with bad odor; bleeding outside menstruation; vulvar pain; dysuria; and tumor formation (in almost 50% of patients). In the initial stages, this carcinoma is observed as an indurated, overelevated lesion; sometimes it can be hyperkeratosic, with variable coloration ranging from erythematous to white. In the initial phases, it can coincide with other lesions, such as lichen sclerosus, vulvar intraepithelial neoplasia (VIN), genital atrophy, squamous cell hyperplasia and overinfection with lichenification from scratching [61]. In more advanced phases, the squamous carcinoma presents as reddish, ulcerated lesions (Figure 14), either polypoid or nodular, or with white coloration, even when associated with palpable inguinal lesions.

Different stages can be differentiated by tumor size, ganglionar affectation and metastatic affectation. Stages IA, IB and II are usually the initial stages of the localized disease, and the most frequently affected zones are the anterior part of the vulva, followed by the labia majora and minora, the clitoris and the vulvar fourchette. In more advanced stages, it frequently propagates to neighboring organs, such as the anus, urethra and vagina. Dissemination to other organs such as bone, liver, lungs and brain is rare [62].

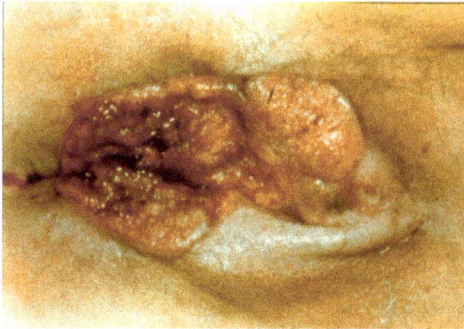

Figure 14. Irregular and ulcerated lesion on the vulva histopathologically compatible with vulval cancer

2.2.3. Penile carcinoma

Penile carcinoma is a rare malignant tumor, but it has a major medical and psychological impact. Amongst the risk factors that influence and contribute to its development are phimosis, balanoposthitis, ultraviolet radiation, smoking, cervical cancer in the partner, sexually transmitted diseases, poor hygiene and human papillomavirus, fundamentally Types 16 and 18, which are highly metastatic.

There are different precursor lesions that carry the risk of developing penile spinocellular cancer or penile squamous-cell invasive carcinoma, such as bowenoid papulosis, balanitis xerotica obliterans, cutaneous horn and Queyrat's erythroplasia that affect the mucous membrane; or Bowen's disease that affects the rest of the genital area.

Penile spinocellular cancer or penile squamous-cell invasive carcinoma is the histological type present in more than 95% of malignant penile invasive neoplasias. Approximately half are well differentiated. They usually metastasize via the lymphatic system, first at the inguinal-femoral level, then at the pelvis; finally, they migrate to distant areas. The hematogenous spread can affect the lungs, liver, brain, pleura, bone, skin and other organs [63].

Clinically, penile carcinoma initially manifests as an elevated papular-type or pustulous lesion that does not resolve with topical treatment and can evolve into an exophytic, polypous or infiltrating lesion (Figure 15). Erythematous and superficial lesions can also appear. They are usually located in the glans and less frequently in the balanopreputial sulcus. If the patient presents phimosis or if the lesion is under the prepuce or is evolved, it protrudes outside the prepuce. These patients can present initially with an inguinal-level adenopathic lesion resulting from an inflammatory or metastatic reaction. The lesions can be single or multiple, fixed or free and can become overinfected.

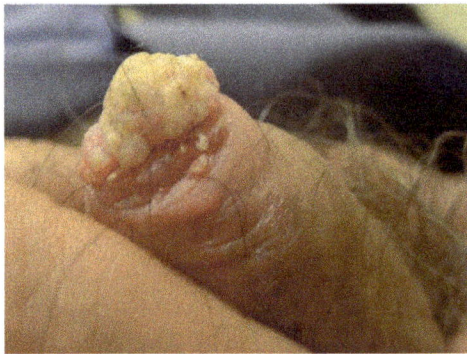

Figure 15. Excrescent lesion on the penis, that after surgery, histological study confirmed penile cancer

The natural clinical evolution of the disease normally progresses through several stages. Initially a papillar lesion appears, gradually ulcerates and overinfects, affecting Buck's fascia and potentially invading the cavernous bodies [64]. In a second stage, the lesion disseminates via the lymphatic pathway, especially at the inguinal level. Finally, the disease produces distant metastases that are uncommon upon initial diagnosis.

2.2.4. Anal carcinoma

Anal carcinoma is not very frequent, representing 1 to 2% of digestive system cancers. Among the risk factors that influence the development and genesis of this cancer, in addition to human papillomavirus (fundamentally, Types 16, 18 and 31), are poor hygiene, chronic anal irritation, smoking, seropositivity for herpes virus, seropositivity for human immunodeficiency virus, sexual promiscuity, passive anal sex, anal fistulas and other less-relevant factors.

Generally, the most frequent type of anal carcinoma associated with papilloma virus is squamous or spinocellular carcinoma. There are also other types, such as basaloid, cloacogenic, basal-squamous, epithelioid, trasitional and mucoepidermoid cancer. As observed with cancer in other locations, there may be premalignant lesions with the potential for developing into anal carcinoma, as in Bowen's disease, Paget's disease, Bowenoid papulosis, leukoplakia and condyloma acuminata [65].

Clinically, anal cancer presents with hemorrhages and constant pain associated with other symptoms, such as changes in defecation, secretion that can be purulent if there is overinfection and pruritus. In more advanced stages, the patient has the sensation of a palpable mass, and the tumor can become ulcerated. In the first stages, during which bleeding, pruritus and pain occur, anal cancer can be easily confused with hemorrhoidal processes, perianal fistulas or anal fissures; thus, it is necessary to carefully explore the area [65, 66].

Exploration of the anal channel must be directed toward identifying the lesion or possible lesions; establishing their size, anatomical limits and relationship with the dentated line; and looking for any other concomitant lesion with different characteristics. Small lesions must be totally resected for study, while bigger lesions require a biopsy.

2.2.5. Cervical cancer

Cancer in the neck of the uterus is the second most common cancer in women (the first is breast cancer). Among the multiple causes related to the development of this neoplasia are smoking, immunosuppression, chlamydia infection, poverty, poor hygienic/dietary conditions, different dietary habits, diethylstilbestrol, promiscuity, early-age pregnancy and infection with human papillomavirus. Different types of human papillomavirus have been implicated in the development of cervical cancer. The most important types are 16, 18, 31, 33 and 45, and the first two are responsible for approximately 2/3 of all cancers in the neck of the uterus.

Cervical cancer can be prevented with cytologic techniques and by applying the Papanicolaou method. The objective is to establish an early diagnosis so that therapy can begin quickly; because the initial stages of this cancer are asymptomatic, frequent and exhaustive reviews are important [67].

As we have previously mentioned, the initial stages of cervical cancer do not produce symptoms; however, when the tumor increases (Figure 16), women present abnormal vaginal bleeding that can occur between menstrual cycles, following sexual relations and after menopause, or the bleeding can prolong menstrual-bleeding periods [68]. Cervical cancer can also be associated with other symptoms, such as pelvic pain and dyspareunia, and it can increase flux and vaginal secretions.

3. Other types of tumors

Next, we will describe other tumoral clinical processes that have been associated with HPV infection. It is important to highlight that the majority of people infected with HPV do not present symptomatology or health-problems related to the infection. In 90% of the cases, the immune system naturally eliminates the virus within two years. However, sometimes HPV infections become chronic, and they can be associated with other lesions or tumors aside from the previously described pathology. These lesions and tumors include warty lesions in the oral

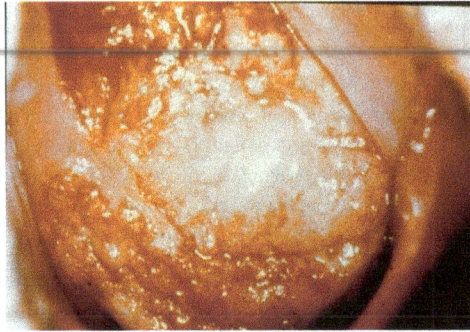

Figure 16. Excrescent ulcerated lesions in cervix clinically compatible with carcinoma

cavity and pharynx (recurrent respiratory papillomatosis [RRP]) and rare but serious cancers such as those of the bladder, lung and oropharynx (the posterior area of the throat, including the base of the tongue and the tonsils).

3.1. Oral and cervical cancer

Eighty-five percent of oral cavity cancers are epidermoid (we will be referring primarily to this type), and their incidence increases progressively with age. HPV 16/18 are the types most frequently associated with oral and cervical cancer, especially in the oropharynx and tonsils [69, 70]. The principal lesions associated with HPV infection in the oral cavity are oral papillomatosis (associated with HPV 6 and 11), focal epithelial hyperplasia (HPV 13 and 32) and erythroplasia (HPV 16).

Causal factors strongly associated with oral and cervical cancer are tobacco and alcoholic beverage consumption. Therefore, investigations to determine the possible etiological role of HPV will need to consider these factors. Several studies that controlled for age, gender, smoking, tobacco chewing and drinking have not observed significant differences among these factors for HPV detection in tumoral tissue, with the exception of smoking. That is, HPV DNA was less likely to be found in the biopsy samples of ex-smokers and smokers than those of people who had never smoked. In comparison, patients with more than a single sexual partner had a higher possibility of HPV DNA detection than those who had a single lifetime sexual partner. Similar observations were obtained when comparing oral sex practitioners versus nonpractitioners. These associations were similar for oral cavity and oropharynx cancer [71].

The clinical manifestations of patients with epidermoid carcinoma are very diverse and depend on the location and size of the lesions. Leukoplakia and erythroplasia are premalignant lesions over which neoplastic lesions can develop. The most common initial presentation is a painful ulcer. Pain appears precociously in lesions that affect the base of the mouth or the gums; however, it is delayed in other locations, such as the base of the tongue. Dysphagia occurs with lesions that affect the oropharynx or that alter the mobility of the tongue. Hemorrhage usually occurs in ulcerated lesions. Other associated symptoms include dysphonia, tooth mobility or loss, anesthesia or trismus. Clinically, the tumor manifests in exophytic, ulcerative or warty forms (Figure 17). It is important to completely explore the entire oral cavity and to obtain a biopsy of the lesion when it is accessible, or a puncture-aspiration with a fine needle when biopsy is difficult. The neck must be carefully explored to detect adenopathies, and a radiologic or endoscopic study should be performed to establish tumoral extension.

The importance of HPV in oropharyngeal carcinoma patients is increasing. It is important to determine the presence or absence of this virus in patients who present epidermoid carcinoma in the oropharynx or who have cervical adenopathy of uncertain origin to obtain information on the patient's therapeutic attitude, prognosis and survival [72].

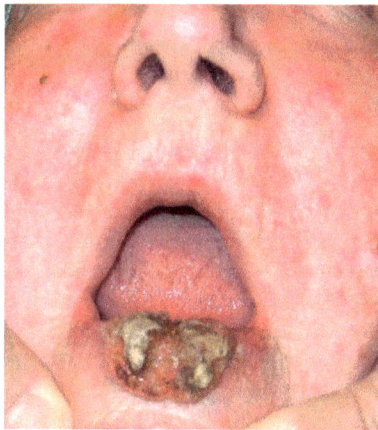

Figure 17. Squamous cell carcinoma of the lip: exophytic, ulcerative, warty tumor of the lower lip.

3.2. Recurrent respiratory papillomatosis and lung cancer

Recurrent respiratory papillomatosis (RRP) is characterized by warty lesions produced by HPV infection of the airways. These lesions can obstruct the airways or cause dysphonia, among other symptoms. Two clinical variants are recognized depending on the patient's age at onset: the juvenile (before 5 years) and the adult form (after 40 years). The juvenile variant is more frequent and severe than the adult form. HPV 6 and 11 are the types most frequently involved in this clinical picture [73]. HPV 11 produces a more severe clinical picture than the other viral variants do, and HPV 11 infection more frequently requires tracheostomy. The transmission mechanisms of the infection are not always clear, but sexual transmission should be considered in adults, and mother-to-child transmission should be considered in the juvenile RRP variant. In this regard, some risk factors associated with this variant have been confirmed. These risk factors include a mother younger than 20 years, vaginal delivery and being firstborn. Sexual abuse should also be suspected in diseased children older than 5 years.

The symptomatology of this disease is varied, and diagnosis is generally delayed because of the disease's rareness. The predominant symptoms are related to upper airway obstruction caused by the frequent involvement of the larynx. These symptoms can occasionally threaten the patient's life. Dyspnea, snoring, dysphonia, the sensation of a foreign body in the throat, coughing or wheezing are common clinical symptoms. The diagnosis should be suspected with these clinical data, and appropriate complementary tests should be requested for diagnosis. Such diagnostic tests include bronchoscopy or laryngoscopy, which will show typical warty images on the airway. HPV serotyping is necessary and has prognostic value.

Lung cancer is one of the most common cancers. It has one of the highest mortality rates among cancers and is particularly associated with smoking. The majority of cancerous lung tumors originate from the bronchial epithelia (bronchogenic carcinomas); the rest derive from other cells and constitute a more heterogeneous group. The maximal incidence is from 40 to 70 years, and the disease is more frequent among men. The diagnosis is usually made late, and only 15% of the patients present a localized disease. Usually there is ganglionar or metastatic disease upon diagnosis. Several histological subtypes have been distinguished and have important prognostic implications. These subtypes are squamous cell carcinoma, adenocarcinoma, large cell carcinoma and microcytic carcinoma.

The most important etiological factors are the substances inhaled when smoking cigarettes;, thus, the risk increases 60- to 70-fold in an individual who smokes two packs per day. The risk diminishes if the habit is abandoned, but it does not become equal to that of nonsmokers. In addition, genetic alterations in lung cancer patients have been widely studied and corroborate the oncogene activation (Ras, Myc, among others) and inactivation of tumor-suppressing genes (p53). The relationship between lung cancer and HPV infection was initially established in 1975 [74]. More recent studies have suggested a 25% HPV infection prevalence associated with lung cancer, with an important variation between countries [75]. High-risk subtypes that have been detected are 16, 18, 31, and 33; the lower-risk subtypes are 6 and 11. Therefore, it has been suggested that HPV infection is the second-most-important risk factor after smoking. The transmission mechanism is not properly known, but it appears that multiple sex partners and oral and anal sex may be among the transmission factors. A higher-than-expected incidence of lung cancer was detected in cervical and anal cancer patients in whom HPV was implicated [76], suggesting a possible hematogenous dissemination of the virus. The action mechanisms that explain the role of HPV in tumor promotion and development are complex. In addition, it has recently been demonstrated that HPV and smoking can have a synergistic effect on tumor promotion [77].

The symptomatology that the disease produces is associated with growth and obstruction of the lung and neighboring structures. Although in some cases the tumors are diagnosed in their asymptomatic phase using radiography, most of the tumors debut with coughing, hemoptysis, wheezing, stridor or dyspnea. If there is eccentric growth, the tumor can irritate the pleura, leading to pain, coughing and restrictive-origin dyspnea. If the tumor grows towards the thorax, it can produce tracheal obstruction, esophageal compression, snoring (by paralyzing the recurrent laryngeal nerve), hemidiaphragm elevation (phrenic nerve paralysis) or Horner's syndrome, Pancoast syndrome or superior vena cava syndrome. Paraneoplastic syndromes can also be detected and are associated with the ectopic production of such hormones as PTH and ACTH by microcytic carcinomas. Eaton-Lambert myasthenic syndrome and Trousseau's migratory thrombophlebitis may also be associated with this clinical presentation, although in very low percentages.

Metastasis is observed in 50% of epidermoid carcinoma patients, 80% of those with adenocarcinoma and up to 95% in microcytic carcinoma patients. The metastases can appear in the brain, bones, bone marrow and liver.

3.3. Bladder cancer

Bladder cancer is the malignant tumor that most frequently affects the urinary tract. Its prognosis is highly variable. It is one of the most common cancers among men. The majority of the tumors are transitional cell carcinomas (90%), which have a high tendency to recur after treatment or become invasive and overwhelm subjacent muscular structures. AS a consequence, it is necessary to periodically control the urothelium. Pure epidermoid carcinoma constitutes 3% of cases, and adenocarcinoma constitutes 2%.

Tobacco consumption also plays an important role in the development of this tumor; it is thought to contribute to up to 50% of urothelial carcinomas. Other risk factors implicated in the development of this tumor are certain drugs, such as cyclophosphamide and phenacetin; infection with Schistosoma haematobium; and external radiotherapy. Genetic alterations have also been detected, including deletions of the RB gene or p53 overexpression. The association between bladder cancer and HPV infection is still controversial, considering that one of the virus's natural reservoirs is the urethra and that it could easily migrate to the bladder. Some authors have strongly implicated the virus in tumors that affect younger patients. A recent meta-analysis of all the published studies on the relationship between HPV and bladder cancer concludes that there is a moderate and clear association amongst both processes and establishes an odds ratio of 2.13 [78]. However, more studies are needed that evaluate the pathogenic relationship between the processes.

The clinical manifestations of this tumor are varied. Hematuria is related to exophytic-growth tumors, whereas irritation symptoms (dysuria, pollakiuria and micturition urgency) are more frequent in patients with localized disease (in situ carcinoma), even though they can also be observed in patients who present tumoral invasion towards the muscle layer of the bladder. However, other important causes of macroscopic and microscopic hematuria must be considered, such as cystitis and prostate problems. When hematuria is found, a complete evaluation should be performed. This evaluation should include urinary cytology, ultrasound (Figure 18) or intravenous pyelogram and cystoscopy. Less common clinical manifestations are pain or nuisance in the renal fossa related to urethral obstruction or pelvic pain and lower extremity edema produced by the obstruction of the iliac vessels. With less frequency, metastatic disease is the first manifestation of these tumors. Once bladder cancer is diagnosed, it is very important to establish whether the muscle layer has been affected. To determine this, ultrasound, CT and nuclear magnetic resonance are of great help.

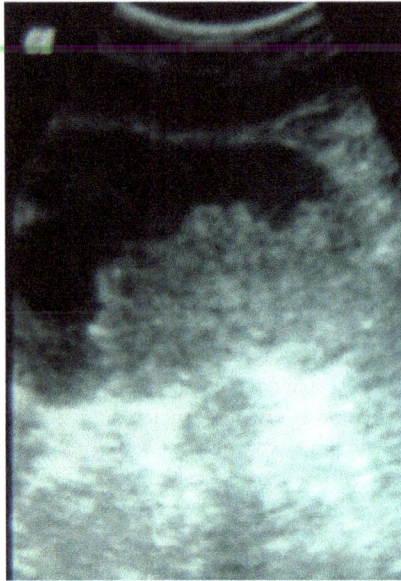

Figure 18. Bladder ultrasound, in which, it can be observed the presence of a lesion that histologically was urothelial cancer.

3.4. Other tumors

Other tumors, including cancers of the larynx, sinonasal tract, nasopharynx, salivary gland, vulva, esophagus and breast, have also been associated with HPV infection [79].

Author details

Miguel Ángel Arrabal-Polo[1], María Sierra Girón-Prieto[2], Jacinto Orgaz-Molina[1],
Sergio Merino-Salas[1], Fernando Lopez-Carmona Pintado[1], Miguel Arrabal-Martin[1] and
Salvador Arias-Santiago[3]

1 San Cecilio University Hospital, Spain

2 Granada District, Spain

3 Baza Hospital. Granada School of Medicine, Spain

References

[1] Kilkenny, M, Merlin, K, Young, R, & Marks, R. . The prevalence of common skin conditions in Australian school students: 1. Common, plane and plantar viral warts. Br J Dermatol. 1998; 138: 840-5.

[2] Beutner, K. R, Becker, T. M, & Stone, K. M. Epidemiology of human papillomavirus infections. Dermatol Clin. (1991). , 9, 211-8.

[3] Chopra, K. F, & Tyring, S. K. The impact of the human immunodeficiency virus on the human papillomavirus epidemic. Arch Dermatol. (1997). , 133, 629-33.

[4] Finkel, M, & Finkel, D. Warts among meat handlers. Arch Dermatol. (1984). , 120, 1314-7.

[5] Keefe, M, Al-ghamdi, A, Coggon, D, et al. Cutaneous warts in butchers. Br J Dermatol. (1994). , 130, 9-14.

[6] Keefe, M, Al-ghamdi, A, Coggon, D, et al. Cutaneous warts in butchers. Br J Dermatol (1994). , 130, 9-14.

[7] Keefe, M, Al-ghamdi, A, Coggon, D, et al. Butchers' warts: no evidence for person to person transmission. Br J Dermatol (1994). , 130, 15-17.

[8] Cobb, M. W. Human papilloma virus infection. J Am Acad Dermatol. (1990). , 22, 547-66.

[9] Dyall-smith, D, Trowell, H, & Dyall-smith, M. L. Benign human papilloma virus infection in renal transplant recipients. Int J Dermatol. (1991). , 30, 785-9.

[10] Milburn, P. B, Brandsma, J. L, Goldsman, C. I, et al. Disseminated warts and evolving squamous cell carcinoma in a patient with acquired immunodeficiency syndrome. J Am Acad Dermatol. (1988). , 19, 401-5.

[11] Kang, S, & Fitzpatrick, T. B. Debilitating verruca vulgaris in a patient infected with human immunodeficiency virus. Arch Dermatol. (1994). , 130, 294-6.

[12] Beutner, K. R, Becker, T. M, & Stone, K. M. Epidemiology of human papillomavirus infections. Derm Clin. (1991). , 9, 211-8.

[13] Zalaudek, I, Giacomel, J, & Cabo, H. Di Stefani A, Ferrara G, Hofmann-Wellenhof R, Malvehy J, Puig S, Stolz W, Argenziano G. Entodermoscopy: a new tool for diagnosing skin infections and infestations. Dermatology. (2008). , 216, 14-23.

[14] Grayson, W, Calonje, E, & Mckee, P. H. Infectious diseases of the skin. In: McKee PH, Calonje E, Granter SR editors. Pathology of the skin with clinical correlation. 3rd ed. England. Elsevier. (2005). , 838-44.

[15] Bae, J. M, Kang, H, Kim, H. O, & Park, Y. M. Differential diagnosis of plantar wart from corn, callus and healed wart with the aid of dermoscopy. Br J Dermatol. (2009). , 160, 220-2.

[16] Prose, N. S, Von Knebel-doeberitz, C, Miller, S, et al. Widespread flat warts associated with human papillomavirus type 5: a cutaneous manifestation of human immunodeficiency virus infection. J Am Acad Dermatol. (1990). , 23, 978-81.

[17] Egawa, K, Honda, Y, Inaba, Y, & Ono, T. Pigmented viral warts: a clinical and histopathological study including human papillomavirus typing. Br J Dermatol. (1998). , 138, 381-9.

[18] Egawa, K. Another viral inclusion wart different from myrmecia. Jpn J Dermatol. (1988). , 98, 1105-12.

[19] Berman, A, Domnitz, J. M, & Winkelmann, R. K. Plantar warts recently turned black: clinical and histopathologic findings. Arch Dermatol. (1982). , 118, 47-51.

[20] Ogino, A, & Ishida, H. Spontaneous regression of generalized molluscum contagiosum turning black. Acta Derm Venereol. (1984). , 64, 83-6.

[21] Egawa, K. New types of human papillomaviruses and intracytoplasmatic inclusion bodies. A classification of inclusion warts according to clinical features, histology and associated HPV types. Br J Dermatol. (1994). , 130, 158-66.

[22] Notarangelo, L, Casanova, J. L, Fischer, A, Puck, J, Rosen, F, Seger, R, & Geha, R. International Union of Immunological Societies Primary Immunodeficiency diseases classification committee. Primary immunodeficiency diseases: an update. J Allergy Clin Immunol. (2004). , 144, 677-87.

[23] Lazarczyk, M, Cassonnet, P, Pons, C, & Jacob, . . The EVER proteins as a natural barrier against papillomaviruses : a new insight into the pathogenesis of human papillomavirus infections. Microbiol Mol Biol Rev. 2009; 73: 348-70.

[24] Burger, B, Kind, F, Spoerri, I, et al. HIV-positive child with epidermodysplasia verruciformis-like lesions and homozygous mutation in TMC6. AIDS. (2010). , 24, 2758-60.

[25] Berthelot, C, Dickerson, M. C, Rady, P, He, Q, Niroomand, F, Tyring, S. K, & Pandya, A. G. Treatment of a patient with epidermodysplasia verruciformis carrying a novel EVER2 mutation with imiquimod. J Am Acad Dermatol. (2007). , 56, 882-6.

[26] Rogers, H. D. MacGregor JL, Nord KM et al. Acquired epidermodysplasia verruciformis. J Am Acad Dermatol. (2009). , 60, 35-20.

[27] Jacobelli, S, Laude, H, Carlotti, A, et al. Epidermodysplasia verruciformis in Human Deficiency Virus-infected patients. A marker of Human Papillomavirus-related disorders not affected by antiretroviral therapy. Arch Dermatol. (2011). , 147, 590-6.

[28] Aceituno-madera, P, Buendía-eisman, A, Arias-santiago, S, & Serrano-ortega, S. Changes in the incidence of skin cancer between 1978 and 2002. Actas Dermosifiliogr. (2010)., 101(1), 39-46.

[29] Cimino-mathews, A, Sharma, R, & Illei, P. B. Detection of human papillomavirus in small cell carcinomas of the anus and rectum. Am J Surg Pathol. (2012)., 36(7), 1087-92.

[30] Iannacone, M. R, Gheit, T, Waterboer, T, Giuliano, A. R, Messina, J. L, Fenske, N. A, et al. Case-control study of cutaneous human papillomaviruses in squamous cell carcinomas of the skin. Cancer Epidemiol Biomarkers Prev. (2012). Jun 15

[31] Alam, M, Caldwell, J. B, & Eliezri, Y. D. Human papillomavirus-associated digital squamous cell carcinoma: literature review and report of 21 new cases. J Am Acad Dermatol. (2003)., 48(3), 385-93.

[32] Iannacone, M. R, Wang, W, Stockwell, H. G, Rourke, O, Giuliano, K, & Sondak, A. R. VK, et al. Sunlight exposure and cutaneous human papillomavirus seroreactivity in Basal cell and squamous cell carcinomas of the skin. J Infect Dis. (2012). Aug;, 206(3), 399-406.

[33] Viarisio, D, Mueller-decker, K, Kloz, U, Aengeneyndt, B, Kopp-schneider, A, & Gröne, H. J. E. and E7 from beta HPV38 cooperate with ultraviolet light in the development of actinic keratosis-like lesions and squamous cell carcinoma in mice. PLoS Pathog. (2011). e1002125

[34] Del Pino M, Bleeker MC, Quint WG, Snijders PJ, Meijer CJ, Steenbergen RD. Comprehensive analysis of human papillomavirus prevalence and the potential role of low-risk types in verrucous carcinoma. Mod Pathol. (2012). Jun 8

[35] Lee, L. A, Huang, C. G, Liao, C. T, Lee, L. Y, Hsueh, C, Chen, T. C, Lin, C. Y, et al. Human papillomavirus-16 infection in advanced oral cavity cancer patients is related to an increased risk of distant metastases and poor survival. PLoS One. (2012). e40767.

[36] Forslund, O, Deangelis, P. M, Beigi, M, Schjølberg, A. R, & Clausen, O. P. Identification of human papillomavirus in keratoacanthomas. J Cutan Pathol. (2003)., 30(7), 423-9.

[37] Masuda, T, Hara, H, Shimojima, H, Suzuki, H, & Tanaka, K. Spontaneous complete regression of multiple Bowen's disease in the web-spaces of the feet. Int J Dermatol. (2006). Jun;, 45(6), 783-5.

[38] Lycka, B. A. owen's disease and internal malignancy. A meta-analysis. Int J Dermatol. (1989)., 28(8), 531-3.

[39] Nakajima, H, Teraishi, M, Tarutani, M, & Sano, S. High prevalence of coinfection with mucosal high-risk type HPV (HR-HPV) and cutaneous HR-HPV in Bowen's disease in the fingers. J Dermatol Sci. (2010)., 60(1), 50-2.

[40] Arias Santiago SAGirón Prieto MS, Aneiros Fernández J, Burkhardt Pérez P, Naranjo Sintes R. Descriptive analysis of basal cell carcinomas in patients aged more than 65 years old undergoing surgery in Hospital Clinic in Granada (Spain) in 2007. Rev Esp Geriatr Gerontol. (2009). , 44(2), 114-5.

[41] Aneiros-fernandez, J, Arias-santiago, S, Garcia-lopez, C, & Valle, O. F. Disfiguring basal cell carcinoma of the nose ("clown nose"). Ear Nose Throat J. (2012). E, 26-7.

[42] Arias-santiago, E l-A. h. m. e. d H, Aneiros-fernández, S, Ruiz-carrascosa, J, Armijo-lozano, J. C, & Naranjo-sintes, R. R. Basal cell carcinoma simulating bilateral cervical adenopathies. Rev Esp Geriatr Gerontol. (2009). , 44(6), 354-5.

[43] Buendía Eisman A, Arias Santiago S, Moreno-Gimenez JC, Cabrera-León A, Prieto L, Castillejo I, Conejo-Mir J. An Internet-based programme to promote adequate UV exposure behaviour in adolescents in Spain. J Eur Acad Dermatol Venereol. 2012 Feb 14. doi:j.(2012). x., 1468-3083.

[44] Paolini, F, Carbone, A, Benevolo, M, Silipo, V, Rollo, F, Covello, R, Piemonte, P, Frascione, P, Capizzi, R, Catricalà, C, & Venuti, A. Human Papillomaviruses, and Akt expression in basal cell carcinoma. J Exp Clin Cancer Res. (2011). , 16INK4a.

[45] Escutia, B, Ledesma, E, Serra-guillen, C, Gimeno, C, Vilata, J. J, Guillén, C, et al. Detection of human papilloma virus in normal skin and in superficial and nodular basal cell carcinomas in immunocompetent subjects. J Eur Acad Dermatol Venereol. (2011). , 25, 832-8.

[46] Ogun, O. A, Ogun, G. O, Bekibele, C. O, & Akang, E. E. Squamous papillomas of the conjunctiva: A retrospective clinicopathological study. Niger J Clin Pract. (2012). , 15(1), 89-92.

[47] Cordova, L, & Jimenez, C. Hiperplasia Epitelial Multifocal, Reporte Familiar Revisión de la Literatura. Revista Latinoamericana de Ortodoncia y Odontopediatria. Ortodoncia.ws edición electrónica mayo (2006). Obtenible en: www.ortodoncia.ws.

[48] Vera-iglesias, E, García-arpa, M, Sánchez-caminero, P, & Romero-aguilera, G. Cortina de la Calle P. Hiperplasia epitelial focal. Actas Dermosifiliogr. (2007). , 98, 621-3.

[49] Delgado, Y, Torrelo, A, Colmenero, I, & Zambrano, A. Focal epithelial hyperplasia]. Actas Dermosifiliogr. (2005). Dec;, 96(10), 697-9.

[50] Patel, R. V, Yanofsky, V. R, & Goldenberg, G. Genital warts: a comprehensive review. J Clin Aesthet Dermatol. (2012). Jun;, 5(6), 25-36.

[51] Anic, G. M, Lee, J. H, Villa, L. L, Lazcano-ponce, E, & Gage, C. José C Silva R, Baggio ML, Quiterio M, Salmerón J, Papenfuss MR, Abrahamsen M, Stockwell H, Rollison DE, Wu Y, Giuliano AR. Risk factors for incident condyloma in a multinational cohort of men: the HIM study. J Infect Dis. (2012). Mar 1;, 205(5), 789-93.

[52] Albero, G, Castellsagué, X, Giuliano, A. R, & Bosch, F. X. Male circumcision and genital human papillomavirus: a systematic review and meta-analysis. Sex Transm Dis.
(2012). Feb;Review., 39(2), 104-13.

[53] Kumaraswamy, K. L, & Vidhya, M. Human papilloma virus and oral infections: an
update. J Cancer Res Ther. (2011). Apr-Jun;Review., 7(2), 120-7.

[54] Trejo Ruiz JJCandela R. Papulosis bowenoide. Rev Cent Dermatol Pascua. (1999). ,
8(3), 147-50.

[55] Cox, D, Greenspan, D, Jordan, R. C, & Greenspan, J. S. Oral bowenoid papulosis in
an HIV-positive male. Oral Surg Oral Med Oral Pathol Oral Radiol Endod. (2006).
Oct;author reply 432., 102(4), 431-2.

[56] Shastry, V, & Betkerur, J. Kushalappa. Bowenoid papulosis of the genitalia successfully treated with topical tazarotene: a report of two cases. Indian J Dermatol. (2009).
Jul;, 54(3), 283-6.

[57] Divakaruni, A. K, Rao, A. V, & Mahabir, B. Erythroplasia of Queyrat with Zoon's balanitis: a diagnostic dilema. Int J STD AIDS. (2008). , 19, 861-3.

[58] Davis-daneshfar, A, & Trüeb, R. M. Bowen's disease of the glans penis (erythroplasia
of Queyrat) in plasma cell balanitis. Cutis. (2000). , 65, 395-8.

[59] Eifel, P. J, Bevek, J. S, & Thigpen, J. T. Cancer of the Cervix, vagina and vulva. Section
2. Cancer Ginecologic cancers. Cancer Principles & Practice of oncology (2000).

[60] Shepherd, J, Sideri, M, & Benedet, J. Carcinoma of the vulva. J Epidemiol Biostat
(1998).

[61] Medeiros, F, Nascimento, A. F, & Crump, C. P. Early vulvar squamous neoplasia: advances in classification, diagnosis and differential diagnosis. Adv Anat Pathol.
(2005). , 12, 20-6.

[62] Deem, S, Keane, T, & Bhavsar, R. Contemporary diagnosis and management of squamous cell carcinoma (SCC) of the penis. BJU Int. (2011). , 108, 1378-92.

[63] Heinlen, J. E, Buethe, D. D, & Culkin, D. J. Advanced penile cancer. Int Urol Nephrol.
(2012). , 44, 139-48.

[64] Simpson, J. A, & Scholefield, J. H. Diagnosis and management of anal intraepithelial
neoplasia and anal cancer. BMJ. (2011). Nov 4;343:d6818. doi:bmj.d6818

[65] Mao, C. Clinical findings among young women with genital human papilomavirus
infection. Am J Obstet Gynecol. (2003). , 188, 677-84.

[66] Solomon, D, Davey, D, Kurman, R, et al. Forum Group Members; Bethesda 2001
Workshop. The 2001 Bethesda System: terminology for reporting results of cervical
cytology. JAMA (2002). , 287, 2114-19.

[67] Evans, M. F, Adamson, C. S, Papillo, J. L, et al. Distribution of human papillomavirus
types in ThinPrep Papanicolaou tests classified according to the Bethesda 2001 termi-

nology and correlations with patient age and biopsy outcomes. Cancer (2006). , 106, 1054-64.

[68] Matuszewski, M, Michajlowski, I, Michajlowski, J, Sokolowska-wojdylo, M, Wlodarc-zyk, A, & Krajka, K. Topical treatment of bowenoid papulosis of the penis with imi-quimod. J Eur Acad Dermatol Venereol. (2009). Aug;, 23(8), 978-9.

[69] Herrero, R, Castellsagué, X, Pawlita, M, Lissowska, J, Kee, F, Balaram, P, et al. IARC Multicenter Oral Cancer Study Group. Human papillomavirus and oral cancer: the International Agency for Research on Cancer multicenter study. J Natl Cancer Inst. (2003). , 95(23), 1772-83.

[70] Pillai, M. R, Phanidhara, A, Kesari, A. L, Nair, P, & Nair, M. K. Cellular manifesta-tions of human papillomavirus infection in the oral mucosa. Journal of Surgical On-cology. (1999). , 71(1), 10-15.

[71] Sanjosé-llongueras, M. J, & García-garcía, A. M. Virus del papiloma humano y cán-cer: epidemiología y prevención. 4ª Monografías de la Sociedad Española de Epide-miología. 69008110

[72] Robinson, M, Schache, A, Sloan, P, & Thavaraj, S. HPV Specific Testing: A Require-ment for Oropharyngeal Squamous Cell Carcinoma Patients. Head Neck Pathol. (2012). Jul;6 Suppl , 1, 83-90.

[73] Omland, T, Akre, H, Vårdal, M, & Brøndbo, K. Epidemiological aspects of recurrent respiratory papillomatosis: A population-based study. Laryngoscope. (2012). , 122(7), 1595-9.

[74] Roglic, M, Jukic, S, & Damjanov, I. Cytology of the solitary papilloma of the bron-chus. Acta Cytologica. (1975). , 19(1), 11-13.

[75] Klein, F. Amin Kotb WFM, Petersen I. Incidence of human papilloma virus in lung cancer. Lung Cancer. (2009). , 65(1), 13-18.

[76] Hennig, E. M, Sou, Z, Karlsen, F, Holm, R, Thoresen, S, & Nesland, J. M. HPV posi-tive bronchopulmonary carcinomas in women with previous high-grade cervical in-traepithelial neoplasia (CIN III) Acta Oncologica. (1999). , 38(5), 639-647.

[77] Muñoz, J. P, González, C, Parra, B, Corvalán, A. H, Tornesello, M. L, Eizuru, Y, et al. Functional Interaction between Human Papillomavirus Type 16 E6 and E7 Oncopro-teins and Cigarette Smoke Components in Lung Epithelial Cells. PLoS One. (2012). e38178.

[78] Jimenez-pacheco, A, Exposito-ruiz, M, Arrabal-polo, M. A, & Lopez-luque, A. J. Meta-analysis of studies analyzing the role of human papillomavirus in the develop-ment of bladder carcinoma. Korean J Urol. (2012). , 53(4), 240-7.

[79] Isayeva, T, Li, Y, Maswahu, D, & Brandwein-gensler, M. Human papillomavirus in non-oropharyngeal head and neck cancers: a systematic literature review. Head Neck Pathol. (2012). Jul;6 Suppl , 1, 104-20.

Chapter 8

Human Papillomavirus Infection and Penile Cancer: Past, Present and Future

João Paulo Oliveira-Costa, Giórgia Gobbi da Silveira,
Danilo Figueiredo Soave,
Andrielle de Castilho Fernandes,
Lucinei Roberto Oliveira, Alfredo Ribeiro-Silva and
Fernando Augusto Soares

Additional information is available at the end of the chapter

1. Introduction

Penile squamous cell carcinoma (PSSC) is an uncommon malignant tumor, which accounts for less than 1% of adult male cancers in North America and Europe, but is markedly higher in developing locations, such as Asia, Africa and South America, representing up to 10% of tumors in men. Human papillomavirus (HPV) infection has shown an important role in penile cancer pathogenesis. In 2009, a systematic review of published literature found that 40% of penile tumors were HPV-related, and that type 16 HPV was the most common subtype in this group (Backes et al., 2009). Another interesting relation between HPV infection and penile cancer is the finding that specific histological subtypes are associated with HPV infection. Penile carcinomas with basaloid differentiation and warty features have shown a strong association with HPV infection, with recent studies showing that HPV infection is present in 76% of basaloid tumors, while the presence in verrucous cancer was 24.5% (Backes et al., 2009).

The recent literature suggests that the oncogenic potential of HPV integration into host DNA genome and their ability to manipulate cell cycle regulators is responsible for the establishment and maintenance of HPV genomes in the squamous epithelium and HPV-related PSCC cancer, which will result in deregulated expression of oncoproteins such as E6 and E7. The oncoprotein E6 is known to induce degradation of the tumor suppressor protein p53 and the oncoprotein E7 binds to retinoblastoma protein (pRb). Thus, the oncoproteins E6/E7 allow cells to evade cell cycle checkpoints and to entrance in S1 phase of cell cycle, leading to disruption of normal cell cycle controls.

Following cell division, infected cells leave the basal layer, migrate towards the suprabasal regions and begin to differentiate. Increased understanding of cervical pathogenesis has led to confirmation of HPV as an etiological agent for several cancers and consequently to the development of preventive vaccines targeting HPV antigens for the control of HPV-related cancers. HPV vaccine was developed as a result of the achievement of core technologies, that are able to produce virus-like particles (VLPs), which, in turn, are able to mimic the natural virus and elicit high-titers of virus neutralizing antibodies. With the progress through advanced stages of clinical trials and further exploration of combinatorial strategies, there is a great promise for significant advances also in the field of therapeutic HPV vaccine development, not only to cervical cancer, but other several malignancies related to HPV infection. Moreover, in this chapter we discuss the current status of HPV vaccines as well as the most common associated factors that might interfere on establishment of strategies that could control the HPV infections and the development of penile carcinoma associated to this infection.

2. Penile cancer

Penile malignancies are thought to arise from the accumulation of multiple mutations that may occur as consequence of progressive genetic instability. This intricate process of genetic instability may be caused by environmental factors, such as history of intense smoking, penile tears, phimosis, and poor genital hygienic habits. (Chaux & Cubilla 2012). In addition, a recent study conducted by Chaux et al. (2011) also described the poor education, penile chronic inflammation, genital warts and Human papillomavirus (related to number of sexual partners during lifetime) as environmental factors to malignant transformation.

There is a worldwide geographic difference in occurrence of penile malignancies that could be caused by differences in socio-economic status, cultural and religious conditions (Bleeker et al. 2009, Chaux & Cubilla, 2012). The higher incidences are frequent in tropical or subtropical regions of Latin America, Asia and Africa but have uncommon incidence rates in Europe, Japan, USA and Israel (Cubilla 2009). Recently, were reported higher incidence rates in underdeveloped regions such as Africa, South America, and Asia (2-4/100000 inhabitants) as compared with North America (United States) and Europe (0.3-1/100000 inhabitants) (Chaux & Cubilla, 2012). Pow-Sang et al. (2010) also described the penile malignancies prevalence rate among different populations. Prevalence rates in developed countries as Israel (0.1/100 000) and United States (0.3-1.8/100 000) and interestingly, compared with underdeveloped countries such as Uganda (2.8/100 000) and Brazil (1.5-3.7/100 000). Once again confirming the disease geographical difference and the influence of country development.

Squamous cell Carcinoma represents vast majority of histological subtype of primary penile malignancies with heterogeneous features due to differences in morphology pathogenesis and prognosis (Hakenberg & Protzel, 2012; Stankiewicz et al., 2012; Syed et al., 2012). Knowledge of origin and progression of penile squamous cell carcinoma depends on an intricate relation between anatomy and histopathology.

The anatomy of the penis is complex and has important implications to define predictive risk model and delineate the prognostic factors (Chaux & Cubilla, 2012). The same authors described 3 anatomical compartments in the penis (Glans, Foreskin and Coronal Sulcus) where the malignant neoplasms may be originated (Fig 1). However, the penile malignant neoplasms have a predilection to originate first on the Gland followed by Foreskin inner mucosa and lastly the Coronal Sulcus is rarely affected by neoplastic entity.

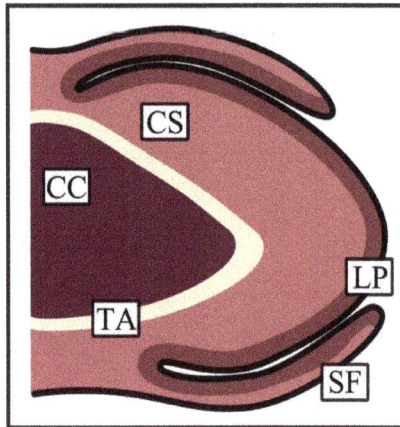

Figure 1. Paraurethral longitudinal section presenting anatomical levels of the Penis. **CC:** Corpus Cavernosum; **CS:** Corpus Spongiosum; **LP:** Lamina Propria; **SF:** Skim of the Foreskim and **TA:** Tunica Albuginea. (Adapted from Chaux & Cubilla 2012).

Recently, Hernandez et al. (2008) performed an epidemiological study with 4967 United States men with the diagnosis of penile squamous cell carcinoma. Thirty four percent of patients (1712) presented neoplasms arising in gland, 13.2% in prepuce, 5.3% in penis shaft, 4.5%, in overlapping of penis, and 42,5% in unspecified site. Lesions generally initiate on the glans and slowly extend to involve completely the glans and shaft of the penis. During the neoplasm progress Buck's fascia act as a natural barrier to local tumor invasion defending the corporal bodies from tumoral expansion (Pow-Sang et al. 2010). This assessment is schematically illustrated in figure 2.

The anatomy of the penis presents a pivotal role in tumor invasion and prognosis of cancer. Moreover, the TNM staging system is based, at least partially, on the commitment of these anatomical levels (Velazquez et al. 2010). The glans can be divided in 4 levels: squamous epithelium, lamina propria, corpus spongiosum, and corpus cavernosum (corpus spongiosum, and corpus cavernosum are subdivided by the tunica albugínea). Anatomical levels in the foreskin, like in glans, are divided in squamous epithelium, lamina propria, dartos muscle, and outer skin (Chaux & Cubilla, 2012).

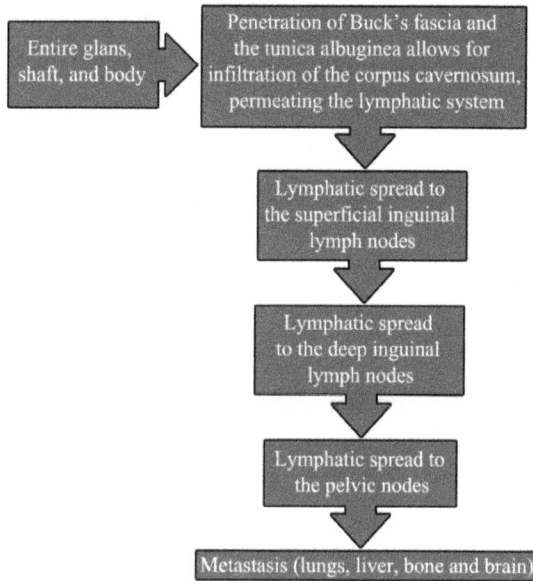

Figure 2. Natural history of penile cancer (Adapted from Pow-Sang et al. 2010).

A previous study suggests that different tumor histological features could be based on anatomical site. This hypothesis is sustained by the histological differences among the urethral segments and their corresponding neoplasms (Velasquez et al. 2005). As discussed previously, Squamous Cell Carcinoma of Usual Type (SCCUT) is the most frequent histopathologic diagnoses in penile malignancies (Chaux & Cubilla, 2012; Stankiewicz et al. 2012) affecting around 48%-65% of all type of penile carcinoma. Additionally, Epstein et al. (2011) reported 11 more subtypes of SCCUT (Table 1). Macroscopic features of SCCUT range from endophytic to irregular exophytic masses, presenting white-to-gray coloration. However, the reddish pigmentation also can be observed (Chaux et al. 2010). Microscopilly, the SCCUT is similar to oral, vulvar and cervical Squamous Cell Carcinomas (Cubilla et al. 2001). SCCUT may vary from well-differentiated tumors to anaplastic entities. Other presented feature is keratinization, ranging from highly keratinized, presented in well-differentiated tumors, until scarce or minimal keratinization observed in anaplastic neoplasm. Chaux et al. (2010)

Evidences from pertinent literature indicate the involvement of groin lymph nodes as the most relevant and unfavorable prognostic factors predicting cancer-specific survival in patients with penile squamous cell carcinoma. Numerically, in the same review, the 5-year cancer-specific survival rate for those presenting cN0 tumors were between 75% and 93%, compared with a 5-year cancer-specific survival rate for those presenting cN3 tumors ranging between 20% and 34%. There is a substantial decrease in the survival rates with N progression (Novara et al. 2007).

Classification of SCCs of the penis	
Subtype	Frequency (%)
Usual SCC	48-65
Basaloid carcinoma	4-10
Warty carcinoma	7-10
Verrucous carcinoma	3-8
Papillary carcinoma	5-15
Sarcomatoid carcinoma	1-3
Mixed carcinomas	9-10
Adenosquamous carcinoma	1-2
Pseudohyperplastic carcinoma	<1
Carcinoma cuniculatum	<1
Pseudoglandular carcinoma	<1
Warty-basaloid carcinoma	9-14

Table 1. Classification of Squamous Cell Carcinomas (SCCs) of the penis (Adapted from Chaux & Cubilla 2012)

Lopes et al. (2002) performed a study that aimed to investigate the p53 in Brazilian patients with PSCC to establish a new prognostic factor for lymph node metastasis and its possible influence on prognosis. This study observed the nodal stage as a factor that influenced survival (independent risk factors) in the univariate and multivariate analyses. Gunia et al. (2012) shown that p16INK4a is a good prognostic marker for penile squamous cell carcinomas, surpassing the prognostic impact of histologically confirmed koilocytosis. In their study, p16INK4a expression predicted better cancer specific survival rates. Furthermore, p16INK4a can be useful in differentiate subtypes of PSCC. According Chaux & Cubilla (2012), warty carcinomas tend to be p16INK4a positive, whereas giant condylomas and papillary and verrucous carcinomas are consistently negative.

Medical record analysis of 145 men with penile squamous cell carcinomas was performed to identify prognostic factors for lymph node involvement (Lopes et al. (1996)). The authors found that lymph node metastasis presents correlation with tumor thickness, lymphatic and vascular embolization. Interestingly, univariate analysis did not reached statistically significant values to pathologic stage of primary tumor, clinical lymph node stage (cN), and histological grade. However, histological grade may be considered an important prognostic factor in penile squamous cell carcinoma. In accord with Cubilla AL. 2009 these prognostic factors are predictive to the nodal spread, metastasis and tumoral dissemination.

Currently, different methods are employed to grade Penile Squamous Cell Carcinomas. For instance, Akhter et al. (2011) uses the Broder's system as histological grade system in Squamous Cell Carcinoma. In the Broder's system Penile Squamous Cell Carcinomas is stratified in 4 grades levels based only in differentiation of the cells: Grade I (well differentiated) presenting <25% undifferentiated cells; Grade II (Moderately differentiated) presenting <50% undifferentiated cells; grade III (Poorly differentiated) presenting <75% undifferentiated cells and grade IV (Anaplastic/Pleomorphic) >75% undifferentiated cells. Cell anaplasia degrees are also pointed as common approach to determine Penile Squamous Cell Carcinomas grading (Mikuz et al. 2004; Slaton et al. 2001), absence of anaplasia (well differentiated cells), grade 1; grade 2, moderately differentiated (<50% anaplastic cells); and grade 3, poorly differentiated (>50% anaplastic cells). Cubilla et al. (2009) reported a method to grade Penile Squamous Cell Carcinomas. Carcinomas with a minimal deviation from normal/hyperplastic morphology of squamous epithelium were considered Grade 1 (extremely well-differentiated). Grade 3 are tumors showing any proportion of anaplastic cells, identified as solid sheets or irregular small aggregates, cords or nests of cells with little or no keratinization, high nuclear cytoplasmic ratio, thick nuclear membrane, nuclear pleomorphism, clumped chromatin, prominent nucleoli and numerous mitosis. Grade 2 is composed by remainder tumors. Grading both extremes of the spectrum is simple and reproducible.

In summary, Penile Squamous Cell Carcinomas represents an aggressive locoregional malignancy with dissemination process may occurring 20-40% (Guimarães et al. 2009), a lethal disorder that often presents after significant delay (Barocas & Chang 2010). Usually, death occurs within 2 years after initial diagnosis (Guimarães et al. 2009). Accurate evaluation of clinical stage, anatomical site, regional lymph nodes, and metastatic disease presents a pivotal role in treatment planning to predict the survival outcome (Barocas & Chang, 2010).

3. HPV

Papillomaviruses are a family of pathogens that infect exclusively the epithelial tissues of amphibians, reptiles, birds and mammals (Franceschi, 2005). The viruses are grouped according to the anatomic site of infection and their preference for either cutaneous or mucosal squamous epithelium. The cutaneous types, or beta papillomaviruses, are usually found in the general population and cause common warts. In contrast, the alpha, or mucosotropic, papillomaviruses have been implicated in mucosal infections (Snow & Laudadio, 2010; Vidal & Gillison, 2008). The mucosotropic group of human papillomavirus comprises 15 species and infects the anogenital tract, upper aerodigestive tract and other head and neck mucosa (Chow et al., 2010). Because they are sexually transmitted and play important roles in diseases, these viruses have received much attention and research and clinical investment (Chow et al., 2010).

As molecular virology is depicted in details in another chapter, here we will only cover penile cancer-related aspects. Currently, over 200 HPV genotypes have been identified (Wang et al., 2012). HPVs with a high affinity for mucosal sites can be classified into non-oncogenic, or low-risk, types or as potentially oncogenic, or high-risk, types. Mucosal and genital HPVs can be divided into low-risk (HPVs 6, 11, 40, 42, 43, 44, 54, 61, 70, 72, 81) and high-risk (HPVs 16, 18, 31, 33, 35, 51, 52) types according to their presence in malignant lesions (Bosch et al., 2002; Muñoz et al., 2003).

The multiplicity of functions of the small papillomavirus oncoproteins, E5, E6 and E7, continues to be studied through last decades, although there are several mechanisms well established. Specifically, more than a dozen protein-protein interactions between E6 and cellular proteins have been shown (Villa et al., 2002). Taken into a carcinogenic point of view, E6 and E7 ORF are considered to play the most important roles, encoding for oncoproteins that allow viral replication and the immortalization and transformation of the epithelial cell that host the HPV DNA (Doorbar et al., 1991).

Proving the importance of p53 and pRb in cell cycle progression, the repression of HPV 16 E6 and E7 expression by dual shRNA transfection has been shown to be capable of restoring the p53 and pRb tumor suppressor pathways and activating apoptosis (Psyrri et al., 2009, Rampias et al., 2009). Thus, the demonstration of this tumor suppressor inactivation by the E6 and E7 HPV oncoproteins has provided a basic explanation for how the high-risk HPV types exert their oncogenic effects on cervical cells, and this explanation are under investigation to be related with other sites of HPV-infection. This is particularly important in penile cancer-associated HPV infection, whereas HPV16 seems to develop a pivotal role, and accounts for more than 60% of HPV-related tumors.

4. HPV impact in squamous cell homeostasis

Different from other viruses, HPV does not infect or replicate in antigen-presenting cells (APCs) of the epithelium nor induce cell lysis, which is a key escape mechanism to avoid that APC recognize and produce antigens derived from the virion, and alerts immune system. About more than 50% of infections present seroconversion in the patients, but the production of antibodies usually occurs only months after the initial infection (Vidal & Gillison, 2008). The life cycle of papillomaviruses is closely tied to the epithelial differentiation process. Infection occurs exclusively in squamous epithelial cells with a preference for the keratinocyte stem cell as the initial target of HPV infection, which will allow the maintenance of viral replication (Vidal & Gillison, 2008). The route of entry for HPV infection is microtraumas or small wounds in the skin or mucosal surface, which are particularly important in penile HPV-infection. These breaks in the epithelial surface allow the virus to access and persist in the nuclei of infected basal layer cells of the epithelium. Until now, no single receptor has been definitively identified and established as being responsible for HPV entry, although is believed that receptors closely related to wound healing might be preferential targets for HPV infection, such as α6 integrin and glycosamioglycan heparin (Vidal & Gillison, 2008).

As most viruses, HPV uses the host cell DNA machinery to maintain the production of viral progeny. This mechanism of viral-induced cell growth is very well known and is analogous to other viruses that disrupt the control of cell growth (Hebner & Laimins, 2006). Following cell division, as the basal cells divide into squamous epithelial cells, HPV establishes its DNA genome in the host cell nuclei, replicates and reaches a high copy number. Infected cells then leave the basal layer, migrate toward the suprabasal regions and begin to differentiate. In the basal layer phase, the HPV genome is maintained at a low copy number, providing a type of stock of viral DNA for further use in cell divisions. At the same time, 'early' viral genes (E5, E6 and E7) are expressed, resulting in enhanced proliferation of the infected cells and their lateral expansion, working to spread infection cells throughout epithelial tissue. While the basal cells and viral DNA divide, some daughter cells may be maintained in the basal layers, whereas other daughter cells move toward the upper layers of the epithelium and begin to differentiate. During this process in which the infected cells enter into the suprabasal layers, the viral genome replicates to a higher copy number; 'late' viral gene (L1 and L2) expression is initiated; and structural proteins, as such capsid proteins, are formed. Subsequently, virions are assembled and released as the upper layer of epithelium is shed (Fehrmann & Laimins, 2003; Scheurer et al., 2005; Vidal & Gillison, 2008).

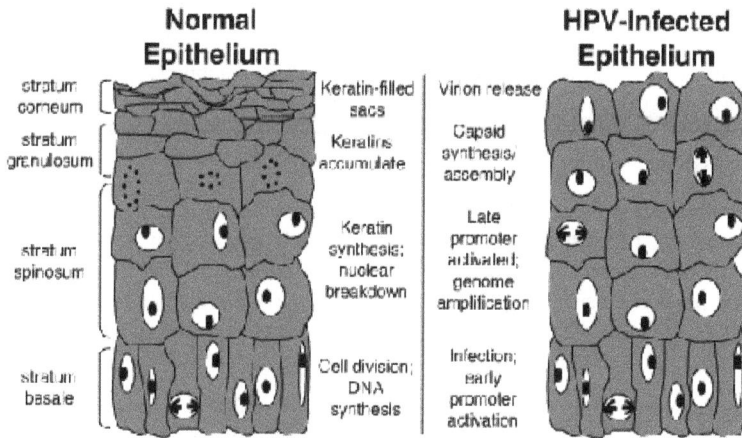

Figure 3. Representation of normal and HPV-infected epithelium according to the cellular differentiation and the differentiation-dependent viral functions (Adapted from Hebner & Laimins, 2006).

This provides an important microenvironment for cellular growth aberrations, and is particularly important in penile pre-neoplastic lesions. Several authors have reported a higher level of HPV detection in PIN, when compared to penile cancer, open field for a HPV importance in the development of tissue growth abnormalities, leading to a soil field for carcinogenesis. In this model, HPV would be an important co-factor in penile pre-neoplastic development. Due to all of his effects in cell growth and lack of cell cycle control, the formation of lesions such as PIN associated to other important factors in penile carcinogenesis (genera hygiene, phimosis, chronic inflammation, high number of sexual partners).

5. Prevalence of HPV infection in penile squamous cell carcinoma and histological considerations

In contrast with the high prevalence of HPV infection in cervix carcinomas, which may be detected in almost 100% of the cases, in penile carcinomas the detection is considerably lower, although it stills an important in penile pathogenesis. According to the current evidences, penile cancer can follow 2 distinct etiologic pathways: one is related to environmental factors, such as phimosis, smoking, poor personal hygiene and chronic inflammation; and other one is the HPV-related penile cancer (Rubin et al., 2001; Cubilla et al., 2010). Several studies have highlighted the prevalence of HPV infection in penile cancer, with an average prevalence of 47% to 48% in more than 60 studies (Backes et al., 2009; Miralles-Guri et al., 2009). Differently from cervix cancer, in penile cancer the prevalence of HPV infection varies according to histological subtypes, being strongly prevalent in basaloid and warty carcinomas, and lesser prevalent in keratinizing variants, such as verrucous, papillary and usual carcinomas (Guimarães et al., 2011). Before understanding the relationship between HPV and specific histological subtypes, a basic knowledge of penile cancer histology is required.

Squamous cell carcinoma of the penis is currently divided in 12 subtypes. Each one of this subtypes shows distinctive outcomes, and this high number of subtypes makes its difficult to characterize the disease. About half of penile cancers are of the usual squamous histology, while the rest is divided through the special types.

Basaloid carcinomas: represent 4-10% of penile tumors. Macroscopically, these tumors show an ulcerative aspect, presenting as a solid, firm invasively neoplasm, with necrosis foci. Microscopically, they present a nesting pattern, with each nest presenting a solid or central necrotic nest (comedonecrosis). Keratinization can be observed, although not pathognomonic. Cells presents as small, basofilic, basaloid, spindle or pleomorphic, with abundance of mitotic and apoptotic figures. Perineural and vascular invasions are often seen.

Warty carcinomas: represent 7-10% of all cases. It can be described as verruciform tumors, with an exoendophytical appearance, although a rare non-invasive exophytic tumor may be found. Histologically, a classical condylomatous papilla is observed, with a arborescent pattern, a central fibrovascular core, and keratinized cells, with presence of superficial and deep pleomorphic koilocytosis. Different from giant condillomas, in warty carcinomas these cells are typically malignant. Also, as a differential diagnosis, low-risk HPV or negative p16INK4a status favors a condilloma diagnosis. Prognosis is often good, with no signs of nodal involvment, although it might be present in deep invasive warty carcinoma (Chaux & Cubilla, 2012).

Verrucous carcinomas: represent 3-8% of the cases. Macroscopically are classically character-ized by exophytic, verrucoid white lesion, with a clear base separating them from the stroma. Microscopically, they are acanthotic, papillomatous neoplasms, with a high degree of difer-entiation. As most well differentiated tumors, they have a good prognosis, only presenting metastasis when they present areas with poor differentiation. However, if it presents large areas of undifferentiation, the tumor is classified as a mixed verrucous carcinoma, as the classical verrucous carcinoma is a classicaly well differentiated tumor.

Papillary carcinoma: represent 9-10% of all cases. It is also a verruciform tumor, diagnosed after excluding the possibility of a verrucous or warty tumor. Macroscopically is observed as an exophytic large tumor, with a clear jagged interface with stroma. Microscopically, papillo-matosis is observed and a low-grade histology is present. Different from verrucous carcinoma, acanthosis is not so prominent, and differently from warty carcinoma, there is no koilocytosis. They have an excellent prognosis with very infrequent metastasis.

Sarcomatoid carcinomas: correspond to 1-3% of cases. Macroscopically, they are hemorrhagic and necrotic, or polypoid tumors. Microscopically, they can mimic several sarcomas, like leiomyosarcomas, osteosarcomas, or fibrosarcomas. They are observed as tumors with two different cellular presentations, with the presence of epithelial and spindle cells. They are typically located in glans, not in corpora cavernosa, and may present foci of associated penile intraepithelial neoplasia. Immunohistochemical stains with high-molecular-weight cytokeratins and p63.

Other mixed tumors are often rare, which makes very difficult to establish their relationship with HPV infection, and comprises several subtypes, such as Pseudohyperplastic Carcinoma, Carcinoma Cunilatum and Pseudoglandular Carcinoma.

As stated before, distinct pathological variants of PSCC are associated with an indolent behavior (eg, verrucous, warty and Buschke-Lowenstein condyloma) and other with more aggressive forms (eg, usual SCC, basaloid and papillary). For basaloid and warty carcinomas, the HPV-infections are present in 80-100% of all cases. It is important to remember that *in situ* SCC seems to be strongly related with HPV-infection (Kayes et al., 2007). Seems plausible then that HPV-infection is far more important as a co-factor that will prepare the soil for a neoplastic malignant transformation, due to the several pathways in which HPV-infection contributes. This is in accordance with the theory of two major pathways in penile cancer development, being one driven by factors such as poor hygiene, presence of phimosis, chronic inflammation, etc), and another one driven by high-risk HPV-infection (Rubin et al., 2001). As discussed above, this represents an astonishing opportunity for a new approach to prevent this disease, as HPV vaccination researches are under constant evolution. As a health problem, the prevention of HPV infection might be able to avoid the development of these subtypes of HPV in men, if the current knowledge of HPV-driven malignancy is right.

6. HPV-status impact on outcome in penile carcinomas

Although there are not many studies investigating a prognostic role for HPV-infection in penile carcinomas, some studies maintain HPV as a controversial factor, in terms either of survival, or local metastasis, and lymph node involvement. From the three more important studies, it is still unknown if HPV alone may have an impact in penile cancer's patients overall survival, as demonstrated in several other solid tumors, such those arising in oral cavity and oropharynx (Lont et al., 2006). In a study conducted by Cubilla et al. (2010), HPV-16 was the most prevalent genotype (72% of all cases), followed by HPV-6 (9%) and HPV-18 (6%). The 16 and 18 genotype (high-risk HPV types) were proposed to be associated with aggressive variants of penile tumors, and to be associated with a poorer outcome in these patients. In several studies, the role of HPV infection in penile cancer could only be observed by indirect means, as the observation that HPV-infected PSCCs were those with more aggressive subtypes, as basaloid and warty tumors. So, it is believed that HPV-infection, specially related to HPV-16 and -18, represented a more aggressive subtype, with a worst survival when compared to HPV-negative PSCCs. But directly comparing HPV expression and survival curves, the most extensive study on high-risk HPV infection was carried out by Lont and colleagues, whom had demonstrated that penile tumors presenting high-risk HPV infection had a better outcome from those tumors where high-risk HPVs were not detected. Interestingly, HIV infection did not correlated (Lont et al., 2006).

7. HPV vaccine

In many countries, vaccines against some HPV types are administered to girls and young women with the goal of protecting them against HPV-induced cervical cancer (Villa et al., 2005; Muñoz et al., 2010). The introduction of HPV vaccines has also drawn more attention to the fact that HPV is associated not only with cervical cancer and genital warts but also with other tumors, such as head and neck and anogenital cancers (Zur Hausen, 2006).

Although the majority of HPV vaccine research has focused on cervical cancer, some vaccine developers have targeted other diseases related to different strains of HPV.

Emerging results from vaccine trials have suggested that some cross-protection is possible. Vaccines against cervical cancer also have the potential to prevent other cancers that are caused by the same types of HPV (Herrero et al., 2003, Kreimer et al., 2005), and half or more of anogenital cancers outside the cervix, including cancer of the vulva, vagina, penis, and anus (Daling et al., 2005, Gross & Pfister 2004). Theoretically, these vaccines should also work against the same viruses at other anatomical sites, which would be of great value for the majority of the patients. Since different HPV-related diseases have share the same contamination basis (eg, HPV contamination in sexual act may happen in anogenital, cervical and even in head and neck areas. Also, almost all HPV-related tumors share individual at risk with the same behavior, and it is believed that this prevent potential directed to several organs could reduce the prevalence of several tumors simultaneously. If proven to do so, this approach would represent a major conceptual breakthrough, not only in prevention of these diseases, but equally importantly, by providing the 'missing link' in the chain of evidence for the final proof of HPV etiology in these tumors (Syrjänen, 2010).

8. The HPV prophylactic vaccines

The current HPV prophylactic vaccines are based on VLPs, with two prophylactic HPV vaccines being commercially available: the bivalent (HPV 16/18) vaccine Cervarix® (GlaxoSmithKline, Middlesex, UK) and the quadrivalent (HPV 6/11/16/18) Gardasil® (Merck, NJ, USA). Licensed globally, these two vaccines have produced great expectations that they will prevent infections and tumors induced by different HPV types (Syrjänen, 2010).

The US Food and Drug Administration (FDA) approved Gardasil for females aged 9–26 in 2006. In October 2009, the FDA approved Cervarix for use in females aged 10–25 and approved

Gardasil for use in males aged 9–26 to prevent genital warts and to prevent the spread of cervical cancer. Moreover, the FDA (2010 and 2010a) has proclaimed that the dosing and administration schedule should be 0.5 mL administered intramuscularly (preferably in a deltoid muscle) on a 3-dose schedule. The second dose should be administered 1 to 2 months later, and the third dose should be administered 6 months after the first dose.

Although clinical trials of Gardasil and Cervarix have been extremely promising, these first generation VLP vaccines may not be the ideal vaccine candidates, especially in already infected patients, and older men and women.

The most recent report from Quadrivalent Human Papillomavirus Vaccine presents important facts about immunization practices, and provides excellent results. The efficacy for prevention of HPV 6-, 11-, 16- and 18-related genital warts was 89.3%, as a profilatic vaccine from those who have take 3 doses and was seronegative at day 1. From males who have received only one dose, regardless of serology or previous infection was of 68.1%. This efficacy was also con firmed by several other trials in female patients, with >98% efficacy in preventing HPV 6-, 11-, 16- and 18-related grade 2 or 3 cervical intraepithelial neoplasia or adenocarcinoma *in situ*(CDC MMWR, 2011).

Another important issue in vaccination process is to determine who are the individuals in more risk populations, in order to a better efficacy, and a reduction of the high costs involved in the vaccine production and distribution. Based on incidence of HPV-infection between several groups, the probabilities of being infected, especially subtypes 16 and 18, are higher in men who have sex with men (MSM) group than in heterosexual men (Heiligenberg, 2010). Several diseases have a higher incidence in MSM group, such as anal intraepithelial neoplasia (AIN), anal cancers, and genital warts (Jin et al., 2007). Another important group which might be benefited by HPV immunization is the HIV-positive patients, although it is not clear whether the immunization could provide a long time antibody titers against HPV 6, 11, 16, and 18, and how immunossupressed patients would react to HPV4 vaccine, in terms of safety and adversely reactions. However, as HPV4 is not a live vaccine, it can be safely administered to person in the most highly risk, such as immunocompromised individuals (like HIV-positive, drug-driven immunossupression, or disease-related immunossupression).

Researchers are now actively working to better develop prophylactic HPV vaccines that may be effective against a broader range of HPV types and have a longer shelf life.

9. The HPV therapeutic vaccines and its perspectives

Immunotherapy offers an attractive alternative treatment strategy because it can address both the underlying HPV infection and the visible lesions. Moreover, immunotherapy can target all HPV-associated lesions, regardless of location, and induce long-lasting immunity, thus preventing recurrence (Chu, 2003; Stanley, 2012).

A judgment of whether therapeutic HPV vaccine candidates have a real effect on disease has been difficult because most trials have not been placebo-controlled, and more important, it stills not clear for how long these patients can maintain high levels of immune response, as they have been already infected. The vaccines have also shown, at best, limited efficacy in eradicating established tumors, although the fact that they have mostly been tested in advanced stage cancer patients with compromised immune systems may have limited their impact (Brinkman et al., 2005).

Perhaps the ideal HPV vaccine strategy calls for a vaccine that possesses both prophylactic and therapeutic properties. A chimeric vaccine of this type could both prevent new HPV infections and clear existing infections. Moreover, such a vaccine would benefit and could be administered to both sexually inexperienced young individuals and older individuals who already harbor HPV (Franceschi, 2005). Of course the costs of the rise of individuals been vaccinated needs to be estimated, in order to not turn HPV vaccine in an expensive waste of health budget. It is important to remember that although some groups are in risk group, not all individuals of this risk group will develop an HPV-related cancer. So, before implementing HPV vaccination to a wide range of patients, it needs to be better classified what populations should be included in vaccination process, and further develop new guidelines to better incorporate in this vaccination individuals that, even in risk groups, still have a higher risk in HPV-infection and spread. Opportunities for primary and secondary prevention should be assessed, including the use of HPV vaccines to prevent infection and therapeutic vaccines in the adjuvant setting for locoregional recurrence and distant disease (Marur et al. 2010). Combined with the fact that no therapeutic vaccines currently exist for other diseases, this goal makes therapeutic HPV vaccine development a challenging task.

The most recent report from Quadrivalent Human Papillomavirus Vaccine (HPV4) presents important facts about immunization practices, and provides excellent results. The efficacy for prevention of HPV 6-, 11-, 16- and 18-related genital warts was 89.3%, as a profilatic vaccine from those who have take 3 doses and was seronegative at day 1. From males who have received only one dose, regardless of serology or previous infection was of 68.1%. This efficacy was also confirmed by several other trials in female patients, with >98% efficacy in preventing HPV 6-, 11-, 16- and 18-related grade 2 or 3 cervical intraepithelial neoplasia or adenocarcinoma *in situ* (CDC MMWR, 2011).

10. Final considerations

Several aspects still remain to be discovered in the field of penile cancers and HPV infection, and although last decade researches were not able to define a causal role for HPV-infection, several progresses have being made in this matter. The genomic detection of HPV DNA, primarily in some subtypes of PSCCs, provides stronger support for a viral etiology in this disease, and corroborates the idea that there are at leas 2 main pathways in penile carcinogenesis, and one of them is closely related to HPV.

Targeted therapy for PSCCs now demands more predictive biomarkers, such as the HPV infection status and mutation status of crucial genes, which could contribute to personalized treatment for each individual and decrease the inherent morbidities. However, for a better understanding of whether the HPV status of tumors has real therapeutic implications in affecting the clinical outcome, upcoming clinical trials should be significantly standardized in their design and performed on PSCC, which have been adequately selected and classified with respect to the different penile carcinoma subtypes. Moreover, we suggest that a more defined consensus in the histological classification in PSCCs should be utilized to improve HPV detection and provides means to compare studies in different populations. This is highly remarkable as is now fully accepted that penile carcinogenesis is quite dependent of local characteristics, and varies worldwide.

We believe that the increasing effects of HPV vaccination in several cancers could help to reduce the number of new PSCC cases, especially in developing countries, with a lower income, and less educated individuals. Although detection of the true effects of HPV vaccination on cancer incidence will probably continue for several decades, monitoring the current effects of HPV vaccination is crucial, not only in cervical cancer, but also in penile cancer.

Author details

João Paulo Oliveira-Costa[1,2], Giórgia Gobbi da Silveira[2], Danilo Figueiredo Soave[2], Andrielle de Castilho Fernandes[2], Lucinei Roberto Oliveira[3], Alfredo Ribeiro-Silva[2] and Fernando Augusto Soares[1]

1 AC Camargo Cancer Hospital - Antonio Prudente Cancer Care Center, Brazil

2 Ribeirão Preto Medical School, University of São Paulo, Brazil

3 Vale do Rio Verde University, Brazil

References

[1] Akhter M, Hossain S, Rahman QB, Molla MR. A study on histological grading of oral squamous cell carcinoma and its co-relationship with regional metastasis. J Oral Maxillofac Pathol. 2011 May;15(2):168-76. PubMed PMID: 22529575. Pubmed Central PMCID: PMC3329698. eng.

[2] Backes DM, Kurman RJ, Pimenta JM, Smith JS. Systematic review of human papillomavirus prevalence in invasive penile cancer. Cancer Causes Control. 2009 May; 20(4):449-57. PubMed PMID: 19082746. eng.

[3] Barocas DA, Chang SS. Penile cancer: clinical presentation, diagnosis, and staging. Urol Clin North Am. 2010 Aug;37(3):343-52. PubMed PMID: 20674691. eng.

[4] Bleeker MC, Heideman DA, Snijders PJ, Horenblas S, Dillner J, Meijer CJ. Penile cancer: epidemiology, pathogenesis and prevention. World J Urol. 2009 Apr;27(2):141-50. PubMed PMID: 18607597. eng.

[5] Bosch FX, Lorincz A, MuÒoz N, Meijer CJ, Shah KV. The causal relation between human papillomavirus and cervical cancer. J Clin Pathol. 2002 Apr;55(4):244-65. PubMed PMID: 11919208. Pubmed Central PMCID: PMC1769629. eng.

[6] Brinkman JA, Caffrey AS, Muderspach LI, Roman LD, Kast WM. The impact of anti HPV vaccination on cervical cancer incidence and HPV induced cervical lesions: consequences for clinical management. Eur J Gynaecol Oncol. 2005;26(2):129-42. PubMed PMID: 15857016. eng.

[7] (CDC) CfDCaP. Recommendations on the use of quadrivalent human papillomavirus vaccine in males--Advisory Committee on Immunization Practices (ACIP), 2011. MMWR Morb Mortal Wkly Rep. 2011 Dec;60(50):1705-8. PubMed PMID: 22189893. eng.

[8] Chaux A, Cubilla AL. Advances in the pathology of penile carcinomas. Hum Pathol. 2012 Jun;43(6):771-89. PubMed PMID: 22595011. eng.

[9] Chaux A, Netto GJ, Rodrìguez IM, Barreto JE, Oertell J, Ocampos S, et al. Epidemiologic profile, sexual history, pathologic features, and human papillomavirus status of 103 patients with penile carcinoma. World J Urol. 2011 Nov. PubMed PMID: 22116602. Pubmed Central PMCID: PMC3292668. ENG.

[10] Chaux A, Velazquez EF, Algaba F, Ayala G, Cubilla AL. Developments in the pathology of penile squamous cell carcinomas. Urology. 2010 Aug;76(2 Suppl 1):S7-S14. PubMed PMID: 20691888. eng.

[11] Chow LT, Broker TR, Steinberg BM. The natural history of human papillomavirus infections of the mucosal epithelia. APMIS. 2010 Jun;118(6-7):422-49. PubMed PMID: 20553526. eng.

[12] Chu NR. Therapeutic vaccination for the treatment of mucosotropic human papillomavirus-associated disease. Expert Opin Biol Ther. 2003 Jun;3(3):477-86. PubMed PMID: 12783616. eng.

[13] Cubilla AL. The role of pathologic prognostic factors in squamous cell carcinoma of the penis. World J Urol. 2009 Apr;27(2):169-77. PubMed PMID: 18766352. eng.

[14] Cubilla AL, Lloveras B, Alejo M, Clavero O, Chaux A, Kasamatsu E, et al. The basaloid cell is the best tissue marker for human papillomavirus in invasive penile squamous cell carcinoma: a study of 202 cases from Paraguay. Am J Surg Pathol. 2010 Jan; 34(1):104-14. PubMed PMID: 20035150. eng.

[15] Cubilla AL, Reuter V, Velazquez E, Piris A, Saito S, Young RH. Histologic classification of penile carcinoma and its relation to outcome in 61 patients with primary resection. Int J Surg Pathol. 2001 Apr;9(2):111-20. PubMed PMID: 11484498. eng.

[16] Daling JR, Madeleine MM, Johnson LG, Schwartz SM, Shera KA, Wurscher MA, et al. Penile cancer: importance of circumcision, human papillomavirus and smoking in in situ and invasive disease. Int J Cancer. 2005 Sep;116(4):606-16. PubMed PMID: 15825185. eng.

[17] Doorbar J, Ely S, Sterling J, McLean C, Crawford L. Specific interaction between HPV-16 E1-E4 and cytokeratins results in collapse of the epithelial cell intermediate filament network. Nature. 1991 Aug;352(6338):824-7. PubMed PMID: 1715519. eng.

[18] Epstein JH, Cubilla AL, Humphrey PA. Tumors of the prostate gland, seminal vesicles, penis, and scrotum. Atlas of tumor pathology. Washington, D.C.: Armed Forces Institute of Pathology; 2011. p. 405-612.

[19] Fehrmann F, Laimins LA. Human papillomaviruses: targeting differentiating epithelial cells for malignant transformation. Oncogene. 2003 Aug;22(33):5201-7. PubMed PMID: 12910257. eng.

[20] Food and Drug Administration (FDA) (2010). Licensure of Bivalent Human Papillomavirus Vaccine (HPV2, Cervarix) for Use in Females and Updated HPV Vaccination Recommendations from the Advisory Committee on Immunization Practices (ACIP). MMWR Morbidity and Mortality Weekly Report., 59, 20, pp. 626-629.

[21] Food and Drug Administration (FDA) (2010a). Licensure of Quadrivalent Human Papillomavirus Vaccine (HPV4, Gardasil) for Use in Males and Guidance from the Advisory Committee on Immunization Practices (ACIP). MMWR Morbidity and Mortality Weekly Report. , 59, 20, pp. 630-632.

[22] Franceschi S. The IARC commitment to cancer prevention: the example of papillomavirus and cervical cancer. Recent Results Cancer Res. 2005;166:277-97. PubMed PMID: 15648196. eng.

[23] Gross G, Pfister H. Role of human papillomavirus in penile cancer, penile intraepithelial squamous cell neoplasias and in genital warts. Med Microbiol Immunol. 2004 Feb;193(1):35-44. PubMed PMID: 12838415. eng.

[24] Guimarães GC, Cunha IW, Soares FA, Lopes A, Torres J, Chaux A, et al. Penile squamous cell carcinoma clinicopathological features, nodal metastasis and outcome in 333 cases. J Urol. 2009 Aug;182(2):528-34; discussion 34. PubMed PMID: 19524964. eng.

[25] Guimarães GC, Rocha RM, Zequi SC, Cunha IW, Soares FA. Penile cancer: epidemiology and treatment. Curr Oncol Rep. 2011 Jun;13(3):231-9. PubMed PMID: 21373986. eng.

[26] Gunia S, Erbersdobler A, Hakenberg OW, Koch S, May M. p16^{INK4a} is a Marker of Good Prognosis for Primary Invasive Penile Squamous Cell Carcinoma: A Multi-Institutional Study. J Urol. 2012 Mar;187:899-907.

[27] Hakenberg OW, Protzel C. Chemotherapy in penile cancer. Ther Adv Urol. 2012 Jun; 4(3):133-8. PubMed PMID: 22654965. Pubmed Central PMCID: PMC3361747. eng.

[28] Hebner CM, Laimins LA. Human papillomaviruses: basic mechanisms of pathogenesis and oncogenicity. Rev Med Virol. 2006 2006 Mar-Apr;16(2):83-97. PubMed PMID: 16287204. eng.

[29] Heiligenberg M; Michael KM; Kramer MA; Pawlita M, Prins M; Coutinho, Roel A, et al. Seroprevalence and Determinants of Eight High-Risk Human Papillomavirus Types in Homosexual Men, Heterosexual Men, and Women: A Population-Based Study in Amsterdam. Sexually Transmitted Diseases. 2010 Nov;37(11):672-80.

[30] Hernandez BY, Barnholtz-Sloan J, German RR, Giuliano A, Goodman MT, King JB, et al. Burden of invasive squamous cell carcinoma of the penis in the United States, 1998-2003. Cancer. 2008 Nov;113(10 Suppl):2883-91. PubMed PMID: 18980292. Pubmed Central PMCID: PMC2693711. eng.

[31] Herrero R, Castellsaguè X, Pawlita M, Lissowska J, Kee F, Balaram P, et al. Human papillomavirus and oral cancer: the International Agency for Research on Cancer multicenter study. J Natl Cancer Inst. 2003 Dec;95(23):1772-83. PubMed PMID: 14652239. eng.

[32] Jin F, Prestage GP, Kippax SC, Pell CM, Donovan B, Templeton DJ, et al. Risk factors for genital and anal warts in a prospective cohort of HIV-negative homosexual men: the HIM study. Sex Transm Dis. 2007 Jul;34(7):488-93. PubMed PMID: 17108849. eng.

[33] Kayes O, Ahmed HU, Arya M, Minhas S. Molecular and genetic pathways in penile cancer. Lancet Oncol. 2007 May;8(5):420-9. PubMed PMID: 17466899. eng.

[34] Kreimer AR, Clifford GM, Boyle P, Franceschi S. Human papillomavirus types in head and neck squamous cell carcinomas worldwide: a systematic review. Cancer Epidemiol Biomarkers Prev. 2005 Feb;14(2):467-75. PubMed PMID: 15734974. eng.

[35] Lont AP, Kroon BK, Horenblas S, Gallee MP, Berkhof J, Meijer CJ, et al. Presence of high-risk human papillomavirus DNA in penile carcinoma predicts favorable outcome in survival. Int J Cancer. 2006 Sep;119(5):1078-81. PubMed PMID: 16570278. eng.

[36] Lopes A, Bezerra AL, Pinto CA, Serrano SV, de MellO CA, Villa LL. p53 as a new prognostic factor for lymph node metastasis in penile carcinoma: analysis of 82 patients treated with amputation and bilateral lymphadenectomy. J Urol. 2002 Jul; 168(1):81-6. PubMed PMID: 12050497. eng.

[37] Lopes A, Hidalgo GS, Kowalski LP, Torloni H, Rossi BM, Fonseca FP. Prognostic factors in carcinoma of the penis: multivariate analysis of 145 patients treated with amputation and lymphadenectomy. J Urol. 1996 Nov;156(5):1637-42. PubMed PMID: 8863559. eng.

[38] Marur S, D'Souza G, Westra WH, Forastiere AA. HPV-associated head and neck cancer: a virus-related cancer epidemic. Lancet Oncol. 2010 Aug;11(8):781-9. PubMed PMID: 20451455. eng.

[39] Mikuz G, Winstanley AM, Schulman CC, Debruyne FM, Parkinson CM. Handling and pathology reporting of circumcision and penectomy specimens. Eur Urol. 2004 Oct;46(4):434-9. PubMed PMID: 15363555. eng.

[40] Miralles-Guri C, Bruni L, Cubilla AL, Castellsaguè X, Bosch FX, de Sanjosè S. Human papillomavirus prevalence and type distribution in penile carcinoma. J Clin Pathol. 2009 Oct;62(10):870-8. PubMed PMID: 19706632. eng.

[41] Muñoz N, Bosch FX, de Sanjosè S, Herrero R, Castellsaguè X, Shah KV, et al. Epidemiologic classification of human papillomavirus types associated with cervical cancer. N Engl J Med. 2003 Feb;348(6):518-27. PubMed PMID: 12571259. eng.

[42] Muñoz N, Kjaer SK, Sigurdsson K, Iversen OE, Hernandez-Avila M, Wheeler CM, et al. Impact of human papillomavirus (HPV)-6/11/16/18 vaccine on all HPV-associated genital diseases in young women. J Natl Cancer Inst. 2010 Mar;102(5):325-39. PubMed PMID: 20139221. eng.

[43] Novara G, Galfano A, De Marco V, Artibani W, Ficarra V. Prognostic factors in squamous cell carcinoma of the penis. Nat Clin Pract Urol. 2007 Mar;4(3):140-6. PubMed PMID: 17347658. eng.

[44] Pow-Sang MR, Ferreira U, Pow-Sang JM, Nardi AC, Destefano V. Epidemiology and natural history of penile cancer. Urology. 2010 Aug;76(2 Suppl 1):S2-6. PubMed PMID: 20691882. eng.

[45] Psyrri A, Gouveris P, Vermorken JB. Human papillomavirus-related head and neck tumors: clinical and research implication. Curr Opin Oncol. 2009 May;21(3):201-5. PubMed PMID: 19370803. eng.

[46] Rampias T, Sasaki C, Weinberger P, Psyrri A. E6 and e7 gene silencing and transformed phenotype of human papillomavirus 16-positive oropharyngeal cancer cells. J Natl Cancer Inst. 2009 Mar;101(6):412-23. PubMed PMID: 19276448. eng.

[47] Rubin MA, Kleter B, Zhou M, Ayala G, Cubilla AL, Quint WG, et al. Detection and typing of human papillomavirus DNA in penile carcinoma: evidence for multiple independent pathways of penile carcinogenesis. Am J Pathol. 2001 Oct;159(4):1211-8. PubMed PMID: 11583947. Pubmed Central PMCID: PMC1850485. eng.

[48] Scheurer ME, Tortolero-Luna G, Adler-Storthz K. Human papillomavirus infection: biology, epidemiology, and prevention. Int J Gynecol Cancer. 2005 2005 Sep-Oct; 15(5):727-46. PubMed PMID: 16174218. eng.

[49] Slaton JW, Morgenstern N, Levy DA, Santos MW, Tamboli P, Ro JY, et al. Tumor stage, vascular invasion and the percentage of poorly differentiated cancer: inde-

pendent prognosticators for inguinal lymph node metastasis in penile squamous cancer. J Urol. 2001 Apr;165(4):1138-42. PubMed PMID: 11257655. eng.

[50] Snow AN, Laudadio J. Human papillomavirus detection in head and neck squamous
      cell carcinomas. Adv Anat Pathol. 2010 Nov;17(6):394-403. PubMed PMID: 20966645.
      eng.

[51] Stankiewicz E, Ng M, Cuzick J, Mesher D, Watkin N, Lam W, et al. The prognostic
      value of Ki-67 expression in penile squamous cell carcinoma. J Clin Pathol. 2012 Jun;
      65(6):534-7. PubMed PMID: 22447920. eng.

[52] Stanley M. Chapter 17: Genital human papillomavirus infections--current and pro-
      spective therapies. J Natl Cancer Inst Monogr. 2003 (31):117-24. PubMed PMID:
      12807955. eng.

[53] Stanley MA. Genital human papillomavirus infections: current and prospective
      therapies. J Gen Virol. 2012 Apr;93(Pt 4):681-91. PubMed PMID: 22323530. eng.

[54] Syed S, Eng TY, Thomas CR, Thompson IM, Weiss GR. Current issues in the manage-
      ment of advanced squamous cell carcinoma of the penis. Urol Oncol. 2003 2003 Nov-
      Dec;21(6):431-8. PubMed PMID: 14693269. eng.

[55] Syrjänen S. The role of human papillomavirus infection in head and neck cancers.
      Ann Oncol. 2010 Oct;21 Suppl 7:vii243-5. PubMed PMID: 20943622. eng.

[56] Velazquez EF, Amin MB, Epstein JI, Grignon DJ, Humphrey PA, Pettaway CA, et al.
      Protocol for the examination of specimens from patients with carcinoma of the penis.
      Arch Pathol Lab Med. 2010 Jun;134(6):923-9. PubMed PMID: 20524869. eng.

[57] Velazquez EF, Soskin A, Bock A, Codas R, Cai G, Barreto JE, et al. Epithelial abnor-
      malities and precancerous lesions of anterior urethra in patients with penile carcino-
      ma: a report of 89 cases. Mod Pathol. 2005 Jul;18(7):917-23. PubMed PMID: 15920559.
      eng.

[58] Vidal L, Gillison ML. Human papillomavirus in HNSCC: recognition of a distinct
      disease type. Hematol Oncol Clin North Am. 2008 Dec;22(6):1125-42, vii. PubMed
      PMID: 19010263. eng.

[59] Villa LL, Bernard HU, Kast M, Hildesheim A, Amestoy G, Franco EL. Past, present,
      and future of HPV research: highlights from the 19th International Papillomavirus
      Conference-HPV2001. Virus Res. 2002 Nov;89(2):163-73. PubMed PMID: 12445656.
      eng.

[60] Villa LL, Costa RL, Petta CA, Andrade RP, Ault KA, Giuliano AR, et al. Prophylactic
      quadrivalent human papillomavirus (types 6, 11, 16, and 18) L1 virus-like particle
      vaccine in young women: a randomised double-blind placebo-controlled multicentre
      phase II efficacy trial. Lancet Oncol. 2005 May;6(5):271-8. PubMed PMID: 15863374.
      eng.

[61] Wang S, Wei H, Wang N, Zhang S, Zhang Y, Ruan Q, et al. The prevalence and role of human papillomavirus genotypes in primary cervical screening in the northeast of China. BMC Cancer. 2012 May;12(160).

[62] Zur Hausen, H. (2006). Infections causing human cancer. Weinheim (Germany): Wiley-VCH Verlag, pp. 145–243.

Chapter 9

Epidemiology of Anogenital Human Papillomavirus Infections

Claudie Laprise and Helen Trottier

Additional information is available at the end of the chapter

1. Introduction

Human papillomaviruses (HPVs) are infectious agents responsible for emergence of anogenital subclinical and clinical infections. HPV infections are the most common sexually transmitted infections worldwide. More than 100 HPV genotypes have been catalogued so far and from these, over 40 genotypes infect mucosa of anogenital tract and other mucosal areas. The epidemiology of anogenital HPV infections has been well described, especially cervical infections in young women and there are also many epidemiologic data among adults of different age and of different regions of the world. HPV is now recognized as a necessary cause for the apparition of cervical cancer in women, and is responsible for a substantial proportion of many other anogenital neoplasms (anal, vaginal, vulvar and penile cancers), and a non-negligible portion of head and neck cancers (oral cavity, pharynx, and larynx). HPV is also responsible for the development of benign lesions such as *condyloma acuminata* (genital warts). Clinical HPV infections are responsible for substantial morbidity and invoke high costs associated with the treatment of clinically relevant lesions. This chapter will review epidemiology of HPV infections affecting the anogenital tract of men and women.

2. Classification and carcinogenicity of HPVs

Papillomaviruses are from the *Papillomaviridae* family and all HPV genotypes share a common structure, L1 protein, that is highly conserved and consequently used for taxonomical purposes[1]. HPVs are classified into 16 genuses (Alpha, Beta, etc.), which are also divided into species. Genus of *Papillomaviridae* share less than 60% nucleotide sequence identity in the L1 protein whereas species within a genus share between 60% and 70% nucleotide identity. A new HPV isolate is recognized as a new genotype when the nucleotide sequence of the L1 gene differs by more than 10% from the genotype with which it has the greatest homology in DNA sequence. More than 100 HPV genotypes have been identified in humans from which over 40 genotypes infect mucosa of anogenital tract and other mucosal areas. As anogenital HPV infections is the interest of this chapter, focus is made on alpha-papillomavirus genus, which include mucosal HPVs (Table 1) [2].

Mucosal HPVs are also classified according to their oncogenic potential: low-oncogenic risk genotypes (LR-HPVs) and high-oncogenic risk genotypes (HR-HPVs). LR-HPVs may cause benign lesions of the anogenital mucosa such as *condylomata acuminata* (genital warts) while HR-HPVs are linked to the development of pre- and malignant lesions. The latest classification published by the World Health Organization's International Agency for Research on Cancer referred genotypes 16, 18, 31, 33, 35, 39, 45, 51, 52, 56, 58 and 59 as HR-HPVs[3, 4]. This classification also included many other genotypes as possibly carcinogenic, such as genotypes 26, 53, 66, 67, 68 70, 73 and 82 (Table 2). These genotypes are referred as possibly carcinogenic because the evidence about their carcinogenicity are more limited. Oncogenic potential classification of HPVs is updated frequently with the occurrence of new epidemiologic evidence[5].

Classification of Human Alpha-Papillomavirus

Genus	Species	HPV Genotypes
Alpha-papillomavirus	Alpha-1	32, 42
	Alpha-2	3, 10, 28,29, 78, 94
	Alpha-3	61, 72, 81, 83, 84, c62 c86, c87, c89
	Alpha-4	2, 27, 57
	Alpha-5	26, 51, 69, 82
	Alpha-6	30, 53, 56, 66
	Alpha-7	18, 39, 45, 59, 68, 70, c85
	Alpha-8	7, 40, 43, c91
	Alpha-9	16, 31, 33, 35, 52, 58, 67
	Alpha-10	6, 11, 13, 44, 55, 74
	Alpha-11	34, 73
	Alpha-12	RhPV1
	Alpha-13	54
	Alpha-14	c90
	Alpha-15	71

*Adapted from De Villiers et al., 2004 [1]

Table 1. Classification of species and genotypes of HPVs among the Alpha genus

Classification of Human Papillomavirus by carcinogenic potential

Oncogenic potential	Genotypes of HPV
High-oncogenic risk	16, 18, 31, 33, 35, 39, 45, 51, 52, 56, 58, 59
Possibly high-oncogenic risk	26, 53, 66, 67, 68, 70, 73, 82,
Low-oncogenic risk	6, 11, 13, 30, 32, 34, 42, 44, 54, 61, 62, 69, 71, 72, 74, 81, 83, 84, 85, 86, 87, 89, 90

*Adapted from Bouvard et al, on behalf of the WHO International Agency for Research on Cancer Monograph Working Group 2009 [3]

Table 2. Classification of HPV genotypes based on carcinogenic potential

3. Routes of transmission

3.1. Primary route of transmission: Sexual contact with an infected partner

Epidemiologic data supports that the primary route of HPVs transmission is via sexual contacts. The most important risk factors for prevalent infection as well as for acquisition or incidence in adults, are related to sexual behaviour variables: age at sexual debut and number of sexual partners, new, recent or lifetime for example [5-7]. Transmission may occur through peno-vaginal intercourse, but also via other sexual practices. Anal intercourse is also associated with HPV infection. History of receptive anal sex has been identified as an important risk factor for anal HPV infection among men [8-12]. Oral sex is also a possible route of HPV transmission as it has been associated with HPV oral infection [13-15]. Furthermore, digital-genital transmission is possible, as genital HPV genotypes have been found on fingers[16]. Insertive sex toys are also a possible of route of transmission[17]. Studies on genital HPV infection between women who have sex with women also suggest that HPV transmission is possible among lesbian partners[18].

3.2. Non-sexual routes of transmission

HPV genital infections can also origin from non-sexual route of transmission. For example, HPV DNA can be detected in genital or oral tract of newborns and children through perinatal/vertical transmission [19-23]. Vertical transmission of HPV from mother to child (perinatal infection) was first reported in 1956 in a case of juvenile laryngeal papillomatosis[24]. Confirmation of the perinatal transmission of HPV in different mucosa (genital, oral) was subsequently supported by several studies although the route of transmission is not well understood[19-23, 25]. Direct maternal transmission during vaginal delivery or at caesarean section following early membrane rupture is possible as well as in utero through semen or ascending infection from mother's genital tract. Transplacental transmission seems possible since HPV DNA has been detected by PCR in amniotic fluid, placenta and cord blood [25, 26].

It is possible that transmission occurs through semen since it has been demonstrated that HPV DNA is found in sperm in a proportion of 8–64% of asymptomatic men[27]. Studies in vitro shown that HPVs may attach to sperm head, and that infected spermatozoids are able to penetrate oocyte and deliver HPV genome into it. Oocyte can actively transcribed HPV genes, for transmission to occur[28].

Other non-sexual skin contact transmission has been documented such as horizontal transmission via fingers, mouth and fomites[5, 17]. For example, it has been shown that HPV infected individuals may have HPVs in genital sample and in their hands showing that they can not only infect their sexual partners but also themselves somewhere else on their body (hands, conjunctive, etc.) as well as other individuals outside sexual contacts[16, 18].

4. Epidemiology of ANOGenital hpv infections

4.1. Anogenital HPV infections in women

4.1.1. Prevalence

Cervical HPV infections

According to a recent meta-analysis that included data from more than 1 million women with normal cytology in 59 countries, the prevalence of cervical HPV infection ranges from 1.6% to 41.9%, with a global prevalence estimated at 11.7% [29]. Sub-Saharan Africa (24.0%), Eastern Europe (21.4%), and Latin America (16.1%) showed the highest prevalences and the regions with the lowest prevalences are: Northern America with 4.7% and Western Asia with 1.7%. Also, it is important to consider that these percentages are probably underestimated as the laboratory methods used to detect HPV do not necessarily included the detection of all HPV genotypes[30]. The 5 most common genotypes worldwide are HPV-16, 18, 52, 31 and 58. Typically, HPV prevalence increases rapidly in adolescence following sexual debut, followed by an age-related decline, and occasionally a second but more modest peak in prevalence among older women in some regions of the world such as in America (Northern, Central and South) and in Europe[31]. Although the reason for this "menopausal" peak is not clear, it could plausibly be attributed to one or more non-mutually exclusive mechanisms, such as reactivation of latent infections acquired earlier in life due to a gradual loss of immunity, or to acquisition of new infections due to sexual contacts with new partners later in life (cohort effect)[5].

Anal HPV infections

Less research has been conducted to determine the prevalence of HPV in anal tract of women. A prevalence of 42% has been observed in healthy women [32] and by contrast to cervical prevalence that shows an age-related decline, the prevalence of anal infection seems relatively steady in all age groups[33]. Some studies also shown that women with cervical HPV infection had more than three fold increased risk of concurrent anal-cervical infection with a high correlation between the concordance of HPV genotypes, indicating a common source of infection[33]. As anal intercourse is not strongly associated with anal HPV infection in women, other important route of transmission have been suggested such as no penetrative sexual contact (for example, involving the fingers or mouth of partner), non-sexual contact, or HPV shedding from the vagina to the anus given the close proximity of these two areas[33, 34].

Vaginal and vulvar HPV infections

It has been suggested that vaginal and vulvar HPV infections are also very common in healthy women although much less data in available for these site specific areas. Some studies have detected HPVs in cervicovaginal samples compare to cervical samples and showed positivity for HPV in cervicovaginal swabs are higher compared to cervical specimens suggesting a higher prevalence HPV in the vagina or vulva than in the cervix only[35]. For example, a prevalence of 42.5% has been observed among females in United States using self-collected cervicovaginal specimen[36].

4.1.2. Incidence

Cervical HPV infections

High rates of incidence of HPV cervical infection are observed especially in young women. Cumulative incidence of more than 40% after 3 years of follow-up has been demonstrated among university students [5, 6, 37]. The highest incidence rates of cervical HPV infection are observed in young women corresponding to age of sexual intercourse debut. Thereafter, incidence in women tends to decline with age, although second peaks are sometimes observed in older women (such as for prevalence data)[5]. For example, in a cohort of women between 13 and 65 years of age in Bogota in Colombia[37], the cumulative incidence of any HPV after five years of follow-up among women aged 15-19, 20-24, 25-29, 30-44 and more than 45 years were 42.5%, 36.9%, 30.0%, 21.9%, and 12.4%,, respectively. The cumulative incidence after 5 years of follow-up in all age groups was 26.3% and infections rate with HR-HPVs were more frequent than infections with LR genotypes (5.0 cases and 2.0 cases/100 woman-years, respectively). Although some studies observed higher incidence of HR-HPV than LR-HPV, these comparisons depend on the assays used. More recent assays detect more types, many of which fall into the LR category.

Anal HPV infections

Cumulative incidence of anal HPV infection in a cohort of women of Hawaii (median age: 40 years old) has been evaluated at almost 70% in an average period of 1.3 years of follow-up. The rate of acquisition of anal HPV infection with any genotype was observed at 46.9 cases per 1000 woman-month. The incidence rate of anal HPV infections with HR-HPVs is also higher than with LR-HPV (such as for cervical infection) with estimates reported by Goodman et al (2008) at 19.5 and 8.2/1000 woman-months for an incident anal HR-HPV and LR-HPV, respectively[32]. Lower risk of acquisition of anal HR-HPV in women over 45 years of age have also been observed compared to women under 25 years of age.

Vaginal and vulvar HPV infections

To our knowledge, there are no estimates on the incidence of vagina and vulvar HPV infection in healthy women.

4.1.3. Special population: HIV-positive women and sex workers

HIV and HPV infection status has been under the projectors during the last years. In a systematic review of HIV-positive women with no cytological abnormalities, prevalence of HPV has been evaluated at 36.3% [38], higher than in worldwide estimated prevalence (11.7%)[29].

More attention was also paid to sex workers in the last years. For example, in a study made in China, prevalence of any HPV genotype was estimated at 38.9% in this population[39]. A recent study in Spain also demonstrated a higher incidence and a higher risk of persistence of HR-HPV infection in sex workers compared to the general population (incidence of 3.98 per 100 women-years relatively to 26.81 per 100 women-years)[40].

4.2. Anogenital HPV infections in men

4.2.1. Prevalence

Depending of the anatomic sites (coronal sulcus, glans, prepuce, shaft, urethra, scrotum, perianal area, anus, semen or urine) that is analysed, HPV prevalence (any genotypes) can vary from 1% to 84% among the general population of men and from 2% to 93% in high-risk men (such as STI clinic attendees, HIV-positive males, and male partners of women with HPV infection or abnormal cytology)[41]. For example, the site specific prevalences of HPV infection in male were estimated between 6.5%-50% in corona and/or glans, 5.6%-51.5% in penile shaft, 24%-50% in prepuce, 7.1%-46.2% in scrotum, and 8.7%-50% in urethra [27]. Contrarily to what is reported in women, HPV prevalence is relatively stable across age groups in men [41, 42]. Prevalence of anal HPV infection in men who have sex with women has been reported to range between 0% and 32.8% [27]. It is important to consider, however, that a high variability in the prevalence estimates may occurred in man due to the variability of sites tested or to the type of specimen used for which the detection method is not completly optimized (such as urine).

4.2.2. Incidence

Few studies have reported HPV infections incidence in men. Cumulative incidence calculated with penile and scrotal sampling, in a cohort of USA men aged between 18-44 years old (mean age: 29.7 years) was 29.3% after a follow-up of 12 months[42]. Incidence rate in this cohort for any HPV genotype infection was 29.4 per 1000 men-months. Incidence rates of HPV-6, 11, 16, and 18 infections were 2.8, 0.5, 4.8, and 0.8 per 1000 men-months, resectively.

4.2.3. Special population: Men who have Sex with Men (MSM) and HIV-positive men

HPV infection is strongly associated with the number of lifetime female sexual partners in men who have sex with women (MSW) and also with the number of male anal-sexual partners in men who have sex with men (MSM) [43]. For MSM, prevalence of any HPV genotype was estimated at 18.5% on the penis, 17.1% on the scrotum, 33.0% on the perineal/perianal region, 42.4% in the anal canal, and 48.0% at any site. The prevalence of HPV infection is high among young sexually active MSM, with the anal canal being the most common site of infection[44]. A study comparing the anal canal HPV prevalence in MSW (12.2%) to MSM (47.2%), confirmed the higher prevalence in MSM[45]. Another example from a cohort of Italy have settled prevalence of anal HPV infection to 74.8% in MSM[8]. As for the general population of men, the incidence of HPV infection does not seem to drop with age in MSM as the prevalence remains high in all age groups[46].

Also, it appears that HIV status increases the risk of HPV infection in MSM. For example, a recent systematic review that compared HPV prevalence in MSM according to HIV status has shown that the anal canal prevalence was higher in HIV-positive individuals: (92.6% for HIV-positive compared to 63.9% for HIV negative men) [47]. HR-HPVs were detected in 73.5% of HIV-positive men whereas it was 37.2% in HIV-negative men. The prevalences of HPV-16 and 18 were also higher in HIV-positive men (35.4% compared to 12.5% for HPV-16 and 18.6% compared to 4.9% for HPV-18).

4.2.4. Circumcision and genital HPV infections

Circumcision has been described to reduce the risk of HPV infections in men. The most recent published meta-analysis shown an inverse association between circumcision and genital HPV prevalence in men with an estimated pooled odds ratio of 0.57 (95% confidence interval: 0.54-0.82)[48]. However, as not many studies have been published on the role of circumcision and HPV infection and as most of them are from observational design, more studies are needed to confirm the protective role of circumcision with HPV anogenital infections in men.

5. Natural history

5.1. Clearance and persistence of HPV infection

5.1.1. Clearance

Although high prevalence of HPV is found in both males and females, most of the HPV infections will be cleared spontaneously. Literature has consistently shown that at least 80 to 90% of cervical HPV infections are transient and are no longer detectable within 1-2 years[49]. HR-HPV infections seem to persist longer than LR-HPV[5]. For example, in cervical swabs of female university students, LR-HPV and HR-HPV infections typically last (in average) 13.4 and 16.3 months, respectively[50]. In a review paper, the median duration (time for 50% of infections to be cleared) of cervical infection reported from published studies ranged from 4 to 20 months, with a tendency for HPV-16 infections to last a little longer[5].

Clearance has also been studied in men. For example, a study on the clearance of HPV infections in penile and scrotum sampling in a cohort of USA men has shown that the median time to clearance of any HPV infection was 5.9 months and that 75% of HPV infections cleared by 12 months[42]. Contrarily to women, LR-HPV and HR-HPV infections durations were almost the same with a median duration of 5.8 months and 6 months respectively. Recent data from a cohort study regrouping men from Brazil, Mexico and USA also supports that median duration of HPV infection is shorter in men than in women with 7.5 months for any HPVs[43].

5.1.2. Persistence

Persistence with an HR-HPV over long periods is an important risk factor for the development and progression of cervical malignant lesion[51]. Approximately between 10% and 20% of women fail to clear HPV infections, resulting in long-term cervical persistent infection[52]. It is not known, however, why some women will develop cervical cancer following persistent infection whereas others do not. Finally, persistence of HPV is recognised as an important step in the etiologic pathway of cervical cancer but it has not been studied in other anogenital cancers in women (vulva, vagina, anal cancer) and in men (penile and anal cancer).

5.2. Multiple HPV infections and reinfection with same or different HPV genotype

5.2.1. Multiple HPV infections

Individuals infected with multiple HPV genotypes are also a very common finding of many epidemiologic studies. For example, among the cohort of Brazilian women, between 1.9% to 3.2% were co-infected with multiples genotypes at a same visit (concurrently infected) whereas when considering cumulatively (period prevalence) during the first year and the first 4 years of follow-up, 12.3% and 22.3% were infected with multiple genotypes, respectively[53]. Coinfection in men have also been studied. In a healthy mexican military cohort, HPV prevalence was 44.6% at one of these sites (urethra, urethral meatus, scrotum, penile, shaft or coronal sulcus) and 51.1% of them had mutiple HPV genotypes[54]. MSM have been studied and are also at high risk of coinfection. For example, Dona et al (2012) in an Italian cohort demonstrated that 65.3% of the HPV-positive MSM had multiple HPV infections[8].

Consequences of multiple HPV infections are still debated, but multiple infections with HR-HPV as well as infection with other agents, such as HIV, may play a critical role in furthering the progression to cervical intraepithelial neoplasia and cervical cancer in women[55]. Co-infection with multiple HPV genotypes is common in women with premalignant lesion but the prevalence of co-infections decreases with the severity of the lesion. It is well recognized that cervical cancer specimen do not frequently harboured multiple HPV genotypes[56]. Although multiple genotypes infection may increase the risk of pre-malignant lesions[53], it is possible that co-infection with multiple HPV genotypes acts as a biomarker of immune failure to clear HPV (which allow HPV-16 to progress more easily) rather than etiologic factors that act synergistically to cause cancer.

5.2.2. Reinfection with same or different HPV genotype

The risk of HPV reinfection with the same genotype is also well debated. What has been shown is that it is possible to see cervical reinfection with the same genotype[57]. However, the provenance of the virus is not well understood in re-infected women. Two hypotheses have been advanced to explain reinfection. The first is based on the assumption that infections acquired at a young age never completely clear but become latent; infections appearing later in life would mostly represent the reactivation of such latent infections acquired many years earlier. The second hypothesis is that infections do clear following an initial immune response, which does not completely protect against future infections by the same HPV genotype, following new exposure via sexual activity later in life[58-60]. Recent studies have shown that reinfection with a same genotype is associated with new sexual partners suggesting that infection in adult women may results not only from reactivation of HPV infections acquired at a young age that never completely cleared, but also from new exposure via sexual activity[37, 57]. There is no available study concerning the probability of reinfection with a same or a different genotype in men.

6. HPV related anogenital diseases

6.1. Low-risk HPV genotypes are associated to non-cancerous anogenital lesions

Condylomata acuminata or genital warts (GWs) in anogenital area are usually caused by low-risk HPV genotypes. Recent studies have shown that about 100% of GWs are caused by either HPV-6 or 11 but that 20–50% of lesions also contain co-infections with HR-HPV genotypes. The majority of individuals who develop genital warts do so approximately 2–3 months after infection[61]. Approximately 30% of all warts will regress within the first four months of infection without any treatment, but recurrence will be see in majority of case, even if adequate treatments have been done[62]. Long-term remission rates remain largely unknown. GWs cause also significant psychological morbidity and substantial healthcare costs. Occasionally, GWs persist for long periods of time and, rarely, such long-standing lesions may progress to malignancy. GWs are highly infectious and contribute significantly to spread of HPV infections[63].

6.2. High-risk HPV genotypes are associated to cancerous anogenital lesions

The viruses cause approximately 15% of human cancers, and of this proportion, nearly half is attributable to HPVs with cervix, vulva, vagina, penis and anal cancers[64]. According to Centers for Disease Control and Prevention (CDC), it has now been accepted that HPV is a necessary cause of cervical cancer as virtually 100% of specimens presents HPV DNA. It is also now accepted that HPV is responsible for 50% of vulvar cancer, 65% of vaginal cancer 35% of penile cancers and 95% of anal cancers[65].

7. Economic and health care system burden of HPV infections

Clinical HPV infections are responsible for substantial morbidity and invoke high costs associated with the treatment of clinically relevant lesions[66]. Currently, two vaccines are available: a bivalent HPV 16/18 AS04-adjuvanted vaccine (GlaxoSmithKline Biologicals, Rixensart, Belgium) and a quadrivalent HPV 6/11/16/18 aluminum-adjuvanted vaccine (Merck and Co., West Point, PA, USA). Both vaccines are designed to protect against the two more prevalent HPV genotypes, HPV-16 and 18, that are responsible together for about 70% of all cervical cancer cases worldwide. The quadrivalent vaccine also offers a protection against

HPV-6 and 11, which cause over 90% of genital warts. These vaccines are likely to have a major impact on the incidence and mortality of cervical cancer in the future as well on the burden of other HPV related diseases. Most of developed countries have national recommendations for the use of HPV vaccines in women and many have implemented publicly funded or co-payment routine vaccination programs[67]. These vaccination programs will have a significant impact on the direct and indirect costs related to HPV infections[68].

7.1. Example of economic burden of HPV-related cancers in U.S.A

Direct and indirect costs related to screening and treatment of HPV-related cancer is substantial. Direct costs include usually costs related to medical services such as appointments with physicians and/or gynaecologists, hospital (including inpatient services), nursing and home care and drug prescriptions and time lost for patients or caregivers. However, indirect costs might also be considered in the evaluation of the burden associated to HPV (loss of productivity, psychological, emotional burden on patient)[68].

A recent study in United States evaluated direct medical cost of the prevention and treatment of pathologies associated with HPV[69]. Most of the annual direct medical costs are attributed to cervical screening and follow-up are estimated at 6.6 billions of U.S. dollars: $5.4 billion for cervical screening routine and $1.2 billion for follow-up costs. Cervical cancer costs $441 millions annually, vulvar and vaginal cancer costing for $37 and $12 millions respectively. Anal cancer and penile cancer treatment costs has been estimated at $155 millions and $7 millions of annual costs respectively.

7.2. Genital warts are also an important economic and health care burden

Direct and indirect costs related to genital warts are also important. Genital warts are known to be resistant to treatment and having high recurrence rates even if the appropriate treatment has been done[62]. This involves repeated physicians visits for treatment and high direct costs. The indirect costs include lower productivity for the patient due to illness as well as psychological and emotional burden such as anger, stress, anxiety, depression, shame, guilt and isolation which are also realities for patients [70, 71]. Chesson et al. evaluated at $288 millions the direct medical costs related to genital warts in United States [69].

8. Conclusion

Anogenital HPV infections are very common and transmitted principally via sexual contacts. High prevalence has been found in both female and male adults. Even if the majority of anogenital infections will clear spontaneously, a small proportion of infection will progress and cause different anogenital cancers. HPV is a necessary cause of cervical cancer and plays a role in other anogenital cancers in men and women. Some subgroups such as MSM, sex workers and HIV individuals are particularly at risk of HPV infections. Clinical HPV infections are responsible for substantial morbidity and invoke high costs associated with the treatment of clinically relevant lesions. Prevention is always preferable to treatment and in this optic,

HPV vaccination, which is currently implanted all over the world, is expected to prevent a substantial proportion of cervical and other HPV-related cancers in the future.

Acknowledgements

Claudie Laprise received a doctoral research award from the Canadian Institutes of Health Research (FRN: 96236) and Helen Trottier received a salary award (chercheur-boursier) from the Fonds de la recherche en santé du Québec.

Author details

Claudie Laprise* and Helen Trottier

*Address all correspondence to: claudielaprise@videotron.ca

Department of Social and Preventive Medicine, University of Montreal, Montreal, Sainte-Justine Hospital Research Center, Montreal, Canada

References

[1] de Villiers EM, Fauquet C, Broker TR, Bernard HU, zur Hausen H. Classification of papillomaviruses. Virology. 2004;324(1):17-27. Epub 2004/06/09.

[2] IARC Working Group. IARC monographs on the evaluation of carcinogenic risks to humans ; v. 100B. 2009: Lyon, France.

[3] Bouvard V, Baan R, Straif K, Grosse Y, Secretan B, El Ghissassi F, et al. A review of human carcinogens--Part B: biological agents. The lancet oncology. 2009;10(4):321-2. Epub 2009/04/08.

[4] IARC Working Group. IARC monographs on the evaluation of carcinogenic risks to humans ; v. 90 Human Papillomaviruses. 2007: Lyon, France.

[5] Trottier H, Franco EL. The epidemiology of genital human papillomavirus infection. Vaccine. 2006;24 Suppl 1:S1-15. Epub 2006/01/13.

[6] Burchell AN, Winer RL, de Sanjose S, Franco EL. Chapter 6: Epidemiology and transmission dynamics of genital HPV infection. Vaccine. 2006;24 Suppl 3:S3/52-61. Epub 2006/09/05.

[7] Tota JE, Chevarie-Davis M, Richardson LA, Devries M, Franco EL. Epidemiology and burden of HPV infection and related diseases: implications for prevention strategies. Preventive medicine. 2011;53 Suppl 1:S12-21. Epub 2011/10/14.

[8] Dona MG, Palamara G, Di Carlo A, Latini A, Vocaturo A, Benevolo M, et al. Prevalence, genotype diversity and determinants of anal HPV infection in HIV-uninfected men having sex with men. Journal of clinical virology : the official publication of the Pan American Society for Clinical Virology. 2012;54(2):185-9. Epub 2012/03/16.

[9] Daling JR, Madeleine MM, Johnson LG, Schwartz SM, Shera KA, Wurscher MA, et al. Human papillomavirus, smoking, and sexual practices in the etiology of anal cancer. Cancer. 2004;101(2):270-80. Epub 2004/07/09.

[10] Guimaraes MD, Grinsztejn B, Melo VH, Rocha GM, Campos LN, Pilotto JH, et al. Anal HPV prevalence and associated factors among HIV-seropositive men under antiretroviral treatment in Brazil. J Acquir Immune Defic Syndr. 2011;57 Suppl 3:S217-24. Epub 2011/09/29.

[11] Piketty C, Darragh TM, Da Costa M, Bruneval P, Heard I, Kazatchkine MD, et al. High prevalence of anal human papillomavirus infection and anal cancer precursors among HIV-infected persons in the absence of anal intercourse. Annals of internal medicine. 2003;138(6):453-9. Epub 2003/03/18.

[12] Wiley DJ, Harper DM, Elashoff D, Silverberg MJ, Kaestle C, Cook RL, et al. How condom use, number of receptive anal intercourse partners and history of external genital warts predict risk for external anal warts. International journal of STD & AIDS. 2005;16(3):203-11. Epub 2005/04/15.

[13] Pickard RK, Xiao W, Broutian TR, He X, Gillison ML. The prevalence and incidence of oral human papillomavirus infection among young men and women, aged 18-30 years. Sexually transmitted diseases. 2012;39(7):559-66. Epub 2012/06/19.

[14] D'Souza G, Agrawal Y, Halpern J, Bodison S, Gillison ML. Oral sexual behaviors associated with prevalent oral human papillomavirus infection. The Journal of infectious diseases. 2009;199(9):1263-9. Epub 2009/03/27.

[15] Kreimer AR, Villa A, Nyitray AG, Abrahamsen M, Papenfuss M, Smith D, et al. The epidemiology of oral HPV infection among a multinational sample of healthy men. Cancer epidemiology, biomarkers & prevention : a publication of the American Association for Cancer Research, cosponsored by the American Society of Preventive Oncology. 2011;20(1):172-82. Epub 2010/12/15.

[16] Sonnex C, Strauss S, Gray JJ. Detection of human papillomavirus DNA on the fingers of patients with genital warts. Sexually transmitted infections. 1999;75(5):317-9. Epub 2000/01/05.

[17] Ferenczy A, Bergeron C, Richart RM. Human papillomavirus DNA in fomites on ob-
     jects used for the management of patients with genital human papillomavirus infec-
     tions. Obstetrics and gynecology. 1989,74(6).950-4. Epub 1909/12/01.

[18] Marrazzo JM, Koutsky LA, Stine KL, Kuypers JM, Grubert TA, Galloway DA, et al.
     Genital human papillomavirus infection in women who have sex with women. The
     Journal of infectious diseases. 1998;178(6):1604-9. Epub 1998/11/17.

[19] Martinelli M, Zappa A, Bianchi S, Frati E, Colzani D, Amendola A, et al. Human pap-
     illomavirus (HPV) infection and genotype frequency in the oral mucosa of newborns
     in Milan, Italy. Clinical microbiology and infection : the official publication of the Eu-
     ropean Society of Clinical Microbiology and Infectious Diseases. 2012;18(6):E197-9.
     Epub 2012/04/12.

[20] Smith EM, Parker MA, Rubenstein LM, Haugen TH, Hamsikova E, Turek LP. Evi-
     dence for vertical transmission of HPV from mothers to infants. Infectious diseases in
     obstetrics and gynecology. 2010;2010:326369. Epub 2010/03/20.

[21] Park H, Lee SW, Lee IH, Ryu HM, Cho AR, Kang YS, et al. Rate of vertical transmis-
     sion of human papillomavirus from mothers to infants: Relationship between infec-
     tion rate and mode of delivery. Virology journal. 2012;9(1):80. Epub 2012/04/14.

[22] Rombaldi RL, Serafini EP, Mandelli J, Zimmermann E, Losquiavo KP. Perinatal
     transmission of human papillomavirus DNA. Virology journal. 2009;6:83. Epub
     2009/06/24.

[23] Medeiros LR, Ethur AB, Hilgert JB, Zanini RR, Berwanger O, Bozzetti MC, et al. Ver-
     tical transmission of the human papillomavirus: a systematic quantitative review.
     Cadernos de saude publica / Ministerio da Saude, Fundacao Oswaldo Cruz, Escola
     Nacional de Saude Publica. 2005;21(4):1006-15. Epub 2005/07/16.

[24] Hajek EF. Contribution to the etiology of laryngeal papilloma in children. The Jour-
     nal of laryngology and otology. 1956;70(3):166-8. Epub 1956/03/01.

[25] Syrjanen S. Current concepts on human papillomavirus infections in children. AP-
     MIS : acta pathologica, microbiologica, et immunologica Scandinavica. 2010;118(6-7):
     494-509. Epub 2010/06/18.

[26] Rombaldi RL, Serafini EP, Mandelli J, Zimmermann E, Losquiavo KP. Transplacental
     transmission of Human Papillomavirus. Virology journal. 2008;5:106. Epub
     2008/09/27.

[27] Dunne EF, Nielson CM, Stone KM, Markowitz LE, Giuliano AR. Prevalence of HPV
     infection among men: A systematic review of the literature. The Journal of infectious
     diseases. 2006;194(8):1044-57. Epub 2006/09/23.

[28] Foresta C, Patassini C, Bertoldo A, Menegazzo M, Francavilla F, Barzon L, et al.
     Mechanism of human papillomavirus binding to human spermatozoa and fertilizing
     ability of infected spermatozoa. PloS one. 2011;6(3):e15036. Epub 2011/03/17.

[29] Bruni L, Diaz M, Castellsague X, Ferrer E, Bosch FX, de Sanjose S. Cervical human papillomavirus prevalence in 5 continents: meta-analysis of 1 million women with normal cytological findings. The Journal of infectious diseases. 2010;202(12):1789-99. Epub 2010/11/12.

[30] Coutlee F, Mayrand MH, Roger M, Franco EL. Detection and typing of human papillomavirus nucleic acids in biological fluids. Public health genomics. 2009;12(5-6): 308-18. Epub 2009/08/18.

[31] de Sanjose S, Diaz M, Castellsague X, Clifford G, Bruni L, Munoz N, et al. Worldwide prevalence and genotype distribution of cervical human papillomavirus DNA in women with normal cytology: a meta-analysis. The Lancet infectious diseases. 2007;7(7):453-9. Epub 2007/06/29.

[32] Goodman MT, Shvetsov YB, McDuffie K, Wilkens LR, Zhu X, Ning L, et al. Acquisition of anal human papillomavirus (HPV) infection in women: the Hawaii HPV Cohort study. The Journal of infectious diseases. 2008;197(7):957-66. Epub 2008/04/23.

[33] Hernandez BY, McDuffie K, Zhu X, Wilkens LR, Killeen J, Kessel B, et al. Anal human papillomavirus infection in women and its relationship with cervical infection. Cancer epidemiology, biomarkers & prevention : a publication of the American Association for Cancer Research, cosponsored by the American Society of Preventive Oncology. 2005;14(11 Pt 1):2550-6. Epub 2005/11/15.

[34] Moscicki AB, Durako SJ, Houser J, Ma Y, Murphy DA, Darragh TM, et al. Human papillomavirus infection and abnormal cytology of the anus in HIV-infected and uninfected adolescents. AIDS. 2003;17(3):311-20. Epub 2003/01/31.

[35] Petignat P, Faltin DL, Bruchim I, Tramer MR, Franco EL, Coutlee F. Are self-collected samples comparable to physician-collected cervical specimens for human papillomavirus DNA testing? A systematic review and meta-analysis. Gynecologic oncology. 2007;105(2):530-5. Epub 2007/03/06.

[36] Hariri S, Unger ER, Sternberg M, Dunne EF, Swan D, Patel S, et al. Prevalence of genital human papillomavirus among females in the United States, the National Health And Nutrition Examination Survey, 2003-2006. The Journal of infectious diseases. 2011;204(4):566-73. Epub 2011/07/28.

[37] Munoz N, Mendez F, Posso H, Molano M, van den Brule AJ, Ronderos M, et al. Incidence, duration, and determinants of cervical human papillomavirus infection in a cohort of Colombian women with normal cytological results. The Journal of infectious diseases. 2004;190(12):2077-87. Epub 2004/11/20.

[38] Clifford GM, Goncalves MA, Franceschi S. Human papillomavirus types among women infected with HIV: a meta-analysis. AIDS. 2006;20(18):2337-44. Epub 2006/11/23.

[39] Li HM, Liang GJ, Yin YP, Wang QQ, Zheng ZJ, Zhou JJ, et al. Prevalence and genotype distribution of human papillomavirus infection among female sex workers in

Guangxi, China: implications for interventions. Journal of medical virology. 2012;84(5):798-803. Epub 2012/03/21.

[40] Gonzalez C, Torres M, Canals J, Fernandez E, Belda J, Ortiz M, et al. Higher incidence and persistence of high-risk human papillomavirus infection in female sex workers compared with women attending family planning. International journal of infectious diseases : IJID : official publication of the International Society for Infectious Diseases. 2011;15(10):e688-94. Epub 2011/07/16.

[41] Smith JS, Gilbert PA, Melendy A, Rana RK, Pimenta JM. Age-specific prevalence of human papillomavirus infection in males: a global review. The Journal of adolescent health : official publication of the Society for Adolescent Medicine. 2011;48(6):540-52. Epub 2011/05/18.

[42] Giuliano AR, Lu B, Nielson CM, Flores R, Papenfuss MR, Lee JH, et al. Age-specific prevalence, incidence, and duration of human papillomavirus infections in a cohort of 290 US men. The Journal of infectious diseases. 2008;198(6):827-35. Epub 2008/07/29.

[43] Giuliano AR, Lee JH, Fulp W, Villa LL, Lazcano E, Papenfuss MR, et al. Incidence and clearance of genital human papillomavirus infection in men (HIM): a cohort study. Lancet. 2011;377(9769):932-40. Epub 2011/03/04.

[44] Goldstone S, Palefsky JM, Giuliano AR, Moreira ED, Jr., Aranda C, Jessen H, et al. Prevalence of and risk factors for human papillomavirus (HPV) infection among HIV-seronegative men who have sex with men. The Journal of infectious diseases. 2011;203(1):66-74. Epub 2010/12/15.

[45] Nyitray AG, Carvalho da Silva RJ, Baggio ML, Lu B, Smith D, Abrahamsen M, et al. Age-specific prevalence of and risk factors for anal human papillomavirus (HPV) among men who have sex with women and men who have sex with men: the HPV in men (HIM) study. The Journal of infectious diseases. 2011;203(1):49-57. Epub 2010/12/15.

[46] Dietz CA, Nyberg CR. Genital, oral, and anal human papillomavirus infection in men who have sex with men. The Journal of the American Osteopathic Association. 2011;111(3 Suppl 2):S19-25. Epub 2011/03/29.

[47] Machalek DA, Poynten M, Jin F, Fairley CK, Farnsworth A, Garland SM, et al. Anal human papillomavirus infection and associated neoplastic lesions in men who have sex with men: a systematic review and meta-analysis. The lancet oncology. 2012;13(5):487-500. Epub 2012/03/27.

[48] Albero G, Castellsague X, Giuliano AR, Bosch FX. Male circumcision and genital human papillomavirus: a systematic review and meta-analysis. Sexually transmitted diseases. 2012;39(2):104-13. Epub 2012/01/18.

[49] Moscicki AB, Schiffman M, Kjaer S, Villa LL. Chapter 5: Updating the natural history of HPV and anogenital cancer. Vaccine. 2006;24 Suppl 3:S3/42-51. Epub 2006/09/05.

[50] Richardson H, Kelsall G, Tellier P, Voyer H, Abrahamowicz M, Ferenczy A, et al. The natural history of type-specific human papillomavirus infections in female university students. Cancer epidemiology, biomarkers & prevention : a publication of the American Association for Cancer Research, cosponsored by the American Society of Preventive Oncology. 2003;12(6):485-90. Epub 2003/06/20.

[51] Bodily J, Laimins LA. Persistence of human papillomavirus infection: keys to malignant progression. Trends in microbiology. 2011;19(1):33-9. Epub 2010/11/06.

[52] Stanley M. Immunobiology of HPV and HPV vaccines. Gynecologic oncology. 2008;109(2 Suppl):S15-21. Epub 2008/06/14.

[53] Trottier H, Mahmud S, Costa MC, Sobrinho JP, Duarte-Franco E, Rohan TE, et al. Human papillomavirus infections with multiple types and risk of cervical neoplasia. Cancer epidemiology, biomarkers & prevention : a publication of the American Association for Cancer Research, cosponsored by the American Society of Preventive Oncology. 2006;15(7):1274-80. Epub 2006/07/13.

[54] Lajous M, Mueller N, Cruz-Valdez A, Aguilar LV, Franceschi S, Hernandez-Avila M, et al. Determinants of prevalence, acquisition, and persistence of human papillomavirus in healthy Mexican military men. Cancer epidemiology, biomarkers & prevention : a publication of the American Association for Cancer Research, cosponsored by the American Society of Preventive Oncology. 2005;14(7):1710-6. Epub 2005/07/21.

[55] de Freitas AC, Gurgel AP, Chagas BS, Coimbra EC, do Amaral CM. Susceptibility to cervical cancer: An overview. Gynecologic oncology. 2012;126(2):304-11. Epub 2012/04/10.

[56] Li N, Franceschi S, Howell-Jones R, Snijders PJ, Clifford GM. Human papillomavirus type distribution in 30,848 invasive cervical cancers worldwide: Variation by geographical region, histological type and year of publication. International journal of cancer Journal international du cancer. 2011;128(4):927-35. Epub 2010/05/18.

[57] Trottier H, Ferreira S, Thomann P, Costa MC, Sobrinho JS, Prado JC, et al. Human papillomavirus infection and reinfection in adult women: the role of sexual activity and natural immunity. Cancer research. 2010;70(21):8569-77. Epub 2010/10/28.

[58] Castle PE, Schiffman M, Herrero R, Hildesheim A, Rodriguez AC, Bratti MC, et al. A prospective study of age trends in cervical human papillomavirus acquisition and persistence in Guanacaste, Costa Rica. The Journal of infectious diseases. 2005;191(11):1808-16. Epub 2005/05/05.

[59] Herrero R, Hildesheim A, Bratti C, Sherman ME, Hutchinson M, Morales J, et al. Population-based study of human papillomavirus infection and cervical neoplasia in

rural Costa Rica. Journal of the National Cancer Institute. 2000;92(6):464-74. Epub 2000/03/16.

[60] Lazcano-Ponce E, Herrero R, Munoz N, Cruz A, Shah KV, Alonso P, et al. Epidemiology of HPV infection among Mexican women with normal cervical cytology. International journal of cancer Journal international du cancer. 2001;91(3):412-20. Epub 2001/02/15.

[61] Stanley M. Pathology and epidemiology of HPV infection in females. Gynecologic oncology. 2010;117(2 Suppl):S5-10. Epub 2011/03/08.

[62] Patel RV, Yanofsky VR, Goldenberg G. Genital warts: a comprehensive review. The Journal of clinical and aesthetic dermatology. 2012;5(6):25-36. Epub 2012/07/07.

[63] Lacey CJ, Lowndes CM, Shah KV. Chapter 4: Burden and management of non-cancerous HPV-related conditions: HPV-6/11 disease. Vaccine. 2006;24 Suppl 3:S3/35-41. Epub 2006/09/05.

[64] Parkin DM, Bray F. Chapter 2: The burden of HPV-related cancers. Vaccine. 2006;24 Suppl 3:S3/11-25. Epub 2006/09/05.

[65] Centers for Disease Control and Prevention. http://www.cdc.gov/hpv/cancer.html (accessed 6 August, 2012).

[66] Insinga RP, Dasbach EJ, Elbasha EH. Assessing the annual economic burden of preventing and treating anogenital human papillomavirus-related disease in the US: analytic framework and review of the literature. PharmacoEconomics. 2005;23(11): 1107-22. Epub 2005/11/10.

[67] Monsonego J, Cortes J, Greppe C, Hampl M, Joura E, Singer A. Benefits of vaccinating young adult women with a prophylactic quadrivalent human papillomavirus (types 6, 11, 16 and 18) vaccine. Vaccine. 2010;28(51):8065-72. Epub 2010/10/26.

[68] Ekwueme DU, Chesson HW, Zhang KB, Balamurugan A. Years of potential life lost and productivity costs because of cancer mortality and for specific cancer sites where human papillomavirus may be a risk factor for carcinogenesis-United States, 2003. Cancer. 2008;113(10 Suppl):2936-45. Epub 2008/11/05.

[69] Chesson HW, Ekwueme DU, Saraiya M, Watson M, Lowy DR, Markowitz LE. Estimates of the annual direct medical costs of the prevention and treatment of disease associated with human papillomavirus in the United States. Vaccine. 2012. Epub 2012/08/08.

[70] Raymakers AJ, Sadatsafavi M, Marra F, Marra CA. Economic and humanistic burden of external genital warts. PharmacoEconomics. 2012;30(1):1-16. Epub 2011/12/29.

[71] Senecal M, Brisson M, Maunsell E, Ferenczy A, Franco EL, Ratnam S, et al. Loss of quality of life associated with genital warts: baseline analyses from a prospective study. Sexually transmitted infections. 2011;87(3):209-15. Epub 2011/02/22.

Chapter 10

Modern Molecular and Clinical Approaches to Eradicate HPV-Mediated Cervical Cancer

Whitney Evans, Maria Filippova, Ron Swensen and
Penelope Duerksen-Hughes

Additional information is available at the end of the chapter

1. Introduction

Cervical cancer was formerly the second most common cancer killer of women worldwide. Following widespread adoption of Papanicolau cytologic screening (Pap test) for cervical cancer in the 1950s, this began to change. Today, advanced cervical cancer is rare in screened populations. Although an uncommon disease in developed nations, internationally about 500,000 women annually are diagnosed with cervical cancer, and about half of those women will die of their disease. In global terms, this ranks second only to breast cancer as a cause of cancer-specific mortality. Over the past three decades the scientific community has witnessed spectacular advances in the understanding of the underlying pathophysiology of cervical cancer, with the most profound discovery being in 1983 of the identification of the human papillomavirus (HPV) within cervical cancer (a discovery that earned Harold Zur-Hausen, M.D the Nobel prize for Medicine and Physiology in 2008). A viral etiology for cervical cancer implied that it may be possible to eradicate cervical cancer through vaccination. This promise was partially fulfilled in 2006 when the United States Food and Drug Administration approved an HPV vaccine for the prevention of HPV-induced cervical dysplasia and/or cancer. These advances, profound though they are, have yet to eradicate cervical cancer. Furthermore, due to the pervasiveness of HPV infection and the timeline of disease progression, it will be a few decades before we will be able to determine the impact preventive practices are having on cancer incidence and prevalence. In addition, those for whom preventative measures are not a solution, including HIV⁺ individuals as well as women already infected with HR-HPV, await an answer.

Over the past several years, developments in innovative imaging, superior surgical technologies, immunotherapies, and molecular therapies have surfaced, making the eradication of cervical cancer a much more achievable goal than in the past. Several areas of cervical cancer research continue to address the challenges posed by the need for appropriate therapeutic alternatives, and progress is occurring at each level of clinical management ranging from detection to the development of small molecule antiviral leads. Because the field is evolving rapidly in all directions and related disciplines, it is helpful to summarize the status of our growth, and to recognize those pioneering efforts that may ultimately contribute to achieving our goal of eliminating cervical cancer. This review seeks to survey the current understanding of cervical cancer etiology and treatment and to review areas requiring additional progress.

2. Prevention, interception and early detection

Disease Burden and Risk: Approximately 20 million Americans are currently infected with HPV, and another 6 million new infections occur annually. In about 90 percent of these cases, the infection is cleared by the immune system within two years [1, 2]. However, a relatively small subset of infections persists, sometimes resulting in viral oncoprotein-mediated perturbation of cell-cycle controls leading to cervical intraepithelial neoplasia (CIN). Approximately 5 percent of Pap specimens are classified as pre-cancerous (CIN 1, 2 or 3) while 0.3 - 0.5 percent are typically diagnosed as carcinoma *in situ* [3].

Occurring in men and women, HPV infection is most commonly transmitted by sexual contact. According to the National Cancer Institute (NCI), a woman's risk of acquiring HPV and subsequently developing cervical cancer is increased when the age of sexual debut occurs at a younger age and when the number of lifetime sexual partners is higher [4]. In addition, it has been shown that prevalence rates of infection are consistently higher by 70 percent in sexually experienced, low-income populations of racial and ethnic diversity compared to the general population [5-7]. Also, the risk of HPV infection progressing to cancer depends on lifestyle. For example [8], at a woman's first Pap test the risk that HPV16 infection is more likely to progress to carcinoma *in situ* is 70 percent higher in women who currently smoke (Relative Risk for current smokers is 1.9) [8-11].

Public Education: Media coverage over the last decade has increased general awareness of HPV infection. However, knowledge regarding how the virus is transmitted and the fact that HPV infection may cause cervical cancer is less well-known, particularly among vulnerable populations [12]. In one survey, when high school students were asked to name a few common sexually transmitted infections (STIs) only 17 percent of students mentioned HPV [13]. A general awareness about HPV infection leading to cervical cancer can be increased through education, but more needs to be done to influence the pre-conceived attitudes about prevention through vaccination and sexual behaviors [14]. For example, HPV infection, like most other STIs, are spread *via* bodily fluids that can be obstructed by condom use [15]. Consequently, this knowledge might heighten the risk-perception (a person's subjective appraisal of danger) of not using a condom during vaginal intercourse encounters and reduce sexually risky behaviors to some appreciable degree.

UNESCO (United Nations Educational, Scientific, and Cultural Organization) has demonstrated the effectiveness of sex education in the global fight against HIV/AIDs. Although HPV does not currently compare to HIV/AIDs in terms of mortality and global magnitude, the need for HPV awareness has grown tremendously and it is speculated that such a plan may prove useful here as well. An increase in consciousness may decrease sexual risk behaviors if populations at high-risk for contracting HPV were actively targeted for education [16, 17]. However, it should be considered that gender inequalities experienced by women in locations like Sub-Saharan Africa, as reported by the Global Health Corps and UNESCO, may negatively impact these initiatives. Furthermore, the cost of such programs compared to other interventional methods has not been determined. But in general, education can be used as a powerful tool in preventing HPV-mediated diseases such as cervical cancer. Ideally, these programs would emphasize risk-perception in both men and women leading to lifestyle modifications, and a further reduction in the incidence of HPV-mediated carcinoma might be realized.

Prophylactic Immune Strategies: Presently, the most effective protective factor against the most prevalent and high-risk types of HPV infection is prophylactic vaccination [18]. It has been seven years since the introduction of the first HPV vaccine [19]. Since then, two vaccines, Gardasil and Cervarix, have been made available to the public to protect against the more common HPV strains [20]. The vaccines induce the production of neutralizing antibodies against HPV L1 capsid virus-like proteins (VLPs), which do not contain virus genetic material. The quadrivalent vaccine, Gardasil, protects against low- and high-risk HPV (LR- and HR-HPV, respectively) types 6, 11, 16, and 18 following full vaccination of all three doses at 0, 1, 2 and 6 months. Alternatively, the bivalent vaccine, Cervarix, prevents infection by HR-HPV types 16 and 18. Both vaccines have been documented to possess compelling prophylactic efficacy in preventing cervical, genital, and anal diseases. This protection is expected to persist for 7 years, or at least during the years of high infection risk for most individuals [20-22].

HPV infections of types other than the four mentioned above are not reliably prevented by vaccination. Also, studies are warranted regarding the vaccine's long-term effects and how they might impact the occurrence of infections by other HPV types. It has already been noted that quadrivalent and bivalent vaccines may exhibit cross-protection against HPV 31 and other types by 75 to 80 percent [23]. However, concerns are emerging that relate to HPV type-replacement. Type-replacement is an increased prevalence of other HPV strains that are not included in the vaccines, while vaccine-type HPV prevalence is decreased. It was recently reported that vaccine-type HPV has been reduced in vaccinated and nonvaccinated women, while nonvaccine-type HPV has slightly increased overall [24]. Researchers do not expect type-replacement to occur frequently. However, studies are becoming more attentive to changes in the prevalence of various HPV types, which are expected to surface first within the sexually experienced population. Such discoveries could encourage the research community to continue seeking multivalent solutions to as many HPV types as possible without eliciting additional harmful results. To date, clinical trials have revealed that the most common adverse response to both vaccines are injection site reactions, which occur more frequently in vaccine groups rather than in participants given placebos [25].

Though most industrialized countries, like Great Britain, have already implemented structured HPV immunization programs, well-functioning programs geared towards adults and young adolescents have yet to be seen in many developing countries. However, there are globally funded systems with strong infrastructure that support the immunization of infants in developing countries [26]. This anomaly is due to several challenges, which include the cost of the vaccines, though the biological, economical, and psychological disease burdens of HPV have also been considered [25, 26]. Therefore, it is no surprise that less developed countries have not made HPV vaccination programs a priority while other issues compete for the same limited governmental resources. The most apparent considerations regarding vaccine distribution in these countries relate to healthcare infrastructure, which can directly affect a country's ability to establish and maintain immunization programs that target the vaccine's intended population – adolescents. Other factors of significant importance comprise how to best promote these programs in a way that does not aggravate ethnic/cultural sensitivities and attitudes about vaccination against an STI [27, 28]. This would further include easing parental concerns about what an STI vaccine might imply if perceived as socially acceptable within the targeted age groups. Perhaps if immunization programs were set up in an educational setting, a stronger risk-perception might be instilled, which would encourage the formation of better habits of awareness. In years to come, these types of educational agendas might also improve adherence to the 3-dose regimen over the six-month vaccination period and increase compliance with screening routines throughout a woman's lifetime [29].

One clear limitation of the HPV vaccines is their lack of efficacy for those who have already been exposed to the virus types included in the vaccines. Of course, this exposure is directly correlated to increasing age and sexual experience [30, 31]. For those who fall into this group, including older women regardless of vaccination status, it is important that screenings continue as outlined by the American Cancer Society (ACS) guidelines for Early Detection of Cervical Neoplasia and Cancer [5]. Therefore, integrated approaches of prevention and detection are required if efforts against HPV-mediated cervical cancer are to be maximized. Another important consideration for vaccination is the immune status of potential vaccine recipients; the immune system must be intact [32]. The immune system's ability to clear antigens depends largely on its strength and competence. Thus, immunocompromised women are especially in peril of HR-HPV infection progressing to cancer [33].

The most common scenarios for compromised immunity are seen in HIV+ individuals and organ transplant beneficiaries. Those infected with HIV have a greater chance of HPV co-infection and progression to invasive cervical cancer as compared to those without HIV [34, 35]. The disparity observed here is most likely due to the immune system's inability to effectively clear virus among this subset due to decreased immune reactivity to HPV antigen [36, 37]. It was also found that HPV infection is prevalent among those receiving organ transplants [38], and that the infection increasingly persisted throughout immunosuppressive therapy to moderate graft rejection [39]. Despite these challenges, researchers agree that previous prophylactic HPV vaccination is still beneficial for organ transplant recipients as well as the HPV/HIV co-infected population who receive HPV vaccination before becoming HIV+. In these cases, any future challenges of HPV infection following vaccination would be neutralized by an earlier developed immunity prior to the individual presenting as HIV$^+$. This is based on the premise that the protection conferred against the viral types represented in the vaccine is expected to last for the same time period as in others who are not infected with HIV. However, what remains unclear is whether the vaccine will prove effective for an individual already infected with HIV, or in any immunocompromised state [37]. The current understanding is that humoral immune responses remain relatively intact following HIV infection. However, in such a state of immune weakness, it is unknown whether protection against HPV can be sustained. Overall, individuals who have been vaccinated prior to becoming immune compromised are expected to benefit from vaccination by maintaining immune competency, because new HPV infections from these specific types and the risk of lesions reactivating from an ongoing, latent HPV infection would be reduced. Of course, they, like other individuals, will only be protected from the vaccine-type strains, and it is imperative to note that questions regarding long-term safety in such vulnerable groups remain unanswered [30, 31, 33, 40, 41].

To this end, it is important that innovative therapeutic approaches to improve immunological surveillance and clearance of HPV continue to develop. It is well-documented that cellular immune components contribute directly to natural clearance of the virus in most people. For instance, CD4+ and CD8+ cytotoxic T cells (CTLs) are thought to target HPV 16 early and late proteins, and active HPV-specific CTLs have been identified in patients with existing infections [42]. Furthermore, researchers have found that in response to a vaccine containing E6 and E7 oncoproteins, CD4+ and CD8+ CTLs were stimulated, thus inducing the regression of HPV-mediated vulvar intraepithelial neoplasia (VIN) in 50 percent of subjects [43]. A variety of other immunotherapy investigations are underway and will be discussed in more detail later in the review.

Physical Barriers: As noted above, the use of condoms can reduce the rate of HPV infection. One study showed that when condoms are used during all vaginal intercourse encounters, HPV transmission/infection is reduced by 70 percent. Even if a condom is used greater than half of the time, the risk of infection is still reduced by 50 percent [44]. Another study similarly reports that condoms benefit users by promoting viral clearance and possible regression of CIN [4]. The use of barrier protectors such as microbicidal and spermicidal gels can also reduce the risk of HPV infection [45, 46]. The recent utilization of pseudoviruses has proven helpful in better understanding HPV invasion into keratinocytes through cell surface proteins. In these pseudovirus studies, carrageenan exhibited a microbicidal function by blocking virus particle attachment to heparin sulphate proteoglycans on cell basement membranes. Beyond its function on tissue surfaces, carrageenan also exhibited post-attachment inhibitory actions. Carrageenan has been used as a thickening agent in sex lubricants and Pap smear gels, and has shown microbicidal function against a host of STI-causing microbes including HPV [46, 47]. Originally derived from red algae, it is structurally similar to heparin but several times more potent. Therefore, it is able to bind virus more effectively than host cells and thereby acts as a decoy receptor [45, 46].

Interception of HPV-Mediated Carcinogenesis: During the decades that frequently occur between HPV infection and cancer development, there exists a window of opportunity to intercept the process. Any interventions that increase viral clearance, for example, would fit into this category. Another possible approach would be to target the process by which viral DNA integrates into the host chromosome, a relatively rare event that greatly increases the incidence of cancer. One study, for example, has postulated that chronic inflammation and the subsequent generation of reactive oxygen/nitrogen species (ROS/RNS) are harbingers of DNA damage, causing high HPV integration rates. Furthermore, smoking, cervical trauma induced by high parity, co-infection with other STDs, and long-term use of oral contraceptives have all been linked to cellular oxidative stress [48]. Thus, breaks in the DNA induced by this oxidative stress increase the probability of viral integration [49]. Interestingly, HR-HPV types integrate more frequently than do LR-HPV. The difference in integration occurrence suggests a distinction in the molecular variation and/or susceptibility between high- and low-grade lesions. Therefore, progression to cervical, and some anogenital, cancers is dependent on the presence of HR-HPV integration into the host genome. Furthermore, scientists are finding certain patterns in HPV integration events. In particular, the E2 ORF region of the viral genome is strongly preferred over other sites of integration, and integration at this site, with its accompanying loss of functional E2 protein, is linked to an increase in E6 and E7 oncogene expression [50, 51]. Consequentially, integration leads to uncontrolled expression of the oncogenes and ultimately to cellular transformation.

The role of chronic inflammation and its link to radical species production in cancer pathogenesis is widely recognized. If increased levels of oxidative stress and ROS do indeed increase the frequency of integration and cancer, one would predict that antioxidant mechanisms that counteract the generation of radical species could therefore exert chemopreventative and chemotherapeutic effects; such mechanisms have indeed been described [52, 53]. In contrast, other groups are studying ways to therapeutically harness the power of oxidative stress for actions against cancer cells. For example, the antimalarial drug, artemisin, was found to induce apoptosis in cervical cancer cells. The mechanism of action involves artemisin interacting with reduced iron to generate oxidative stress through ROS, as well as the destabilization of mitochondrial oxidative mechanisms [45, 54]. These discoveries merit further research that continues to seek ways of preventing HPV-mediated oncogenesis.

Screening for HPV and Cervical Cancer: The ultimate goal of cervical cancer screening, as outlined by the American Cancer Society (ACS) guidelines for the prevention and early detection of cervical cancer, is to prevent morbidity and mortality by determining appropriate treatment plans. In detecting the presence of HPV in the cervix, screening methods should serve to distinguish transient from persistent infections, and to effectively diagnose disease while minimizing or avoiding unnecessary complications induced by these techniques. Because 50 percent of women diagnosed with cervical cancer in the U.S. have never been screened, the importance of diligent watchfulness cannot be over-stated. Moreover, when HIV+ women comply with regular detection methods and schedules, their otherwise 10-fold higher risk of progression to invasive cervical carcinoma is diminished [30, 31, 55]. Earlier detection corresponds to better prognosis [56]. Thus, it is ideal for precancerous women who are at significantly higher risk for invasive cervical carcinoma to be promptly identified and to undergo intervention. Generally, it is recommended that cervical cancer screening start no earlier than age 21 for both non-vaccinated and vaccinated women, implying that cervical monitoring is an integral component of preventing invasive disease at all stages [5]. Because cervical cancer detection programs are the most expensive preventive measure in developed countries, enhancements to existing screening techniques, or the development of completely innovative and economical methods would be beneficial.

The most utilized and successful of screening methods in lowering cervical cancer incidence rates (by 70 percent) is exfoliative cervicovaginal cytology, or the Pap test. The Pap test satisfies the aforementioned objectives for reducing the occurrence of squamous cervical carcinoma through appropriate screening [5]. Pap tests are recommended for all sexually active women and/or women ages 21 and older. Now, a modified liquid-based version of the Pap smear is available. In a liquid-based Pap test such as Cytoscreen or Thinprep, the cells are first filtered and fixed in preservative. Then the specimen is smeared on a glass slide, which is slightly in contrast to the conventional method of directly smearing a sample onto a microscope slide. Other tests such as visual inspection with acetic acid (VIA) are useful in resource-limited settings. Further modifications of VIA include magnified visual inspection with acetic acid (VIAM) and visual inspection with Lugol's iodine solution (VILI) [57]. Colposcopy, though considered more diagnostic, also allows a magnified visualization of abnormal cervical cells [56]. Other cervical cancer screening tests may also be applied: pelvic examination – involving internal palpation of the reproductive organs; automated cervical screening techniques – supplemental imaging that reduces false positives from the cytological tests; computer imaging; polar probe – measuring the differences in electrical stimulation between normal and abnormal cervical tissue; laser-induced fluorescence – measuring spectroscopic differences in florescence between normal and diseased cervix; speculoscopy – cervical inspection using acetic acid with chemiluminescent light; and cervicography – photo development while using acetic acid [56].

Complementing the Pap test is the detection of HPV DNA. The direct testing for HPV DNA is becoming standard in many cervical cancer screening regimens, as its combined use with liquid-based cytology has generated results with even better sensitivity (up to 100 percent) for predicting high-grade cervical dysplasia [58]. HPV DNA is usually obtained from cervical scrapes and/or biopsy specimens, and recent clinical studies continue to assert the unique value of HPV-DNA testing over cytology [59-61]. Nevertheless, only time will tell the extent to which the Pap test will be replaced by the more economically appealing HPV-DNA test. To date, the FDA has approved five HPV-DNA tests: the Hybrid Capture 2 HPV DNA test, the Cervista HPV HR test, the Cervista HPV16/18 test, the Cobas 4800 HPV test, and the Aptima HPV assay. Other commonly used assays not approved by the FDA include PCR and Southern Blot hybridization, the latter being the laboratory gold standard. Some other recent innovative HPV detection methods are complete HPV genotyping, HPV mRNA detection, HPV load quantitation, identifying HPV integration, p16 ELISA, methylation profiles, and the E6 Strip test [62, 63].

Cervical cancer incidence and mortality seem to be on a downward swing in the U.S., primarily due to cytological gynecologic screening through the Pap test. Nevertheless, the global burden of HPV infection remains. Because no single detection method is optimal for every situation, it is essential that novel techniques to identify cervical cancer and HPV infection be continuously developed. Ideally, these new procedures/assays would allow clinicians to easily distinguish between low-risk and high-risk HPV status without causing undue concern in patients with transient infection. However, the cost of cervical cancer screening programs, even in developed countries, may hamper the implementation of these new advances.

3. Current clinical treatmemts

Staging and Treatment Options: Despite prevention initiatives to stay the tide of carcinogenesis caused by HR-HPV, thousands worldwide still require treatment. Currently, the most effective course of managing cervical carcinoma involves surgery and/or radiation. However, surgery provides the management team better insight into the extent of the disease because it allows the assessment of lymph node involvement [64, 65]. The surgical options available range from total removal of the cervix (radical hysterectomy) to less extreme options that preserve the fertility of the patient (radical trachelectomy), and are somewhat contingent upon disease progression. Other procedures such as chemotherapy, radiotherapy, or a combination thereof are routinely used, and their utilization depends on cancer stage as well. Factors further impacting the course of management include pregnancy; disease recurrence; fertility preservation; cervical location of the lesion; cancer type; age and general physical health. But the most important treatment determinant for cervical cancer is stage of disease, and years of clinical trials and case studies have formed the standard by which each stage is managed.

The staging of cervical cancer is based on the physical examination and is established by the International Federation of Gynecology and Obstetrics (FIGO). The World Health Organization reaffirms the FIGO organization of cervical carcinoma progression into four stages (I-IV):

Stage I: cancer found only in the cervix.

Stage II: cancer found beyond the cervix in the vagina, but has not spread to the pelvic wall and excludes the lower third of the vagina.

Stage III: cancer has spread to the lower third of the vagina and/or pelvic sidewall, and includes cases with kidney involvement.

Stage IV: cancer has grown beyond the pelvis and involves tissue of the rectum, bladder, and/or distal sites of metastasis.

The four main stages are then organized into sub-categories that further describe the extent of growth, adjacent tissue involvement, local organ participation, and metastasis to distal sites through the lymphatic system [66]. Present challenges to the optimal clinical staging of cervical cancer include complications associated with parametrial invasion, tumor location/size variation, and lymph node metastases, but developments in imaging are changing the tide [67, 68]. The ACS asserts that individuals diagnosed with cervical cancer from the early stages through late stage II actually have a survival rate greater than 50 percent. Cancers diagnosed at stage III and IV yield 30 and 15 percent survival rates, respectively. However, survival rates approach 100 percent if the cancer is caught early enough. The tools used in the process of staging and subsequent treatment of cervical cancer are numerous and will be mentioned only as they fit the scope of this review. Therefore, the sections below are not intended to represent a comprehensive discussion of these modalities.

Imaging: One of the most important aspects of cervical cancer treatment is identifying and evaluating abnormal tissue morphology using radiological technologies such as magnetic resonance imaging (MRI), x-ray computed tomography (CT scan), and positron emission tomography (PET). Because the effectiveness of these devices depends on clinical expertise and equipment, diagnostic imaging possesses several inherent discrepancies [64]. However, many researchers have begun studies that will help to improve these methods and/or to enable clinicians to draw better conclusions. Advancements in the functionality of diagnostic imaging are making it easier than ever to assess and exploit tumor parameters such as cellularity, blood flow, and glucose metabolism. Recent studies are showing that the glucose analogue, fluorine-labeled fluoro-2-deoxy-D-glucose (FDG), is particularly useful in gauging tumor metabolic activity. When combined with PET (FDG-PET), FDG is considered to have high sensitivity in detecting primary cervical tumors [69]. Additionally, combining PET and CT is becoming more acceptable as a way to eliminate the guesswork involved in evaluating metastasis to lymph nodes [70]. However, MRI is the preferred imaging method in managing cervical cancer due to the high quality of anatomic resolution it provides in the pelvis; this enhances its ability to evaluate primary tumor volume [67, 71]. New developments in MRI technology such as diffusion-weighted MRI (DWI) compare normal and abnormal tissues based on the Brownian motion of water molecules, the movement of which impacts cellular membrane integrity. However, these features may not be as distinct or reliable in excessively necrotic tumors. Another derivative of MRI is dynamic contrast-enhanced MRI (DCE-MRI), which provides an unprecedented appraisal of tumor vasculature through contrast distribution over time. Therefore, DCE-MRI may prove to be distinctly helpful in ascertaining a tumor's unique response to therapies [67, 72].

Surgery: Surgery is the advised treatment for cervical carcinoma at stages I and II. The preferred procedure, radical hysterectomy (RH), has a 75 to 80 percent cure rate according to the NCI and is the gold standard of treatment. RH is the complete removal of the uterus, cervix, and upper portion of the vagina, and involves measuring metastasis to the parametrial and pelvic lymph nodes [73, 74]. Other procedures, such as total and subtotal hysterectomies, do not require the removal of the vagina and cervix, respectively. At the early phase of stage I, less invasive techniques labeled *excisional* therapies selectively remove pathologic tissue [75, 76]. Large loop loop excision of the transformation zone (LLETZ) and cold knife conization procedures are classified as excisional therapies and are used without great risk of the cancer recurring. Conical biopsies, or the removal and microscopic examination of presumably abnormal tissue, may suffice in some situations. *Ablative* therapies such as laser and cryosurgery are utilized in expunging carcinomas *in situ* of lesser risk. This distinction between therapies is supported by studies showing that lesions from more progressed carcinomas return at a higher rate when treated with ablative techniques as compared to excisional ones [76]. In some instances, neither excision nor ablative therapies are suitable for the grade of disease, and hysterectomy is recommended. Indeed, patients not interested in fertility loss or those with lymph and vascular space involvement (LVSI) should elect for RH (RH). Nonetheless, for nulliparous women radical trachelectomy, or the removal of the uterine cervix only, with lymphadenectomy is always an option up to late stage I (Ib1) [77-79]. According to the ACS, RH is always optional for those diagnosed with early stage squamous cell cervical carcinoma, but it is strongly suggested for adenocarcinoma cervical cancer.

Surgery is immensely valuable for determining lymph node status, which is strongly correlated to survival [80]. The risk of lymph node metastasis is increased by 10 percent if tumor invasion reaches between 3 and 5 mm beyond the primary lesion. If this occurs, the NCI recommends that a modified RH comprising pelvic lymph node dissection be performed even in early disease stages. Furthermore, if metastasis to the lymph nodes or parametria is found, their removal is indicated as well as radiotherapy or chemo radiotherapy post-operatively. Post-surgery radiotherapy is also indicated if the tissue collected during surgery has a positive margin, which alludes to residual cancer and commonly occurs in late stage I. Though it is advisable to use radio and chemotherapies in stage II, some experts also support hysterectomy following these procedures. In summation, surgery yields its most potent benefits in the earlier stages of cervical carcinoma, though this fact can be viewed as a great limitation in the case of advanced disease. Other limitations of surgery include pelvic sepsis and thrombosis as well as vesicovaginal fistulas. However, opting for surgery in the management of cervical cancer may prevent vaginal stenosis, spare ovarian function, and protect local organs from future complications. There is no doubt that surgery is vital in the prospective treatment planning of the patient following operation because it allows the delineation of tumor metastasis [65]. However, surgical options are contingent upon early detection, and thus time will always be one of the most important factors in predicting a prognosis. Fortunately, advances in the field of surgery have given patients better alternatives that are less invasive (i.e. laparoscopic surgery), and these procedures, together with non-invasive therapies, will continue to benefit those for whom preventive measures have failed.

Radiotherapy: More advanced cervical cancer (stage IIb and higher) is treated with radiotherapy (RT), chemotherapy, or a combination of the two. However, surgery and RT both aim to completely eradicate malignancy and have equally positive results in attenuating disease in the initial phases. RT is generally substituted for surgery when circumstances render an operation less than optimal as in the case of elderly patients, obese patients, or patients with several co-morbidities [80, 81]. Usually younger patients elect for surgery in order to preserve sexual function and to avoid side effects such as vaginal dryness and narrowing caused by scar tissue (as described by the ACS). Elderly patients (65+ years), who account for 20 percent of cervical cancer cases, usually choose the less invasive RT [82]. Cancer cells are more susceptible to radiation than are normal cells because radiation uses high-energy particles to target and kill rapidly dividing cells through DNA damage. In general, there are two main types of radiation therapy: external beam radiation, and internal (implant) radiation usually referred to as intracavitary brachytherapy (BT). External beam radiation therapy (EBRT) is aimed wholly at the pelvis, much like a regular x-ray, and is often accompanied by cisplatin chemotherapy. The chemotherapy is added to enhance the effectiveness of the radiation and to treat metastasis to lymph nodes [83]. The selectivity of EBRT for cervical sites is enhanced by combining its use with a CT scan via 3-D conformal radiation therapy (3-D

CRT), which better concentrates radiation to specific regions of interest. BT involves the placement of a radioactive device in the uterus or vagina. Low or high-doses of radiation are given over long or short periods of time, respectively, and in accordance with the Manchester triple source system. Also, BT is a highly specialized method of radiotherapy requiring costly equipment and extensive technical training, as device positioning is very important in treatment success [84].

Maximum dose toleration by adjacent tissues such as vaginal tissue is a major limiting factor in all radiotherapy procedures. Therefore, many strategies attempt to radiosensitize the appropriate tissues (*See Neoadjuvant and Combination therapies,* below) before exposing them to radiation. Intensity modulated radiation therapy (IMRT) offers a unique advantage through the virtual mapping of tumors so that the delivery of radiation is focused and minimal tissue damage occurs to the surrounding vital structures. Supplemental techniques to improve the localization of radiation such as hyperthermia, neutron therapy, and hypoxic cell sensitizers still need refinement, and are not routinely utilized [85, 86]. Despite potential high levels of toxicity necessitating close patient monitoring, RT is a powerful tool in managing cervical cancer. The side effects of RT that have caused the greatest concern include hematologic imbalances, GI distress, GU complications due to hydronephrosis, and secondary malignancy. Future improvements in the field of RT to treat cervical cancer must first rectify the issues of maximum dose tolerance by exploiting radiosensitizing methods in order to compensate for the systemic and potentially oncologic risks associated with radiation.

Chemotherapy: Chemotherapy is the principal treatment option for recurrent and metastatic cervical cancer, and it is recommended by the ACS for the management of late stage I of cervical cancer or higher. Chemotherapy can be curative or palliative. In early cervical disease, chemotherapy can be curative, but may also be given in more advanced stages (stage IV and recurrence) to alleviate the ravaging effects of the cancer itself and its related symptoms. Chemotherapy may also be given in the later stages to postpone the toxicities associated with it until absolutely necessary. Thus, designing optimal regimens suited for each case is essential to attaining both patient comfort and treatment success. Chemotherapy can also be given adjunctively to strengthen the effects of primary treatment, or provided post-operatively [87]. In fact, the ways in which chemotherapy can be administered are numerous, ranging from single, doublet, triplet, or quartlet-agent regimens to combined chemoradiation routines. However, a few agents such as cisplatin, paclitaxel, and ifosfamide are distinguished for being somewhat autonomously potent [88]. The success of single-agent chemotherapy generally depends on histology. For example, although cisplatin is most effective for treating squamous cell carcinomas (SCC), paclitaxel has been shown to improve the median survival of non-SCC type patients as compared to others who did not receive paclitaxel [89]. Furthermore, paclitaxel yielded a response rate (RR) of 33 percent, surpassing other single agents in non-SCC type cervical cancer treatment [88, 89].

Cisplatin, a platinum-based agent, is the accepted standard of chemotherapy for cervical cancer, and it improves survival in chemoradiation recipients as compared to the use of other chemotherapeutic drugs [90-94]. However, its adequacy in improving survival and quality of life in palliative management has been questioned. Some tumor cells acquire resistance to cisplatin, and so non-platinum chemotherapy or higher doses of cisplatin, in these cases, are indicated [81, 91]. In the cases of cisplatin resistance or disease recurrence, non-platinum-based agents such as topotecan, vinorelbine, irinotecan, paclitaxel, mitomycin c, and ifosfamide are sometimes combined with cisplatin. Topotecan and 5-fluorouracil (5-FU), among other combinations, seem to produce an additive effect with cisplatin to reduce its toxicity, increasing its RR from 20 to 50 percent [90, 91, 95]. Similarly, when paclitaxel is combined with cisplatin, a high RR of 46 percent is reached for late stage IV cervical cancer and is accompanied by decreased hematologic complications. However, a Gynecologic Oncologic group study reported that consistent, weekly schedules of cisplatin alone are less toxic than cisplatin combined with other agents, particularly 5-FU [92, 96]. Sanazol and tirapazamine are relatively new chemotherapeutic agents that specifically target and destroy hypoxic tissue by dissociating into free radicals that cause DNA damage. Therefore, drug selectivity for hypoxic tissue will result in greater cytotoxicity among malignant cervical cells [81]. Multiple-agent regimens may also include the use of antibodies targeting a tumor's peculiar characteristics. For example, if a particular tumor markedly over-expresses EGFR-1, it would be appropriate to include Cetuximab in treatment, or Bevacizumab in the case of extreme vascularity [95].

Combination Therapies: Multidisciplinary treatment might be indicated throughout any of the stages of cervical carcinoma, mainly depending on its aggressiveness. In fact, it is quite common for treatment schedules to include chemotherapy, radiation therapy, and surgery [81]. The concurrent use of chemotherapy and radiation therapy is reported by the NCI to reduce cervical cancer mortality by 30 to 50 percent, particularly in late stage II. Alternatively, neoadjuvant therapy, defined as a specific sequence for delivering any treatment before a definitive therapy such as surgery or radiotherapy, may be employed. Neoadjuvant therapy is intended to prime the target tissue, thus making it more susceptible to primary treatment [71, 93]. Neoadjuvant chemotherapy (NACT) is often administered before radiation in order to radiosensitize solid tumor cells and to decrease tumor size and hypoxic cell numbers. In few instances, NACT could potentially provide patients with the option of surgery even though it may have been unfeasible prior to NACT. Moreover, researchers are finding that patients who receive sequential NACT-RH have a 10 to 15 percent survival advantage five years after treatment [97]. In cases when surgery does not completely remove all traces of abnormal tissue as anticipated, chemotherapy or radiation must be given post-operatively to inhibit local and distal metastasis through the lymphatic system. Hence, there is no doubt that concurrent chemotherapy and radiation therapy can improve survival in women with locally advanced cervical cancer or recurrent cancer [93, 98]. Radiation treatment alone does not contain cancer in 35 to 90 percent of patients, but chemotherapy given with radiation treatment yields much higher survival rates. The chemotherapeutic drugs most commonly used with radiation are cisplatin, 5-FU, mitomycin C, and hydroxyurea, though cisplatin produces the largest increase in survival by reducing mortality and recurrence [93, 94]. Many times, the sensitizing effects of drugs are needed to accentuate the value of other treatment methods, as is the case with histone deacetylase inhibitors, decitabine and valproic acid, that radiosensitize tumors for RT [81]. Thus, researchers may build and forge new applications through trials that study combination therapies.

4. Molecular therapies in development

Therapeutic Immune Strategies: The development of the prophylactic vaccine has forever changed the course of HPV-mediated cervical disease. Nevertheless, it is clear that there is still an immense need for therapeutic options, especially in developing countries where the positive, yet costly measures of preventative initiatives remain to be implemented. In contrast to prophylactic vaccines that target the L1 and L2 proteins and are protective against HPV infections, therapeutic vaccines would ideally target molecules such as E6 and/or E7 post-infection, which are directly linked to HPV-mediated carcinogenesis [99]. Therapeutic vaccines may be constructed in a variety of ways, as described below [100].

Live, vector-based vaccines, bacterial and viral, can generate very robust cell-mediated and adaptive immune responses, and because of this they are preferred over peptide/protein vaccines. Specifically, bacterial vectors function well when they are packaged with antigen (genes or proteins), thereby alerting antigen-presenting cells (APCs) to initiate an immune response. Though several bacterial vectors have been tested, *L. monocytogenes* is a prototypic example. Simply, *L. monocytogenes* stimulates antigen-specific CD8+ and CD4+ T cell responses following its evasion of immune destruction by releasing *Lm* toxin to avoid phagosomal lysis. However, the most appealing factor of the *L. monocytogenes* vector is that the immune response can be easily controlled by antibiotics should the body react adversely to *Lm* [101-104]. With regards to viral vectors, a few viruses, such as the vaccinia virus, adenovirus, vesicular stomatitis virus, and alphavirus, have distinguished themselves and show great promise. In fact, researchers have discovered that when an adenovirus vector is used to deliver calreticulin and HPV E7 antigens, the size of E7-expressing tumors in mice decrease [105]. A highly anticipated viral vaccine candidate is the TA-HPV vaccine, consisting of both HPV16 and HPV18 E6 and E7 antigens and a vaccinia virus vector. TA-HPV is safe and efficient in stimulating either a specific CTL response or a serological response, which might depend on the epigenetic patterns of each individual [106]. Similarly, the MVA E2 vaccine is also packaged with the vaccinia virus, and uses the bovine papillomavirus E2 protein to repress E6 and E7 transcription. MVA-HPV-IL2, currently undergoing a phase III clinical trial for CIN 2-3 treatment, utilizes a modified vaccinia Ankara viral vector, and uniquely contains HPV16 E6 and E7 DNA as well as IL-2 [99, 107]. The co-expression of a cytokine with HPV antigens induces a stronger immune response by stimulating dendritic cell maturation, though the refinement of viral vector tools must include solutions for overcoming pre-existing immunity. To rectify this, Cox-2 inhibitors are presently being tested to offset such immune interferences, thus allowing greater exploitation of a potentially powerful treatment. However, safety factors remain a high priority when viral vectors are considered, and these vectors must be properly constructed for use in both immunocompetent and immunocompromised individuals [100].

In peptide-based vaccines, antigens from HPV are directly administered to elicit a response from dendritic cells (DCs) *via* toll-like receptor (TLR) activation [108]. The peptide vaccine platform is ideal for mass production, but the breadth of its efficacy is limited by the expression of only one major histocompatibility complex I (MHC I) phenotype; protein-based vaccines are not encumbered in the same way. However, if the specific immunogenic epitopes on peptides could be identified it would greatly remedy this difficulty. Some investigators are taking a different approach by overlapping peptides with a broad range of different epitopes to obtain a greater immune response [109]. Meanwhile, other researchers have focused on the development of vaccines that utilize a synthetic E7 peptide component to clear HPV-mediated tumors in mice, such as TriVax [110]. Unfortunately, a limitation of both peptide- and protein-based vaccines is low immunogenicity. This challenge, however, is no longer intractable with the advent of various immunomodulatory adjuvant agents such as TLR ligands, cytokines, and lipids, all of which help to stimulate a robust immune response. Another recently popular strategy thought to increase protein/peptide vaccine potency involves the Pan HLA-DR epitope peptide (PADRE), which binds MHC class II molecules with much stronger affinity [108]. Following the success of PADRE and other similar technologies, more potent enhancers of peptide vaccines such as 4-1BB ligand, CpG oligodeoxynucleotide, mutant cholera toxin, and lipopeptides are now emerging [111].

In general, protein-based therapeutic vaccines, like peptide-based vaccines, are advantageous for safety and tolerability. Although protein-based vaccines are not restricted by MHC compatibility, they cannot directly stimulate cytotoxic T lymphocytes. Protein vaccine adjuvants that are considered to compensate for this weakness in protein vector therapy include liposome-polycation-DNA and the saponin-based ISCOMATRIX. The ISCOMATRIX is an adjuvant complex consisting of phospholipids and cholesterols, and it causes a rapid innate immune cell response [112]. In general, any strategy that increases antigen uptake by APCs, antigen presentation, or the CTL response is expected to improve the immunogenicity of a protein. One protein-based therapeutic vaccine in clinical trials is TA-CIN. Essentially, TA-CIN is a mixture of L2, E6, and E7 proteins from HPV16. The L2 antigen launches a humoral response, and the E6 and E7 proteins induce T cell responses. However, further investigation revealed that TA-CIN is even more powerful when combined with the TA-HPV vaccine [113-115]. Another strong protein-based vaccine candidate, due to its safety and ability to induce lesion regression in various HPV-related diseases, is HspE7 [116]. HspE7 is a fusion product of HPV16 E7 and the *Mycobacterium bovis* Hsp65 proteins. Another potential strategy to improve immunogenicity in protein-based therapeutic vaccines is the use of the Fve adjuvant, which is derived from a fungal protein originating in the *Flammulina velutipes* species, and has been shown to produce potent humoral and cellular immune responses. The antitumor effects of Fve in HPV-mediated cancers are attributed to its ability to induce IFN-gamma secretion and to stimulate T helper and CTLs in tumor-bearing mice [117]. Our knowledge about how to apply protein and peptide therapeutic vaccines against cervical cancer is steadily increasing. The immediate next step is to follow up with successful clinical trials, and to implement the most useful of these methods, or a combination thereof.

One advantage of DNA-based vaccination is its capacity to increase immunological memory through constant antigen production. Because the immune response itself is not anti-vector, multiple vaccinations are possible. Moreover, the antigens produced by DNA vaccines can be delivered in a variety of ways, resulting in stimulation of both APCs and T lymphocyte immune defenses [118, 119]. However, DNA vaccines also present the challenge of overcoming low immunogenicity due to limited APC specificity. Therefore, future developments must focus on antigen modifications so as to elicit a stronger DC adaptive immune response. One such strategy increases the number of HPV DNA plasmid transfection events in DCs. These DCs will then present antigen to, and ultimately activate, naive CD4+ and CD8+ lymphocytes [119]. However, researchers still must determine the most efficient and effective way to deliver HPV DNA to DCs. A fairly recent investigation discusses a novel method to administer a dose-driven vaccine by gene gun technology, which forms a DNA-coated stream of gold particles targeting Langerhans cells in the skin [120]. Other studies justify the use of cell membrane permeabilization by electroporation, thereby causing cells to experience an electric shock and maximizing cellular uptake of DNA [121, 122].

Electroporation also leads to inflammation and cytokine recruitment, thus enhancing the immune environment. Additionally, electroporation was found to be particularly effective against E7-expressing tumors. The VGX-3100 plasmid DNA vaccine, targeting E6 and E7 antigens of HPV16 and 18, seemed to have great efficacy when it was combined with electroporation administration [123]. Furthermore, clinical trials attest to the value of this particular method of treatment delivery in CIN 2 and 3 lesions. Strategies that increase transfection efficiency are continuously being sought through experimentation with diverse routes of vaccine administration, such as intramuscular *versus* intradermal techniques. The efficient intramuscular administration of DNA is achieved *via* microencapsulation, which uses a biopolymer that surrounds the plasmid to prevent degradation by nucleases. Conversely, intradermal administration involves skin patch tattooing using microneedles [124]. One encapsulated DNA-based vaccine that has been tested with both administrative routes is the amolimogene bepiplasmid (also known as ZYC101a), which contains T cell epitopes and HPV16 and 18 E6/E7 viral protein fragments [125, 126]. In this study, it was concluded that intramuscular methods were more effective [127, 128].

Another strategy to strengthen DNA-based vaccines focuses on improving DC antigen processing. Those cells that have become transfected with HPV DNA material may be prompted to generate a more potent immune response through codon optimization or demethylation techniques that will increase gene translation efficiency [100]. These methods work to improve antigen translation and expression in cells with HPV DNA. Additionally, DNA vaccination with the MHC class I chaperone molecule, calreticulin, was shown to increase the CD8+ immune response, thereby leading to an antitumor effect [129]. It is also possible to improve antigen processing through the MHC class II pathway. For instance, the E7/LAMP-1 vaccine allows antigen to be further sorted in endosomal and lysosomal compartments, thus priming CD4+ and CD8+ lymphocytes for a greater response as compared to the administration of E7 alone [130]. Substitution of the MHC class II peptide, CLIP (Class II-associated peptide), for the PADRE peptide in the invariant chain is a promising strategy to not only increase antigen presentation, but also to secrete cytokines that stimulate T cell proliferation, thus resulting in greater CD4+ lymphocyte activity [131, 132]. Other methods of improving antigen presentation include cross-presentation by extracellular proteins like HSP 70, up-regulation of MHC II expression on the surface of DCs, and single chain trimer technology (SCT). SCT involves the fusion of HPV antigen to the MHC class I molecule, beta-2 microglobulin, resulting in the appropriate recognition of antigen and action against an E6-expressing tumor [133, 134].

RNA replicon-based vaccines have some advantages over DNA vaccines: 1) they are less likely to integrate into the host genome, thus decreasing the risk of cell transformation and 2) they can potentially generate more protein than can DNA methods. Of course, RNA replicon-based vaccines may be introduced into the host as DNA. From here, the cell can then transcribe the DNA molecule into RNA, but without the structural genes needed to construct viral particles. Therefore, no antibodies are produced against viral immunologic molecules and administration can be repeated. One significant limitation of using replicons is that RNA is inherently unstable. However, the use of a DNA-launched RNA replicon could surmount this difficulty, and concerns of gene integration could be addressed by designing the DNA to self-destruct following gene expression. Because immunologic cells undergo apoptosis in this process, it is necessary to fuse the HPV antigen to an anti-apoptotic protein, otherwise DC numbers will be drastically reduced [100, 135, 136]. The Kunjin flavivirus has the potential to accomplish the same goal by delivering the desired antigens into cells without immediately inducing apoptosis, thus prolonging the window of time for antigen presentation by transfected cells and improving overall immunogenicity [137-139].

Dendritic cell-based vaccines can be prepared in several ways: by introducing exogenous HPV antigen via endocytosis in to DCs; by infusing DCs with E6/E7 DNA or RNA through electroporation; or, the antigen may be packaged together with liposomes or nanoparticles to be delivered into DCs [140]. DC interactions with T cells and the subsequent perpetuation of the immune signal are essential features that determine whether an organism will demonstrate a strong immune response, or whether it will exhibit immune tolerance (e.g. if the DCs are immature) [141, 142]. Essentially, DCs activate T cells and T cells, in turn, mediate DC apoptosis. Therefore, it has been proposed that prolonging DC survival may strengthen and lengthen the initial T cell stimulation [143]. However, because the idea of combining HPV vaccines with anti-apoptotic proteins has not gained much popularity due to the possibility of cellular transformation, other approaches such as co-administering vaccines with siRNAs targeting pro-apoptotic proteins are gaining traction. Designing shRNAs directed at FasL produced by DCs to promote T cell apoptosis, for example, could increase the number of T cells stimulated [144]. DC activation can also be prolonged by deactivating the negative regulation of cytokine signaling through SOCS-1, which acts on the Jak-Stat pathway [132, 145, 146].

Because tumor cell-based vaccines have shown promise in malignancies like melanoma, colon and prostate cancers, many subscribe to this paradigm as the key to solving the cervical carcinoma dilemma. The idea of manipulating tumor cells into becoming more discernible by the immune system is based on their expression of immunomodulatory cytokines like IL-2 and IL-12 [147]. Other studies have found that engineering tumor cells to secrete pro-immune cytokines such as GM-CSF produces antitumor immunity as well [148]. The advantage of using tumor cell-based vaccines is that multiple antigens can be targeted on the surface of a tumor, thus increasing the chance that a single cell or group of cells expressing those antigens will be eliminated by the immune system. As can be expected, such an individualized treatment is costly and may border on the impractical as compared to other recent advances in the field of cervical cancer vaccination. Furthermore, patients who qualify for tumor cell-based vaccination would be at greater risk in the receipt of new cancer cells than if they were to employ a treatment plan composed of existing therapies [149].

Of course, every approach has its advantages and disadvantages, but combining several therapeutic vaccines into a single regimen may offer synergy and thus strengthen treatment efficacy. For example, one preclinical study tested a prime-boost vaccination model. The immune system was first primed with a DNA vaccine consisting of HPV16 E7 and LAMP-1 (Sig/E7/LAMP-1). Then, a booster dose of Sig/E7/LAMP-1 was given again to maintain and increase the T-cell response over a longer period [150]. Because several prime-boost studies have yielded continuous positive results in safety and efficacy, we can expect to see similar combinatory therapeutic trials in the future.

RNA-based Therapy: RNAs have the unique ability to form double-stranded molecules by hybridizing with complementary antisense RNA. It was established years ago that antisense E6/E7 RNAs in a plasmid could stagnate cellular growth [151]. More recently, the ability to design antisense oligodeoxynucleotides (ODNs) that specifically bind E6/E7 RNA molecules at the translation initiation region with high affinity have made the use of translation inhibition more feasible for achieving cervical carcinoma treatment goals. Later studies have confirmed these results, and suggest that stronger, additive effects may also occur when antisense ODNs are designed with adjacent mRNA targets in mind [152, 153].

Tristetrapolin (TTP) is an RNA-binding protein with anti-cancer properties, and yields its effects by binding to AU rich regions of mRNA and promoting their destruction. These AU-rich elements (AREs) of mRNA, located in the untranslated region of the strand, are naturally involved in regulating cellular growth and inflammation *via* mediators such as TNF-alpha and COX-2. Therefore, the affinity with which TTP binds these elements makes this interaction an attractive point of intervention. For example, HPV$^+$ HeLa cells exposed to TTP demonstrated higher levels of p53 as compared to untreated cells. Additionally, in the presence of TTP, these same cells acquired the ability to inhibit E6-AP expression, suggesting a possible mechanism for the rescue of p53 [154]. Other RNA-based methods targeting HPV include the use of siRNAs directed against E6 and E7. siRNAs cause the cleavage and degradation of homologous sequences through their participation in the RNA-induced Silencing Complex (RISC). Researchers are now investigating the use of vehicles such as shRNAs to target and destroy RNAs of interest. However, better systems for delivering shRNAs to the nuclei, and better ways to access cellular uptake mechanisms for siRNAs, are needed [155].

Antibody-based Therapy: The use of monoclonal antibodies in cancer treatment is an appealing concept due to the selectivity and specificity with which an antibody can bind to the molecule of interest. Molecules participating in tumor progression can be targeted by antibodies through three general mechanisms: 1) Recognition of specific tumor-associated receptors, such as EGFR; 2) Binding to immune effector cells, and 3) Binding to tumor-promoting molecules such as VEGF. Though no monoclonal antibodies have been approved for the treatment of cervical cancer, researchers are accruing more convincing evidence of their value [156]. As with most cancers, cervical carcinomas possess a dynamic vascular network. Thus, much investigation has gone into developing biologic agents that target molecular pathways associated with vascularization, such as those involving vascular endothelial growth factor (VEGF). Bevacizumab is an angiogenesis inhibitor that ultimately delays vasculogenic processes, and has long been used effectively in the treatment of other malignancies such as colorectal cancer. The discovery of Bevacizumab's anti-angiogenic properties in recurrent cervical cancer during a phase II clinical trial has now warranted further investigation within the context of both single-agent and combination therapies [157]. Another antibody, Cetuximab, has a high affinity for epidermal growth factor receptor (EGFR), which is influential in cell differentiation processes. However, Cetuximab has distinguished itself as effective only against growths of squamous cell origin. Thus, other EGFR inhibitors such as gefitinib, erlotinib, and lapatinib are being investigated [158, 159]. In one research model, Cetuximab was shown to inhibit tumor cell growth following exposure to ionizing radiation, which induced EGFR pathway activation and VEGF over-expression [160]. Though others have reported Cetuximab to be more limited in activity in some populations [158], the roles of both VEGF and EGFR in cervical cancer remain under intense study. Another unique approach in helping to further define molecular targets using antibodies is to structure them against a particular domain of an HPV oncoprotein. By designing mAbs against HPV16 E6 zinc-binding domains researchers are able to map key peptide sequences, and potentially interfere with cell transformation mechanisms affecting p53 tumor suppressor levels [161].

Small Molecule Inhibitors and Antiviral Leads: As the field of prevention continues to advance (e.g. through the development of prophylactic vaccines), one might ask why additional resources should be directed towards the discovery of small molecule HPV inhibitors. The short answer is that due to the timeline of disease progression, it will be a few decades before these preventative measures will make a significant impact on the disease burden. In the meantime, infected women and others who do not benefit from these approaches have access to only a limited, and frequently inadequate, set of options such as lesion removal. In addition to the obvious drawbacks of surgical treatment, such as invasiveness and cytodestruction, it is well established that viral persistence is mainly responsible for disease, especially among the elderly and the immunodeficient [162]. Hence, lesions do frequently recur. In addition to these concerns, as previously stated, a low risk perception might further short circuit preventive measures, thus increasing the need to contain HPV therapeutically. Moreover, the fact that one-third of all cervical cancers are caused by types of HPV that are not included in the current vaccines [163] should maintain a sense of urgency with regards to developing more comprehensive and long-lasting approaches. Though no small molecule inhibitor of HPV has yet been approved, a significant amount of antiviral agent research has focused on five major potential targets for intervention: 1) Inhibition of E1/E2 interactions, 2) E6 and E7 oncoprotein blockade, 3) Direct interference with E6AP-mediated p53 degradation, 4) Interference with interactions between HPV and other apoptotic factors (i.e. Bax and FADD), and 5) Stalling the ubiquitin proteasome system to reduce the degradation of anti-tumor proteins. The following sections will discuss these topics in greater detail.

Studies have revealed that certain host proteins are co-opted by the virus and used to carry out viral functions. For instance, the bromodomain protein, Brd4, which normally serves as a regulator of cell growth and transcription, has been implicated in the tethering of bovine papillomavirus (BPV) episomes to chromosomes in dividing cells [164, 165]. Also, it was recently published that Brd4 not only binds to the HPV regulatory protein, E2, aiding in many of its functions, but also stabilizes it [166, 167]. Although the ways in which Brd4 can interact with the bovine and human papillomaviruses may differ, the concern that Brd4 may play a key role in viral replication appears to be substantiated. Regarding PV E2, research has indicated that its N-terminal transactivation domain is quite conserved among the papillomaviruses [168]. Thus, many of the properties of the PV E2 protein are likely to be shared between many PVs [166]. Origin-specific viral DNA replication is overseen by E2 once the viral helicase, E1, has been loaded successfully onto the origin of replication by E2. E2 also represses the expression of E6/E7 oncoproteins at the transcriptional level, in addition to performing other regulatory tasks. Therefore, it could be quite detrimental to the intracellular establishment of the virus, its subsequent replication and cellular transformation if the interactions between E2 and its cellular partners could be targeted. For example, while Brd4 is bound to E2, E2 is unable to engage P-TEFB, a transcription elongation factor, and this affects the expression of downstream genes such as E6 and E7 from the integrated viral genome [169]. Future studies are expected to provide more conclusive data regarding P-TEFB, the roles of Brd4, and their association with HPV proteins. But as a key regulatory protein, the importance of E2 on HPV viability and replication makes it a prime target for intervention.

E1 is the only enzymatic product of the viral genome, coding for an ATPase, and is thus an appealing target for molecular intervention. Indeed, if E1's binding and helicase properties could be blocked, DNA replication would be halted. Inevitably, impeding this process would also thwart the hijacking of cellular replication machinery for viral genome multiplication. Because the virus uses cellular replication factors derived from the host, current antiviral agents that block viral proteases and polymerases are ineffective in opposing HPV. DNA helicase unwinding is powered by the energy provided through ATP hydrolysis *via* the ATPase. ATP acts not only as the substrate, but also as an E1-E2 allosteric modulator [170]. As such, inhibitors sensitive to ATP concentrations, such as biphenylsulfonacetic acid, seem quite promising, in part because this agent does not directly bind ATP. Adding amides to certain positions of the biphenyl group enhances the compound's affinity for HPV6 E1, increasing its specificity [171]. However, whether biphenyl inhibitors can be applied to other HPV types remains undetermined. Furthermore, researchers have struggled to demonstrate inhibitory activity in cell-based assays [172]. In summary, future small inhibitors of E1 must directly target the enzyme's binding pocket, thereby conferring greater binding strength and specificity to E1-inhibitor complexes.

Small molecular inhibitors called indandiones are recognized as the first class of molecules to block HPV DNA replication by interrupting E1-E2 binding. The presence of indandiones induces conformational changes in E2, forming a deep binding pocket through which the small molecule modifies protein activity [173]. The success of preliminary trials attests to the great potential and need of inhibitors intended for binding pockets. Repaglinides operate similarly to indandiones in disrupting E1-E2 binding, though their effect is reversible, and they are reported to occupy a larger area of the binding pocket than do their indandione counterparts. One limitation for these classes of compounds is the poor binding frequently observed between small molecules and a large protein interface. However, these studies have demonstrated that designing small molecules to target large protein interfaces might actually be necessary in order to disclose pockets thought not to exist, or to create new ones. Another factor that must be considered is the fact that viral integration into the host genome frequently leads to loss of E1/E2 gene expression, meaning that established cancers are likely to have lost the molecules targeted by inhibitors of E1 and/or E2, thereby limiting their usefulness [174, 175].

In contrast, E6 and E7 are frequently over-expressed in established cancers, making these two proteins quite attractive as targets. E6 and E7 are the zinc finger-containing proteins primarily responsible for the malignant alterations and de-differentiation of keratinocytes observed during cell transformation. These changes occur following integration of the HPV genome into host DNA [163, 176]. During this process, the regulators of viral replication, E1 and E2, are frequently disrupted, allowing over-expression of E6 and E7. HR-HPV types induce cell immortalization and transformation primarily through the over-expression of E6 and/or E7, which are best known for their ability to accelerate the degradation of the p53 and retinoblastoma proteins (pRB), respectively. The E6-mediated loss of p53 function leads to an insensitivity to apoptotic signals as well as to a loss of cell cycle regulation at the G1/S checkpoint in response to DNA damage. E7 contributes to the hyperplasia crisis by accelerating the degradation of pRB and thereby stimulating cells in Interphase to re-enter the cell cycle at S phase [177-179]. Together, over-expression of the E6 and E7 oncoproteins, decrease apoptosis and increase cell division, setting the stage for cancer [180]. Antiviral agents that can partially, if not fully, inhibit E6 and/or E7 functions clearly have the potential to negatively impact the carcinogenic process. One group, for example, proposed such a strategy in their study of the HPV16 E7-antagonizing peptide, Pep-7 [181]. Pep-7 was originally introduced as a short peptide component of the vacuole/lysosomal pathway [182]. However, Pep-7 was later shown not only to reduce the viability of HPV-positive cells *in vitro*, but it also decreased expression of E7 in SiHa cells in a xenograft model. It is conjectured that the selective mechanism Pep-7 uses to suppress cell proliferation may hinge on its ability to obstruct E7-pRB associations, even releasing pRB from E7 [181].

In contrast to E7, which appears to act primarily by increasing the ability of expressing cells to replicate, E6 acts by reducing the ability of expressing cells to undergo apoptosis. Apoptosis is a natural, cell-mediated death response to irreparable DNA damage. One target of E6 is the p53 tumor suppressor, which is degraded following association of E6 with the ubiquitin protein ligase, E6AP. The E6/E6AP complex binds to p53 and initiates its ubiquitination and consequent proteolytic destruction [183]. This means that the downstream targets of p53, which mediate cell cycle arrest and apoptosis, are not activated. Therefore, interference with the E6/E6AP-mediated proteasomal degradation of p53 has been seen as another possible strategy for treatment. The ubiquitination proteasome system (UPS) begins with the ubiquitin activating E1 molecules interacting with E2 conjugating enzymes, followed by catalyzation of the polyubiquitination cascade onto target proteins by E3 enzymes [184]. A subset of E3s, called RING-finger E3s, are a group of ubiquitin ligases that have domains to which ubiquitination substrates bind, and it is thought that by inhibiting this interaction, p53 might be preserved. One prominent p53-related RING-finger ubiquitin ligase is MDM2. MDM2 is normally expressed in a negative feedback manner to regulate p53 levels. Three dominant trains of thought have guided approaches seeking ways in which the negative effects of MDM2 might be neutralized: 1) Blocking activation domains on p53, 2) Increasing nuclear export of p53 so as not to activate MDM2 transcription, and 3) Inhibiting MDM2. Of these, the third approach has received the most attention. In one such study, small molecules were screened and selected based on their MDM2 inhibitory properties, and a class called the Nutlins was discovered. Nutlins competitively bind MDM2 at the same site typically occupied by p53, and structurally interpose themselves between p53 and MDM2 [185]. In contrast, another molecule labeled RITA actually binds to p53 and stabilizes it against degradation by inhibiting p53 from interacting with most of its binding partners, including MDM2 [186]. A more recent addition to the MDM2 inhibitor group is TRIAD1, a RING-finger bearing molecule, that functions similarly to RITA in that it binds p53 (at the C-terminus), and also intercepts ubiquitination triggered by MDM2 [187].

One well-established inhibitor of the UPS is Bortezomib. Bortezomib targets and reversibly blocks 26S proteasome activity, and has already been FDA-approved for the treatment of multiple myeloma and lymphoma [188]. Though its use has been proposed for the treatment of many diseases, from non-small cell lung cancer to pancreatic cancer, an equivalent and thorough exploration in the context of cervical carcinoma is still needed [189]. This suggestion is solidly founded on the observed sensitization of cervical cancer cells to apoptosis by another protease inhibitor (PI), MG132 [190]. A final set of PIs are those that inhibit the HIV protease. The anti-oncogenic properties of HIV PIs were first noted with respect to the 20S proteasome, and further investigation explicitly demonstrated Lopinavir active against E6-induced p53 degradation. Though Lopinavir also stabilizes p53, it exhibits low potency and virus is not fully cleared. The value of HIV PIs in cervical cancer treatment could be potentiated by its current availability as an antiviral agent, which might expedite the clinical trial process [191-193].

While p53 and the proteins to which it is connected are clearly targets worth exploring, other pro-apoptotic targets could prove just as important in halting the progression of HPV-mediated disease. HPV16 E6 binds to several additional signaling molecules in the intrinsic and extrinsic apoptotic pathways, including Bax, FADD, and procaspase-8, thus blocking their ability to interact with their normal partners and leading to their premature disposal by the proteasome. Not only does HPV16 E6 indirectly affect Bax *via* the degradation of p53, but Bax mRNA levels are decreased and the protein itself is destabilized in the presence of E6. Therefore, apoptotic cascades involving Bax and p53 represent a compelling site at which antiviral therapy could be targeted [194, 195]. It has also been reported that HPV16 E6 binds to both FADD and caspase 8 *via* DED residues, and a peptide corresponding to the binding site of FADD blocked both of these interactions. Expression of this peptide in HPV+ cells was able to re-sensitize those cells to apoptosis triggered through the extrinsic pathway [196, 197]. A search for small molecules capable of interfering with these interactions was conducted and several candidates were identified, primarily among the flavones and flavonols. Of these compounds, myricetin generated the lowest IC_{50} in assays designed to detect inhibition of E6-procaspase 8 binding [198]. More research is needed to optimize and test these small molecule leads.

5. Final remarks

In summary, the scientific community has witnessed tremendous progress in the recent years towards the goal of eradicating HPV-mediated cervical carcinoma. Of these endeavors, routine Pap testing and the prophylactic vaccines, Gardasil and Cervarix, are particularly noteworthy for their documented and anticipated progress in decreasing the burden of this disease. Improved vaccines are under development, as are better methods for early detection. Additionally, recent discoveries pertaining to the HPV life cycle, viral infection, and immune clearance have provided guidance toward educating the public about the biological and behavioral risk factors linked to cervical cancer. However, awareness among the populations of greatest risk, in both developed and underdeveloped countries, is lacking. Although high-risk individuals may belong to diverse ethnic groups and/or have lower socioeconomic standing, they may not all benefit equally from any single approach, necessitating the importance of targeted education and intervention. Thus, future initiatives for the prevention of cervical cancer must aim to decrease existing inequalities, with a strong emphasis on educating about HPV transmission and screening throughout a woman's lifetime, particularly in groups where incidence and death rates are disproportionate. The hope is that these preventive methods – and in particular, the vaccine – will significantly reduce the HPV disease burden for future generations.

While progress in prevention must continue, complementary approaches that can provide better treatment options to populations that cannot directly benefit from vaccine-associated therapies must also be developed. These groups include women who are already infected with HPV, immunocompromised individuals such as those with HPV/HIV co-infections, and organ transplant patients. In treating these individuals, the prognosis and treatment of cervical cancer depends on our ability to medically diagnose and assign a disease stage. Therefore, improvements in diagnostic imaging, surgery, radiation therapy, chemotherapy, or a combination thereof are being studied to give women more options and to enhance each patient's ability to make better-informed decisions.

Along with clinical treatment, molecular therapies that target cervical cancer processes are also anticipated to contribute to the elimination of cervical cancer. Research focusing on HPV early proteins will continue to provide insights regarding the viral mechanisms used to take control over cellular processes. Of these viral components, the E6 and E7 oncoproteins have long been recognized as the main mediators of HPV-associated malignancies. Therefore, the idea that approaches targeting these two oncoproteins are likely to act in an anti-oncogenic manner is quite reasonable. Such discoveries have the potential to exert a broad impact in the field of virology, as they will enable researchers to more fully understand virus-host interactions and how to better equip the body to respond to or even prevent infection.

In conclusion, cervical cancer research has come a long way, but there is still much more to be done to ensure that our accomplishments are not overshadowed by failures to educate, vaccinate, improve clinical management, and strengthen our knowledge about HPV. Indeed, it is quite possible that the challenge of HPV-mediated cervical cancer can be overcome in this generation, given the abundance of advancements, ideas and potential avenues that have been discussed here.

Acknowledgements

This work was partially supported by a grant from the National Institutes of Health 5R25GM060507, which provided support to WE.

Author details

Whitney Evans[1,3], Maria Filippova[1], Ron Swensen[2] and Penelope Duerksen-Hughes[1]

1 Department of Basic Science, Loma Linda University School of Medicine, Loma Linda, CA, USA

2 Department of Gynecology and Obstetrics, Loma Linda University School of Medicine, Loma Linda, CA, USA

3 Center for Health Disparities and Molecular Medicine, Loma Linda University School of Medicine, Loma Linda, CA, USA

References

[1] Braaten KP, Laufer MR. Human Papillomavirus (HPV), HPV-Related Disease, and the HPV Vaccine. Reviews in obstetrics and gynecology. 2008;1(1):2-10. Epub 2008/08/15.

[2] Dunne EF, Markowitz LE. Genital human papillomavirus infection. Clin Infect Dis. 2006;43(5):624-9. Epub 2006/08/04.

[3] Banik U, Bhattacharjee P, Ahamad SU, Rahman Z. Pattern of epithelial cell abnormality in Pap smear: A clinicopathological and demographic correlation. Cytojournal. 2011;8:8. Epub 2011/06/30.

[4] Hogewoning CJ, Bleeker MC, van den Brule AJ, Voorhorst FJ, Snijders PJ, Berkhof J, et al. Condom use promotes regression of cervical intraepithelial neoplasia and clearance of human papillomavirus: a randomized clinical trial. Int J Cancer. 2003;107(5): 811-6. Epub 2003/10/21.

[5] Saslow D, Solomon D, Lawson HW, Killackey M, Kulasingam SL, Cain JM, et al. American Cancer Society, American Society for Colposcopy and Cervical Pathology, and American Society for Clinical Pathology Screening Guidelines for the Prevention and Early Detection of Cervical Cancer. J Low Genit Tract Dis. 2012;16(3):175-204. Epub 2012/03/16.

[6] Downs LS, Smith JS, Scarinci I, Flowers L, Parham G. The disparity of cervical cancer in diverse populations. Gynecol Oncol. 2008;109(2 Suppl):S22-30. Epub 2008/06/14.

[7] Shikary T, Bernstein DI, Jin Y, Zimet GD, Rosenthal SL, Kahn JA. Epidemiology and risk factors for human papillomavirus infection in a diverse sample of low-income young women. J Clin Virol. 2009;46(2):107-11. Epub 2009/08/12.

[8] Gunnell AS, Tran TN, Torrang A, Dickman PW, Sparen P, Palmgren J, et al. Synergy between cigarette smoking and human papillomavirus type 16 in cervical cancer in

situ development. Cancer epidemiology, biomarkers & prevention : a publication of the American Association for Cancer Research, cosponsored by the American Society of Preventive Oncology. 2006;15(11):2141-7. Epub 2006/10/24.

[9]   Fonseca-Moutinho JA. Smoking and cervical cancer. ISRN Obstet Gynecol. 2011;2011:847684. Epub 2011/07/26.

[10] Gonzalez P, Hildesheim A, Rodriguez AC, Schiffman M, Porras C, Wacholder S, et al. Behavioral/lifestyle and immunologic factors associated with HPV infection among women older than 45 years. Cancer Epidemiol Biomarkers Prev. 2010;19(12): 3044-54. Epub 2010/10/19.

[11] Jones CJ, Brinton LA, Hamman RF, Stolley PD, Lehman HF, Levine RS, et al. Risk factors for in situ cervical cancer: results from a case-control study. Cancer research. 1990;50(12):3657-62. Epub 1990/06/15.

[12] Marlow LA, Waller J, Wardle J. Public awareness that HPV is a risk factor for cervical cancer. Br J Cancer. 2007;97(5):691-4. Epub 2007/08/10.

[13] Marek E, Dergez T, Rebek-Nagy G, Kricskovics A, Kovacs K, Bozsa S, et al. Adolescents' awareness of HPV infections and attitudes towards HPV vaccination 3 years following the introduction of the HPV vaccine in Hungary. Vaccine. 2011;29(47): 8591-8. Epub 2011/09/24.

[14] Marek E, Dergez T, Rebek-Nagy G, Szilard I, Kiss I, Ember I, et al. Effect of an educational intervention on Hungarian adolescents' awareness, beliefs and attitudes on the prevention of cervical cancer. Vaccine. 2012;30(48):6824-32. Epub 2012/09/25.

[15] Christopher A. Hearing addresses condoms for HPV prevention. J Natl Cancer Inst. 2004;96(13):985. Epub 2004/07/09.

[16] Lauby JL, Batson H, Milnamow M. Effects of drug use on sexual risk behavior: results of an HIV outreach and education program. J Evid Based Soc Work. 2010;7(1): 88-102. Epub 2010/02/24.

[17] Calsyn DA, Saxon AJ, Wells EA, Greenberg DM. Longitudinal sexual behavior changes in injecting drug users. AIDS. 1992;6(10):1207-11. Epub 1992/10/01.

[18] Rambout L, Hopkins L, Hutton B, Fergusson D. Prophylactic vaccination against human papillomavirus infection and disease in women: a systematic review of randomized controlled trials. CMAJ. 2007;177(5):469-79. Epub 2007/08/03.

[19] Lowy DR, Schiller JT. Prophylactic human papillomavirus vaccines. J Clin Invest. 2006;116(5):1167-73. Epub 2006/05/04.

[20] Saslow D, Castle PE. American Cancer Society Guideline for Human Papillomavirus (HPV) Vaccine Use to Prevent Cervical Cancer and Its Precursors. 2006.

[21] Future II SG. Quadrivalent vaccine against human papillomavirus to prevent high-grade cervical lesions. The New England journal of medicine. 2007, May;356(19): 1915-27. Epub 2007/05/15.

[22] Future II SG. Prophylactic efficacy of a quadrivalent human papillomavirus (HPV) vaccine in women with virological evidence of HPV infection. The Journal of infectious diseases. 2007, November;196(10):1438-46. Epub 2007/11/17.

[23] Garland SM. Can cervical cancer be eradicated by prophylactic HPV vaccination? Challenges to vaccine implementation. Indian J Med Res. 2009;130(3):311-21. Epub 2009/11/11.

[24] Kahn JA, Brown DR, Ding L, Widdice LE, Shew ML, Glynn S, et al. Vaccine-Type Human Papillomavirus and Evidence of Herd Protection After Vaccine Introduction. Pediatrics. 2012. Epub 2012/07/11.

[25] Villa LL. HPV prophylactic vaccination: The first years and what to expect from now. Cancer Lett. 2011;305(2):106-12. Epub 2010/12/31.

[26] Kane MA, Serrano B, de Sanjose S, Wittet S. Implementation of human papillomavirus immunization in the developing world. Vaccine. 2012;30 Suppl 5:F192-200. Epub 2012/12/05.

[27] Agoston I, Sandor J, Karpati K, Pentek M. Economic considerations of HPV vaccination. Prev Med. 2010;50(1-2):93. Epub 2009/12/17.

[28] Katz IT, Ware NC, Gray G, Haberer JE, Mellins CA, Bangsberg DR. Scaling up human papillomavirus vaccination: a conceptual framework of vaccine adherence. Sex Health. 2010;7(3):279-86. Epub 2010/08/20.

[29] Adams M, Jasani B, Fiander A. Human papilloma virus (HPV) prophylactic vaccination: challenges for public health and implications for screening. Vaccine. 2007;25(16): 3007-13. Epub 2007/02/13.

[30] Massad LS, Evans CT, Weber KM, Goderre JL, Hessol NA, Henry D, et al. Changes in knowledge of cervical cancer prevention and human papillomavirus among women with human immunodeficiency virus. Obstet Gynecol. 2010;116(4):941-7. Epub 2010/09/23.

[31] Massad LS, Evans CT, Wilson TE, Goderre JL, Hessol NA, Henry D, et al. Knowledge of cervical cancer prevention and human papillomavirus among women with HIV. Gynecol Oncol. 2010;117(1):70-6. Epub 2010/01/29.

[32] Bergot A, Kassianos A. New Approaches to Immunotherapy for HPV Associated Cancer. Cancers. 2011(3):3461-95.

[33] Palefsky JM, Gillison ML, Strickler HD. Chapter 16: HPV vaccines in immunocompromised women and men. Vaccine. 2006;24 Suppl 3:S3/140-6. Epub 2006/09/05.

[34] Auvert B, Marais D, Lissouba P, Zarca K, Ramjee G, Williamson AL. High-risk human papillomavirus is associated with HIV acquisition among South African female sex workers. Infect Dis Obstet Gynecol. 2011;2011:692012. Epub 2011/08/02.

[35] Fitzgerald DW, Bezak K, Ocheretina O, Riviere C, Wright TC, Milne GL, et al. The effect of HIV and HPV coinfection on cervical COX-2 expression and systemic prostaglandin E2 levels. Cancer Prev Res (Phila). 2012;5(1):34-40. Epub 2011/12/03.

[36] Stanley M. Immune responses to human papillomavirus. Vaccine. 2006;24 Suppl 1:S16-22. Epub 2005/10/13.

[37] Gormley RH, Kovarik CL. Human papillomavirus-related genital disease in the immunocompromised host: Part II. Journal of the American Academy of Dermatology. 2012;66(6):883 e1-17; quiz 99-900. Epub 2012/05/16.

[38] Ghazizadeh S, Lessan-Pezeshki M, Nahayati MA. Human papilloma virus infection in female kidney transplant recipients. Saudi journal of kidney diseases and transplantation : an official publication of the Saudi Center for Organ Transplantation, Saudi Arabia. 2011;22(3):433-6. Epub 2011/05/14.

[39] Palefsky J. HPV infection and HPV-associated neoplasia in immunocompromised women. International Journal of Gynecology and Obstetrics. 2006, November; 94:556-64.

[40] Massad LS, Evans CT, Minkoff H, Watts DH, Strickler HD, Darragh T, et al. Natural history of grade 1 cervical intraepithelial neoplasia in women with human immunodeficiency virus. Obstet Gynecol. 2004;104(5 Pt 1):1077-85. Epub 2004/11/02.

[41] Melmed GY. Vaccinations and the Utilization of Immunosuppressive IBD Therapy. Gastroenterology & Hepatology. 2008;4(12):859-61.

[42] Nimako M, Fiander AN, Wilkinson GW, Borysiewicz LK, Man S. Human papillomavirus-specific cytotoxic T lymphocytes in patients with cervical intraepithelial neoplasia grade III. Cancer Res. 1997;57(21):4855-61. Epub 1997/11/14.

[43] Kenter GG, Welters MJ, Valentijn AR, Lowik MJ, Berends-van der Meer DM, Vloon AP, et al. Vaccination against HPV-16 oncoproteins for vulvar intraepithelial neoplasia. N Engl J Med. 2009;361(19):1838-47. Epub 2009/11/06.

[44] Winer RL, Hughes JP, Feng Q, O'Reilly S, Kiviat NB, Holmes KK, et al. Condom use and the risk of genital human papillomavirus infection in young women. N Engl J Med. 2006;354(25):2645-54. Epub 2006/06/23.

[45] Fradet-Turcotte A, Archambault J. Recent advances in the search for antiviral agents against human papillomaviruses. Antivir Ther. 2007;12(4):431-51. Epub 2007/08/03.

[46] Buck CB, Thompson CD, Roberts JN, Muller M, Lowy DR, Schiller JT. Carrageenan is a potent inhibitor of papillomavirus infection. PLoS Pathog. 2006;2(7):e69. Epub 2006/07/15.

[47] Roberts JN, Buck CB, Thompson CD, Kines R, Bernardo M, Choyke PL, et al. Genital transmission of HPV in a mouse model is potentiated by nonoxynol-9 and inhibited by carrageenan. Nat Med. 2007;13(7):857-61. Epub 2007/07/03.

[48] Castle PE, Giuliano AR. Chapter 4: Genital tract infections, cervical inflammation, and antioxidant nutrients--assessing their roles as human papillomavirus cofactors. J Natl Cancer Inst Monogr. 2003(31):29-34. Epub 2003/06/17.

[49] Williams VM, Filippova M, Soto U, Duerksen-Hughes PJ. HPV-DNA integration and carcinogenesis: putative roles for inflammation and oxidative stress. Future Virol. 2011;6(1):45-57. Epub 2011/02/15.

[50] Morrison MA, Morreale RJ, Akunuru S, Kofron M, Zheng Y, Wells SI. Targeting the human papillomavirus E6 and E7 oncogenes through expression of the bovine papillomavirus type 1 E2 protein stimulates cellular motility. J Virol. 2011;85(20):10487-98. Epub 2011/08/13.

[51] Sanchez-Perez AM, Soriano S, Clarke AR, Gaston K. Disruption of the human papillomavirus type 16 E2 gene protects cervical carcinoma cells from E2F-induced apoptosis. J Gen Virol. 1997;78 (Pt 11):3009-18. Epub 1997/11/21.

[52] Srivastava S, Natu SM, Gupta A, Pal KA, Singh U, Agarwal GG, et al. Lipid peroxidation and antioxidants in different stages of cervical cancer: Prognostic significance. Indian J Cancer. 2009;46(4):297-302. Epub 2009/09/15.

[53] Di Domenico F, Foppoli C, Coccia R, Perluigi M. Antioxidants in cervical cancer: Chemopreventive and chemotherapeutic effects of polyphenols. Biochim Biophys Acta. 2012;1822(5):737-47. Epub 2011/10/25.

[54] Crespo-Ortiz MP, Wei MQ. Antitumor activity of artemisinin and its derivatives: from a well-known antimalarial agent to a potential anticancer drug. J Biomed Biotechnol. 2012;2012:247597. Epub 2011/12/17.

[55] anderson j. Cervical Cancer Screening & Prevention for HIV-infected Women In the DevelopingWorld. 2010.

[56] Duraisamy K. Methods of Detecting Cervical Cancer. Advances in Biological Research. 2011;5(4):226-32.

[57] Chen C, Yang Z, Li Z, Li L. Accuracy of several cervical screening strategies for early detection of cervical cancer: a meta-analysis. Int J Gynecol Cancer. 2012;22(6):908-21. Epub 2012/06/08.

[58] Clavel C, Masure M, Bory JP, Putaud I, Mangeonjean C, Lorenzato M, et al. Human papillomavirus testing in primary screening for the detection of high-grade cervical lesions: a study of 7932 women. Br J Cancer. 2001;84(12):1616-23. Epub 2001/06/13.

[59] Flores YN, Bishai DM, Lorincz A, Shah KV, Lazcano-Ponce E, Hernandez M, et al. HPV testing for cervical cancer screening appears more cost-effective than Papanicolau cytology in Mexico. Cancer Causes Control. 2011;22(2):261-72. Epub 2010/12/21.

[60] Ronco G, Cuzick J, Pierotti P, Cariaggi MP, Dalla Palma P, Naldoni C, et al. Accuracy of liquid based versus conventional cytology: overall results of new technologies for cervical cancer screening: randomised controlled trial. BMJ. 2007;335(7609):28. Epub 2007/05/23.

[61] Origoni M, Cristoforoni P, Costa S, Mariani L, Scirpa P, Lorincz A, et al. HPV-DNA testing for cervical cancer precursors: from evidence to clinical practice. Ecancermedicalscience. 2012;6:258. Epub 2012/07/11.

[62] Gravitt PE, Coutlee F, Iftner T, Sellors JW, Quint WG, Wheeler CM. New technologies in cervical cancer screening. Vaccine. 2008;26 Suppl 10:K42-52. Epub 2008/10/14.

[63] Brown AJ, Trimble CL. New technologies for cervical cancer screening. Best Pract Res Clin Obstet Gynaecol. 2012;26(2):233-42. Epub 2011/11/29.

[64] James RM, Cruickshank ME, Siddiqui N. Management of cervical cancer: summary of SIGN guidelines. BMJ. 2008;336(7634):41-3. Epub 2008/01/05.

[65] Blomfield P. Management of cervical cancer. Aust Fam Physician. 2007;36(3):122-5. Epub 2007/03/07.

[66] I. AJ. The current management of cervical cancer. 6. 2004:196-202.

[67] Alvarez Moreno E, Jimenez de la Pena M, Cano Alonso R. Role of New Functional MRI Techniques in the Diagnosis, Staging, and Followup of Gynecological Cancer: Comparison with PET-CT. Radiol Res Pract. 2012;2012:219546. Epub 2012/02/09.

[68] Bell DJ, Pannu HK. Radiological assessment of gynecologic malignancies. Obstet Gynecol Clin North Am. 2011;38(1):45-68, vii. Epub 2011/03/23.

[69] Magne N, Chargari C, Vicenzi L, Gillion N, Messai T, Magne J, et al. New trends in the evaluation and treatment of cervix cancer: the role of FDG-PET. Cancer Treat Rev. 2008;34(8):671-81. Epub 2008/10/14.

[70] Herzog TJ. New approaches for the management of cervical cancer. Gynecol Oncol. 2003;90(3 Pt 2):S22-7. Epub 2003/09/18.

[71] Moore DH. Cervical cancer. Obstet Gynecol. 2006;107(5):1152-61. Epub 2006/05/02.

[72] Kundu S, Chopra S, Verma A, Mahantshetty U, Engineer R, Shrivastava SK. Functional magnetic resonance imaging in cervical cancer: current evidence and future directions. J Cancer Res Ther. 2012;8(1):11-8. Epub 2012/04/26.

[73] Trimble EL. Cervical cancer state-of-the-clinical-science meeting on pretreatment evaluation and prognostic factors, September 27-28, 2007: proceedings and recommendations. Gynecol Oncol. 2009;114(2):145-50. Epub 2009/07/03.

[74] Greggi S, Scaffa C. Surgical Management of Early Cervical Cancer: The Shape of Future Studies. Curr Oncol Rep. 2012. Epub 2012/09/05.

[75] Rapiti E, Usel M, Neyroud-Caspar I, Merglen A, Verkooijen HM, Vlastos AT, et al. Omission of excisional therapy is associated with an increased risk of invasive cervical cancer after cervical intraepithelial neoplasia III. Eur J Cancer. 2012;48(6):845-52. Epub 2011/06/11.

[76] Wilkinson EJ. Women with cervical intraepithelial neoplasia: requirement for active long-term surveillance after therapy. J Natl Cancer Inst. 2009;101(10):696-7. Epub 2009/05/14.

[77] Chen Y, Xu H, Zhang Q, Li Y, Wang D, Liang Z. A fertility-preserving option in early cervical carcinoma: laparoscopy-assisted vaginal radical trachelectomy and pelvic lymphadenectomy. Eur J Obstet Gynecol Reprod Biol. 2008;136(1):90-3. Epub 2006/12/02.

[78] Ribeiro Cubal AF, Ferreira Carvalho JI, Costa MF, Branco AP. Fertility-sparing surgery for early-stage cervical cancer. Int J Surg Oncol. 2012;2012:936534. Epub 2012/07/26.

[79] Marchiole P, Benchaib M, Buenerd A, Lazlo E, Dargent D, Mathevet P. Oncological safety of laparoscopic-assisted vaginal radical trachelectomy (LARVT or Dargent's operation): a comparative study with laparoscopic-assisted vaginal radical hysterectomy (LARVH). Gynecol Oncol. 2007;106(1):132-41. Epub 2007/05/12.

[80] Bansal N, Herzog TJ, Shaw RE, Burke WM, Deutsch I, Wright JD. Primary therapy for early-stage cervical cancer: radical hysterectomy vs radiation. Am J Obstet Gynecol. 2009;201(5):485 e1-9. Epub 2009/11/03.

[81] Movva S, Rodriguez L, Arias-Pulido H, Verschraegen C. Novel chemotherapy approaches for cervical cancer. Cancer. 2009;115(14):3166-80. Epub 2009/05/20.

[82] Yoshida K, Sasaki R, Nishimura H, Miyawaki D, Kawabe T, Okamoto Y, et al. Radiotherapy for Japanese elderly patients with cervical cancer: preliminary survival outcomes and evaluation of treatment-related toxicity. Arch Gynecol Obstet. 2011;284(4): 1007-14. Epub 2010/12/01.

[83] Tan LT, Jones B, Shaw JE. Radical radiotherapy for carcinoma of the uterine cervix using external beam radiotherapy and a single line source brachytherapy technique: the Clatterbridge technique. Br J Radiol. 1997;70(840):1252-8. Epub 1998/03/20.

[84] Viani GA, Manta GB, Stefano EJ, de Fendi LI. Brachytherapy for cervix cancer: low-dose rate or high-dose rate brachytherapy - a meta-analysis of clinical trials. J Exp Clin Cancer Res. 2009;28:47. Epub 2009/04/07.

[85] Singh TT, Singh IY, Sharma DT, Singh NR. Role of chemoradiation in advanced cervical cancer. Indian J Cancer. 2003;40(3):101-7. Epub 2004/01/13.

[86] Pearcey R, Brundage M, Drouin P, Jeffrey J, Johnston D, Lukka H, et al. Phase III trial comparing radical radiotherapy with and without cisplatin chemotherapy in patients with advanced squamous cell cancer of the cervix. J Clin Oncol. 2002;20(4):966-72. Epub 2002/02/15.

[87] Sivanesaratnam V. The role of chemotherapy in cervical cancer--a review. Singapore Med J. 1988;29(4):397-401. Epub 1988/08/01.

[88] Tao X, Hu W, Ramirez PT, Kavanagh JJ. Chemotherapy for recurrent and metastatic cervical cancer. Gynecol Oncol. 2008;110(3 Suppl 2):S67-71. Epub 2008/06/06.

[89] Gien LT, Beauchemin MC, Thomas G. Adenocarcinoma: a unique cervical cancer. Gynecol Oncol. 2010;116(1):140-6. Epub 2009/11/03.

[90] Friedlander M, Grogan M. Guidelines for the treatment of recurrent and metastatic cervical cancer. Oncologist. 2002;7(4):342-7. Epub 2002/08/20.

[91] Tewari KS, Monk BJ. The rationale for the use of non-platinum chemotherapy doublets for metastatic and recurrent cervical carcinoma. Clin Adv Hematol Oncol. 2010;8(2):108-15. Epub 2010/04/14.

[92] Waggoner SE. Cervical cancer. Lancet. 2003;361(9376):2217-25. Epub 2003/07/05.

[93] Rose PG. Combined-modality therapy of locally advanced cervical cancer. J Clin Oncol. 2003;21(10 Suppl):211s-7s. Epub 2003/05/14.

[94] Rose PG, Ali S, Watkins E, Thigpen JT, Deppe G, Clarke-Pearson DL, et al. Long-term follow-up of a randomized trial comparing concurrent single agent cisplatin, cisplatin-based combination chemotherapy, or hydroxyurea during pelvic irradiation for locally advanced cervical cancer: a Gynecologic Oncology Group Study. J Clin Oncol. 2007;25(19):2804-10. Epub 2007/05/16.

[95] Cadron I, Van Gorp T, Amant F, Leunen K, Neven P, Vergote I. Chemotherapy for recurrent cervical cancer. Gynecol Oncol. 2007;107(1 Suppl 1):S113-8. Epub 2007/09/07.

[96] Rose PG, Bundy BN, Watkins EB, Thigpen JT, Deppe G, Maiman MA, et al. Concurrent cisplatin-based radiotherapy and chemotherapy for locally advanced cervical cancer. N Engl J Med. 1999;340(15):1144-53. Epub 1999/04/15.

[97] Benedetti-Panici P, Greggi S, Colombo A, Amoroso M, Smaniotto D, Giannarelli D, et al. Neoadjuvant chemotherapy and radical surgery versus exclusive radiotherapy in locally advanced squamous cell cervical cancer: results from the Italian multicenter randomized study. J Clin Oncol. 2002;20(1):179-88. Epub 2002/01/05.

[98] Hockel M. Laterally extended endopelvic resection. Novel surgical treatment of locally recurrent cervical carcinoma involving the pelvic side wall. Gynecol Oncol. 2003;91(2):369-77. Epub 2003/11/06.

[99]   Ma B. HPV and Therapeutic Vaccines: Where are We in 2010? Current Cancer Therapy Reviews. 2010;6:81-103.

[100] Lin K, Roosinovich E, Ma B, Hung CF, Wu TC. Therapeutic HPV DNA vaccines. Immunol Res. 2010;47(1-3):86-112. Epub 2010/01/13.

[101] Mustafa W, Maciag PC, Pan ZK, Weaver JR, Xiao Y, Isaacs SN, et al. Listeria monocytogenes delivery of HPV-16 major capsid protein L1 induces systemic and mucosal cell-mediated CD4+ and CD8+ T-cell responses after oral immunization. Viral Immunol. 2009;22(3):195-204. Epub 2009/05/14.

[102] Hussain SF, Paterson Y. What is needed for effective antitumor immunotherapy? Lessons learned using Listeria monocytogenes as a live vector for HPV-associated tumors. Cancer Immunol Immunother. 2005;54(6):577-86. Epub 2005/01/15.

[103] Sewell DA, Douven D, Pan ZK, Rodriguez A, Paterson Y. Regression of HPV-positive tumors treated with a new Listeria monocytogenes vaccine. Arch Otolaryngol Head Neck Surg. 2004;130(1):92-7. Epub 2004/01/21.

[104] Lin CW, Lee JY, Tsao YP, Shen CP, Lai HC, Chen SL. Oral vaccination with recombinant Listeria monocytogenes expressing human papillomavirus type 16 E7 can cause tumor growth in mice to regress. Int J Cancer. 2002;102(6):629-37. Epub 2002/11/26.

[105] Zhao KJ, Cheng H, Zhu KJ, Xu Y, Chen ML, Zhang X, et al. Recombined DNA vaccines encoding calreticulin linked to HPV6bE7 enhance immune response and inhibit angiogenic activity in B16 melanoma mouse model expressing HPV 6bE7 antigen. Arch Dermatol Res. 2006;298(2):64-72. Epub 2006/05/20.

[106] Kaufmann AM, Stern PL, Rankin EM, Sommer H, Nuessler V, Schneider A, et al. Safety and immunogenicity of TA-HPV, a recombinant vaccinia virus expressing modified human papillomavirus (HPV)-16 and HPV-18 E6 and E7 genes, in women with progressive cervical cancer. Clin Cancer Res. 2002;8(12):3676-85. Epub 2002/12/11.

[107] Liu M, Acres B, Balloul JM, Bizouarne N, Paul S, Slos P, et al. Gene-based vaccines and immunotherapeutics. Proc Natl Acad Sci U S A. 2004;101 Suppl 2:14567-71. Epub 2004/08/31.

[108] Wu CY, Monie A, Pang X, Hung CF, Wu TC. Improving therapeutic HPV peptide-based vaccine potency by enhancing CD4+ T help and dendritic cell activation. J Biomed Sci. 2010;17:88. Epub 2010/11/26.

[109] Mirshahidi S, Kramer VG, Whitney JB, Essono S, Lee S, Dranoff G, et al. Overlapping synthetic peptides encoding TPD52 as breast cancer vaccine in mice: prolonged survival. Vaccine. 2009;27(12):1825-33. Epub 2009/02/10.

[110] Barrios K. Moffitt Cancer Center Researchers Develop and Test New Anti-Cancer Vaccine press release. 2012. Epub June 8, 2012.

[111] Cho HI, Celis E. Overcoming doubts and other obstacles in the development of effec-
       tive peptide-based therapeutic vaccines against cancer. Expert Rev Vaccines.
       2010;9(4):343-5. Epub 2010/04/08.

[112] Wilson NS, Yang B, Morelli AB, Koernig S, Yang A, Loeser S, et al. ISCOMATRIX
       vaccines mediate CD8+ T-cell cross-priming by a MyD88-dependent signaling path-
       way. Immunol Cell Biol. 2012;90(5):540-52. Epub 2011/09/07.

[113] Hung CF, Ma B, Monie A, Tsen SW, Wu TC. Therapeutic human papillomavirus vac-
       cines: current clinical trials and future directions. Expert Opin Biol Ther. 2008;8(4):
       421-39. Epub 2008/03/21.

[114] Pearse MJ, Drane D. ISCOMATRIX adjuvant: a potent inducer of humoral and cellu-
       lar immune responses. Vaccine. 2004;22(19):2391-5. Epub 2004/06/15.

[115] Maraskovsky E, Sjolander S, Drane DP, Schnurr M, Le TT, Mateo L, et al. NY-ESO-1
       protein formulated in ISCOMATRIX adjuvant is a potent anticancer vaccine inducing
       both humoral and CD8+ t-cell-mediated immunity and protection against NY-
       ESO-1+ tumors. Clin Cancer Res. 2004;10(8):2879-90. Epub 2004/04/23.

[116] Einstein MH, Kadish AS, Burk RD, Kim MY, Wadler S, Streicher H, et al. Heat shock
       fusion protein-based immunotherapy for treatment of cervical intraepithelial neopla-
       sia III. Gynecol Oncol. 2007;106(3):453-60. Epub 2007/06/26.

[117] Ding Y, Seow SV, Huang CH, Liew LM, Lim YC, Kuo IC, et al. Coadministration of
       the fungal immunomodulatory protein FIP-Fve and a tumour-associated antigen en-
       hanced antitumour immunity. Immunology. 2009;128(1 Suppl):e881-94. Epub
       2009/09/25.

[118] Huang CF, Monie A, Weng WH, Wu T. DNA vaccines for cervical cancer. Am J
       Transl Res. 2010;2(1):75-87. Epub 2010/02/26.

[119] Hung CF, Monie A, Alvarez RD, Wu TC. DNA vaccines for cervical cancer: from
       bench to bedside. Exp Mol Med. 2007;39(6):679-89. Epub 2007/12/28.

[120] Best SR, Peng S, Juang CM, Hung CF, Hannaman D, Saunders JR, et al. Administra-
       tion of HPV DNA vaccine via electroporation elicits the strongest CD8+ T cell im-
       mune responses compared to intramuscular injection and intradermal gene gun
       delivery. Vaccine. 2009;27(40):5450-9. Epub 2009/07/23.

[121] Chen CA, Chang MC, Sun WZ, Chen YL, Chiang YC, Hsieh CY, et al. Noncarrier
       naked antigen-specific DNA vaccine generates potent antigen-specific immunologic
       responses and antitumor effects. Gene Ther. 2009;16(6):776-87. Epub 2009/04/10.

[122] Trimble C, Lin CT, Hung CF, Pai S, Juang J, He L, et al. Comparison of the CD8+ T
       cell responses and antitumor effects generated by DNA vaccine administered
       through gene gun, biojector, and syringe. Vaccine. 2003;21(25-26):4036-42. Epub
       2003/08/19.

[123] Bodles-Brakhop AM, Heller R, Draghia-Akli R. Electroporation for the delivery of DNA-based vaccines and immunotherapeutics: current clinical developments. Mol Ther. 2009;17(4):585-92. Epub 2009/02/19.

[124] van den Berg JH, Nujien B, Beijnen JH, Vincent A, van Tinteren H, Kluge J, et al. Optimization of intradermal vaccination by DNA tattooing in human skin. Hum Gene Ther. 2009;20(3):181-9. Epub 2009/03/21.

[125] Garcia F, Petry KU, Muderspach LI. ZYC101a for Treatment of High-Grade Cervical Intraepithelial Neoplasia: A Randomized Controlled Trial. American College of Obstetricians and Gynecologists. 2004;103(2):317-26.

[126] Matijevic M, Hedley ML, Urban RG, Chicz RM, Lajoie C, Luby TM. Immunization with a poly (lactide co-glycolide) encapsulated plasmid DNA expressing antigenic regions of HPV 16 and 18 results in an increase in the precursor frequency of T cells that respond to epitopes from HPV 16, 18, 6 and 11. Cell Immunol. 2011;270(1):62-9. Epub 2011/05/10.

[127] Alvarez-Salas LM. Amolimogene bepiplasmid, a DNA-based therapeutic encoding the E6 and E7 epitopes from HPV, for cervical and anal dysplasia. Curr Opin Mol Ther. 2008;10(6):622-8. Epub 2008/12/04.

[128] Sheets EE, Urban RG, Crum CP, Hedley ML, Politch JA, Gold MA, et al. Immunotherapy of human cervical high-grade cervical intraepithelial neoplasia with microparticle-delivered human papillomavirus 16 E7 plasmid DNA. Am J Obstet Gynecol. 2003;188(4):916-26. Epub 2003/04/25.

[129] Cheng WF, Hung CF, Chai CY, Hsu KF, He L, Ling M, et al. Tumor-specific immunity and antiangiogenesis generated by a DNA vaccine encoding calreticulin linked to a tumor antigen. J Clin Invest. 2001;108(5):669-78. Epub 2001/09/07.

[130] Chen CH, Ji H, Suh KW, Choti MA, Pardoll DM, Wu TC. Gene gun-mediated DNA vaccination induces antitumor immunity against human papillomavirus type 16 E7-expressing murine tumor metastases in the liver and lungs. Gene therapy. 1999;6(12): 1972-81. Epub 2000/01/19.

[131] Hung CF, Tsai YC, He L, Wu TC. DNA vaccines encoding Ii-PADRE generates potent PADRE-specific CD4+ T-cell immune responses and enhances vaccine potency. Molecular therapy : the journal of the American Society of Gene Therapy. 2007;15(6): 1211-9. Epub 2007/03/16.

[132] Tsen SW, Paik AH, Hung CF, Wu TC. Enhancing DNA vaccine potency by modifying the properties of antigen-presenting cells. Expert review of vaccines. 2007;6(2): 227-39. Epub 2007/04/06.

[133] Bolhassani A, Zahedifard F, Taghikhani M, Rafati S. Enhanced immunogenicity of HPV16E7 accompanied by Gp96 as an adjuvant in two vaccination strategies. Vaccine. 2008;26(26):3362-70. Epub 2008/05/13.

[134] Kim D, Hoory T, Monie A, Ting JP, Hung CF, Wu TC. Enhancement of DNA vaccine potency through coadministration of CIITA DNA with DNA vaccines via gene gun. J Immunol. 2008;180(10):7019-27. Epub 2008/05/06.

[135] Hsu KF, Hung CF, Cheng WF, He L, Slater LA, Ling M, et al. Enhancement of suicidal DNA vaccine potency by linking Mycobacterium tuberculosis heat shock protein 70 to an antigen. Gene Ther. 2001;8(5):376-83. Epub 2001/04/21.

[136] Kim TW, Hung CF, Juang J, He L, Hardwick JM, Wu TC. Enhancement of suicidal DNA vaccine potency by delaying suicidal DNA-induced cell death. Gene Ther. 2004;11(3):336-42. Epub 2004/01/23.

[137] Harvey TJ, Anraku I, Linedale R, Harrich D, Mackenzie J, Suhrbier A, et al. Kunjin virus replicon vectors for human immunodeficiency virus vaccine development. J Virol. 2003;77(14):7796-803. Epub 2003/06/28.

[138] Anraku I, Harvey TJ, Linedale R, Gardner J, Harrich D, Suhrbier A, et al. Kunjin virus replicon vaccine vectors induce protective CD8+ T-cell immunity. J Virol. 2002;76(8):3791-9. Epub 2002/03/22.

[139] Varnavski AN, Young PR, Khromykh AA. Stable high-level expression of heterologous genes in vitro and in vivo by noncytopathic DNA-based Kunjin virus replicon vectors. J Virol. 2000;74(9):4394-403. Epub 2001/02/07.

[140] Bolhassani A, Safaiyan S, Rafati S. Improvement of different vaccine delivery systems for cancer therapy. Mol Cancer. 2011;10:3. Epub 2011/01/08.

[141] Tan JK, O'Neill HC. Maturation requirements for dendritic cells in T cell stimulation leading to tolerance versus immunity. J Leukoc Biol. 2005;78(2):319-24. Epub 2005/04/06.

[142] Lesterhuis WJ, de Vries IJ, Adema GJ, Punt CJ. Dendritic cell-based vaccines in cancer immunotherapy: an update on clinical and immunological results. Ann Oncol. 2004;15 Suppl 4:iv145-51. Epub 2004/10/13.

[143] Cella M, Scheidegger D, Palmer-Lehmann K, Lane P, Lanzavecchia A, Alber G. Ligation of CD40 on dendritic cells triggers production of high levels of interleukin-12 and enhances T cell stimulatory capacity: T-T help via APC activation. J Exp Med. 1996;184(2):747-52. Epub 1996/08/01.

[144] Huang B, Mao CP, Peng S, Hung CF, Wu TC. RNA interference-mediated in vivo silencing of fas ligand as a strategy for the enhancement of DNA vaccine potency. Hum Gene Ther. 2008;19(8):763-73. Epub 2008/07/17.

[145] Kim TW, Lee JH, He L, Boyd DA, Hardwick JM, Hung CF, et al. Modification of professional antigen-presenting cells with small interfering RNA in vivo to enhance cancer vaccine potency. Cancer Res. 2005;65(1):309-16. Epub 2005/01/25.

[146] Song XT, Evel-Kabler K, Rollins L, Aldrich M, Gao F, Huang XF, et al. An alternative and effective HIV vaccination approach based on inhibition of antigen presentation attenuators in dendritic cells. PLoS Med. 2006;3(1):e11. Epub 2005/12/31.

[147] Weiss JM, Subleski JJ, Wigginton JM, Wiltrout RH. Immunotherapy of cancer by IL-12-based cytokine combinations. Expert Opin Biol Ther. 2007;7(11):1705-21. Epub 2007/10/27.

[148] Borrello I, Sotomayor EM, Cooke S, Levitsky HI. A universal granulocyte-macrophage colony-stimulating factor-producing bystander cell line for use in the formulation of autologous tumor cell-based vaccines. Hum Gene Ther. 1999;10(12):1983-91. Epub 1999/08/31.

[149] de Gruijl TD, van den Eertwegh AJ, Pinedo HM, Scheper RJ. Whole-cell cancer vaccination: from autologous to allogeneic tumor- and dendritic cell-based vaccines. Cancer Immunol Immunother. 2008;57(10):1569-77. Epub 2008/06/05.

[150] Chen CH, Wang TL, Hung CF, Pardoll DM, Wu TC. Boosting with recombinant vaccinia increases HPV-16 E7-specific T cell precursor frequencies of HPV-16 E7-expressing DNA vaccines. Vaccine. 2000;18(19):2015-22. Epub 2002/04/09.

[151] Rorke EA. Antisense human papillomavirus (HPV) E6/E7 expression, reduced stability of epidermal growth factor, and diminished growth of HPV-positive tumor cells. J Natl Cancer Inst. 1997;89(17):1243-6. Epub 1997/09/18.

[152] Marquez-Gutierrez MA, Benitez-Hess ML, DiPaolo JA, Alvarez-Salas LM. Effect of combined antisense oligodeoxynucleotides directed against the human papillomavirus type 16 on cervical carcinoma cells. Archives of medical research. 2007;38(7): 730-8. Epub 2007/09/12.

[153] Alvarez-Salas LM, Arpawong TE, DiPaolo JA. Growth inhibition of cervical tumor cells by antisense oligodeoxynucleotides directed to the human papillomavirus type 16 E6 gene. Antisense & nucleic acid drug development. 1999;9(5):441-50. Epub 1999/11/11.

[154] Sanduja S, Kaza V, Dixon DA. The mRNA decay factor tristetraprolin (TTP) induces senescence in human papillomavirus-transformed cervical cancer cells by targeting E6-AP ubiquitin ligase. Aging (Albany NY). 2009;1(9):803-17. Epub 2010/02/17.

[155] Bousarghin L, Touze A, Gaud G, Iochmann S, Alvarez E, Reverdiau P, et al. Inhibition of cervical cancer cell growth by human papillomavirus virus-like particles packaged with human papillomavirus oncoprotein short hairpin RNAs. Mol Cancer Ther. 2009;8(2):357-65. Epub 2009/01/29.

[156] Bellati F, Napoletano C, Gasparri ML, Visconti V, Zizzari IG, Ruscito I, et al. Monoclonal antibodies in gynecological cancer: a critical point of view. Clin Dev Immunol. 2011;2011:890758. Epub 2012/01/12.

[157] Monk BJ, Sill MW, Burger RA, Gray HJ, Buekers TE, Roman LD. Phase II trial of bevacizumab in the treatment of persistent or recurrent squamous cell carcinoma of the

cervix: a gynecologic oncology group study. J Clin Oncol. 2009;27(7):1069-74. Epub 2009/01/14.

[158] Santin AD, Sill MW, McMeekin DS, Leitao MM, Jr., Brown J, Sutton GP, et al. Phase II trial of cetuximab in the treatment of persistent or recurrent squamous or non-squamous cell carcinoma of the cervix: a Gynecologic Oncology Group study. Gynecol Oncol. 2011;122(3):495-500. Epub 2011/06/21.

[159] del Campo JM, Prat A, Gil-Moreno A, Perez J, Parera M. Update on novel therapeutic agents for cervical cancer. Gynecol Oncol. 2008;110(3 Suppl 2):S72-6. Epub 2008/06/12.

[160] Pueyo G, Mesia R, Figueras A, Lozano A, Baro M, Vazquez S, et al. Cetuximab may inhibit tumor growth and angiogenesis induced by ionizing radiation: a preclinical rationale for maintenance treatment after radiotherapy. Oncologist. 2010;15(9):976-86. Epub 2010/08/28.

[161] Lagrange M, Charbonnier S, Orfanoudakis G, Robinson P, Zanier K, Masson M, et al. Binding of human papillomavirus 16 E6 to p53 and E6AP is impaired by monoclonal antibodies directed against the second zinc-binding domain of E6. J Gen Virol. 2005;86(Pt 4):1001-7. Epub 2005/03/24.

[162] Costa S, De Simone P, Venturoli S, Cricca M, Zerbini ML, Musiani M, et al. Factors predicting human papillomavirus clearance in cervical intraepithelial neoplasia lesions treated by conization. Gynecol Oncol. 2003;90(2):358-65. Epub 2003/08/02.

[163] D'Abramo CM, Archambault J. Small molecule inhibitors of human papillomavirus protein - protein interactions. Open Virol J. 2011;5:80-95. Epub 2011/07/20.

[164] Abbate EA, Voitenleitner C, Botchan MR. Structure of the papillomavirus DNA-tethering complex E2:Brd4 and a peptide that ablates HPV chromosomal association. Mol Cell. 2006;24(6):877-89. Epub 2006/12/26.

[165] You J, Croyle JL, Nishimura A, Ozato K, Howley PM. Interaction of the bovine papillomavirus E2 protein with Brd4 tethers the viral DNA to host mitotic chromosomes. Cell. 2004;117(3):349-60. Epub 2004/04/28.

[166] Zheng G, Schweiger MR, Martinez-Noel G, Zheng L, Smith JA, Harper JW, et al. Brd4 regulation of papillomavirus protein E2 stability. J Virol. 2009;83(17):8683-92. Epub 2009/06/26.

[167] Lee AY, Chiang CM. Chromatin adaptor Brd4 modulates E2 transcription activity and protein stability. The Journal of biological chemistry. 2009;284(5):2778-86. Epub 2008/11/29.

[168] Steger G, Schnabel C, Schmidt HM. The hinge region of the human papillomavirus type 8 E2 protein activates the human p21(WAF1/CIP1) promoter via interaction with Sp1. The Journal of general virology. 2002;83(Pt 3):503-10. Epub 2002/02/14.

[169] Yan J, Li Q, Lievens S, Tavernier J, You J. Abrogation of the Brd4-positive transcrip-
       tion elongation factor B complex by papillomavirus E2 protein contributes to viral
       oncogene repression. J Virol. 2010;84(1):76-87. Epub 2009/10/23.

[170] White PW, Pelletier A, Brault K, Titolo S, Welchner E, Thauvette L, et al. Characteri-
       zation of recombinant HPV6 and 11 E1 helicases: effect of ATP on the interaction of
       E1 with E2 and mapping of a minimal helicase domain. J Biol Chem. 2001;276(25):
       22426-38. Epub 2001/04/17.

[171] White PW, Faucher AM, Massariol MJ, Welchner E, Rancourt J, Cartier M, et al. Bi-
       phenylsulfonacetic acid inhibitors of the human papillomavirus type 6 E1 helicase in-
       hibit ATP hydrolysis by an allosteric mechanism involving tyrosine 486. Antimicrob
       Agents Chemother. 2005;49(12):4834-42. Epub 2005/11/24.

[172] Faucher AM, White PW, Brochu C, Grand-Maitre C, Rancourt J, Fazal G. Discovery
       of small-molecule inhibitors of the ATPase activity of human papillomavirus E1 heli-
       case. J Med Chem. 2004;47(1):18-21. Epub 2003/12/30.

[173] White PW, Titolo S, Brault K, Thauvette L, Pelletier A, Welchner E, et al. Inhibition of
       human papillomavirus DNA replication by small molecule antagonists of the E1-E2
       protein interaction. J Biol Chem. 2003;278(29):26765-72. Epub 2003/05/06.

[174] Hafner N, Driesch C, Gajda M, Jansen L, Kirchmayr R, Runnebaum IB, et al. Integra-
       tion of the HPV16 genome does not invariably result in high levels of viral oncogene
       transcripts. Oncogene. 2008;27(11):1610-7. Epub 2007/09/11.

[175] White PW, Faucher AM, Goudreau N. Small molecule inhibitors of the human papil-
       lomavirus E1-E2 interaction. Curr Top Microbiol Immunol. 2011;348:61-88. Epub
       2010/08/03.

[176] Hudson JB, Bedell MA, McCance DJ, Laiminis LA. Immortalization and altered dif-
       ferentiation of human keratinocytes in vitro by the E6 and E7 open reading frames of
       human papillomavirus type 18. J Virol. 1990;64(2):519-26. Epub 1990/02/01.

[177] Song S, Liem A, Miller JA, Lambert PF. Human papillomavirus types 16 E6 and E7
       contribute differently to carcinogenesis. Virology. 2000;267(2):141-50. Epub
       2000/02/09.

[178] Song S, Pitot HC, Lambert PF. The human papillomavirus type 16 E6 gene alone is
       sufficient to induce carcinomas in transgenic animals. J Virol. 1999;73(7):5887-93.
       Epub 1999/06/11.

[179] Song S, Gulliver GA, Lambert PF. Human papillomavirus type 16 E6 and E7 onco-
       genes abrogate radiation-induced DNA damage responses in vivo through p53-de-
       pendent and p53-independent pathways. Proc Natl Acad Sci U S A. 1998;95(5):
       2290-5. Epub 1998/04/16.

[180] Tan S, de Vries EG, van der Zee AG, de Jong S. Anticancer drugs aimed at E6 and E7 activity in HPV-positive cervical cancer. Curr Cancer Drug Targets. 2012;12(2): 170-84. Epub 2011/12/15.

[181] Guo CP, Liu KW, Luo HB, Chen HB, Zheng Y, Sun SN, et al. Potent anti-tumor effect generated by a novel human papillomavirus (HPV) antagonist peptide reactivating the pRb/E2F pathway. PLoS One. 2011;6(3):e17734. Epub 2011/03/23.

[182] Webb GC, Zhang J, Garlow SJ, Wesp A, Riezman H, Jones EW. Pep7p provides a novel protein that functions in vesicle-mediated transport between the yeast Golgi and endosome. Mol Biol Cell. 1997;8(5):871-95. Epub 1997/05/01.

[183] Talis AL, Huibregtse JM, Howley PM. The role of E6AP in the regulation of p53 protein levels in human papillomavirus (HPV)-positive and HPV-negative cells. J Biol Chem. 1998;273(11):6439-45. Epub 1998/04/16.

[184] Mani A, Gelmann EP. The ubiquitin-proteasome pathway and its role in cancer. J Clin Oncol. 2005;23(21):4776-89. Epub 2005/07/22.

[185] Kojima K, Konopleva M, McQueen T, O'Brien S, Plunkett W, Andreeff M. Mdm2 inhibitor Nutlin-3a induces p53-mediated apoptosis by transcription-dependent and transcription-independent mechanisms and may overcome Atm-mediated resistance to fludarabine in chronic lymphocytic leukemia. Blood. 2006;108(3):993-1000. Epub 2006/03/18.

[186] Nalepa G, Rolfe M, Harper JW. Drug discovery in the ubiquitin-proteasome system. Nat Rev Drug Discov. 2006;5(7):596-613. Epub 2006/07/04.

[187] Bae S, Jung JH, Kim K, An IS, Kim SY, Lee JH, et al. TRIAD1 inhibits MDM2-mediated p53 ubiquitination and degradation. FEBS Lett. 2012. Epub 2012/07/24.

[188] Chen D, Frezza M, Schmitt S, Kanwar J, Dou QP. Bortezomib as the first proteasome inhibitor anticancer drug: current status and future perspectives. Curr Cancer Drug Targets. 2011;11(3):239-53. Epub 2011/01/21.

[189] Nawrocki ST, Carew JS, Pino MS, Highshaw RA, Andtbacka RH, Dunner K, Jr., et al. Aggresome disruption: a novel strategy to enhance bortezomib-induced apoptosis in pancreatic cancer cells. Cancer Res. 2006;66(7):3773-81. Epub 2006/04/06.

[190] Hougardy BM, Maduro JH, van der Zee AG, de Groot DJ, van den Heuvel FA, de Vries EG, et al. Proteasome inhibitor MG132 sensitizes HPV-positive human cervical cancer cells to rhTRAIL-induced apoptosis. Int J Cancer. 2006;118(8):1892-900. Epub 2005/11/16.

[191] Hampson L, Kitchener HC, Hampson IN. Specific HIV protease inhibitors inhibit the ability of HPV16 E6 to degrade p53 and selectively kill E6-dependent cervical carcinoma cells in vitro. Antivir Ther. 2006;11(6):813-25. Epub 2007/02/22.

[192] Bernstein WB, Dennis PA. Repositioning HIV protease inhibitors as cancer therapeutics. Curr Opin HIV AIDS. 2008;3(6):666-75. Epub 2009/04/18.

[193] Gaedicke S, Firat-Geier E, Constantiniu O, Lucchiari-Hartz M, Freudenberg M, Galanos C, et al. Antitumor effect of the human immunodeficiency virus protease inhibitor ritonavir: induction of tumor-cell apoptosis associated with perturbation of proteasomal proteolysis. Cancer Res. 2002;62(23):6901-8. Epub 2002/12/04.

[194] Magal SS, Jackman A, Ish-Shalom S, Botzer LE, Gonen P, Schlegel R, et al. Downregulation of Bax mRNA expression and protein stability by the E6 protein of human papillomavirus 16. J Gen Virol. 2005;86(Pt 3):611-21. Epub 2005/02/22.

[195] Vogt M, Butz K, Dymalla S, Semzow J, Hoppe-Seyler F. Inhibition of Bax activity is crucial for the antiapoptotic function of the human papillomavirus E6 oncoprotein. Oncogene. 2006;25(29):4009-15. Epub 2006/02/08.

[196] Tungteakkhun SS, Filippova M, Neidigh JW, Fodor N, Duerksen-Hughes PJ. The interaction between human papillomavirus type 16 and FADD is mediated by a novel E6 binding domain. J Virol. 2008;82(19):9600-14. Epub 2008/07/18.

[197] Tungteakkhun SS, Filippova M, Fodor N, Duerksen-Hughes PJ. The full-length isoform of human papillomavirus 16 E6 and its splice variant E6* bind to different sites on the procaspase 8 death effector domain. J Virol. 2010;84(3):1453-63. Epub 2009/11/13.

[198] Yuan CH, Filippova M, Tungteakkhun SS, Duerksen-Hughes PJ, Krstenansky JL. Small molecule inhibitors of the HPV16-E6 interaction with caspase 8. Bioorg Med Chem Lett. 2012;22(5):2125-9. Epub 2012/02/04.

Chapter 11

The Role of Human Papillomavirus In Pre-Cancerous Lesions and Oral Cancers

Danilo Figueiredo Soave, Mara Rubia Nunes Celes, João Paulo Oliveira-Costa, Giorgia Gobbi da Silveira, Bruna Riedo Zanetti, Lucinei Roberto Oliveira and Alfredo Ribeiro-Silva

Additional information is available at the end of the chapter

1. Introduction

The head and neck squamous cell carcinomas (HNSCC) are the sixth most frequent malignancy worldwide. It is properly established as heterogeneous solid tumor, composed by cells with different phenotypic features with malignant potential. Oral squamous cell carcinoma (OSCC) is a significant subset of the worldwide burden of HNSCCs. It is essential the understanding of the OSCC biology and biological behavior of pre-cancerous conditions and pre-cancerous lesions that may be responsible for malignant transformation. Heterogeneity in prevalence and anatomic distribution are associated to demographic differences in the habits of exposure tobacco and alcohol. The use of tobacco and alcohol are often established as risk factors for OSCC, but this phenomenon could also emerge in individuals not exposed to them. As OSCC, the pre-cancerous lesions also present a strict connection to tobacco consumption. However, a relationship between alcohol carcinogenic effect and pre-cancer lesions are not clear. These populations that develop the pre-cancer lesions or OSCC in the absence of prior contact with risk factors suggest that others factors can play a role in head and neck carcinogenesis. There is a longstanding analysis, over the past 2 decades, whether the human papilloma virus (HPV) infection could have a role in the OSCC carcinogenesis. HPV were first established as cancer development agent in cervical cancer, succeeding reports established the HPV infection in mucosal tissues of the oral cavity upper gastrointestinal tract, anogenital tract. In cervical cancer the categorization subdivided the HPV types into low-risk high-risk types, only the types 16, 18, 31, 33, 35, 39, 45, 51, 52, 56, and 58 are consistently grouped as high risk. The high-risk types 16 and 18, as in the cervical and anogenital cancer, are the most common entities detected in pre-cancerous and HNSCC lesions. Miller & Johnstone [1] describe that likelihood of detecting HPV, comparing pre-cancerous lesions and HNSCC to normal epithelium, was three times higher in pre-cancerous lesions and four a five times higher in HNSCC. In despite of large number of studies, the accurate role of HPV in the HNSCC development and progression has been controversial so as in OSCC. HPVs are a circular virion enclosed in a small capsid. The carcinogenic process occurs through the HPV-DNA integration into host cell. Usually, the viral oncoproteins codified by HPV-DNA, leads a functional alteration in p53 and pRb pathways, and consequently genomic instability. However, the oncoproteins expression alone is not sufficient to induce neoplastic transformation suggesting the requirement of supplementary genetic modifications. Increased understanding of the role of HPV antigens in neoplastic pathogenesis confirms the HPV as an etiological agent for cancers and, the knowledge of HPV cancer biology consequently will provide the development of preventive vaccines and antiviral treatment. The HPV vaccines have been formulated as a result of core technologies implementation that is able to construct virus-like particles (VLPs) equivalent to natural virions but, at the same time, are not capable to induce an infectious process. In addition, in this chapter we will discuss the HPV relationship with the pre-cancerous lesions and OSCC. The present data summarize the knowledge regarding the epidemiology, behavior, biology, malignant transformation mechanisms, and prognosis of HPV infection.

2. A brief history of papillomavirus and cancer

Human Papillomavirus infection was firstly identified from the embalmed body of a 12th century B.C. ancient Egyptian worker [2]. During the mummy necropsy procedure Scientists observed a wart on the sole of his foot. This evidences demonstrated that HPV infection occurred [3]. Medical literary tidings regard skin and genital warts were described in classical Greek and Roman literature [2]. However, association between viral origin of warts and sexual transmission was only confirmed in 19th century [2]. Rigoni-Stern (1842) hypothesized that cervical cancer could be promoted through sexual contacts. The Italian physician postulated this conception through the observation of high rates on cervical cancer in sexually active women, in comparison with non-sexually active women. [4]. Essays to establish relationship between cervical cancer and HPV-infections were initiated in 1972, this hypothesis was supported by a rare description of condylomata acuminate malignant transformation into squamous cell carcinomas highlighting the carcinogenic potential of hpv [4]. Harald zur Hausen, in 1975 [5], published that HPV could have a pivotal role in human cervix carcinogenesis. Eight year after, Hausen et al. identified the subtypes HPV16 and 18 on cervix cancer.

HPV infection was well established as etiologic factor of almost 100% of cervical malignancies [6]. After this appointment, several studies have addressed to find presence and prevalence of HPV infection in different tumor sites, including skin, urethra, nasal cavity, paranasal sinus, larynx, tracheobronchial mucosa and oral cavity [7]. In 1983, a series of studies presented by Syrjänen et al. [8] highlighted the possible correlation between HPV and oral lesions (non-neoplastic, benignant and malignant lesions). At the same year, a light microcopy study provided by Syrjänen et al. [9-11] firstly suggested a link among HPV infection, HNSCC and OSCC, through the examination of 40 biopsy specimens. These authors described morpho-logical alterations caused by HPV infection in 16 cases; this observation gives supports to HPV involvement in the development of OSCC. However, the confirmatory evidence of HPV-DNA in the oral lesions was presented only in 1985 [6,12]. Although the presence of HPV DNA has been suggested as a possible etiologic factor of oral pre-cancer and cancer, this association has not been as reliable as in cervical cancers.

3. HPV biology: General considerations

HPV represent a group of DNA viruses that was recently recognized to form their own family, Papillomaviridae that initially, together with polyomaviruses, was grouped in the Papova-viridae family [13]. They are an ancient family of pathogens and are known to infect epithelial tissues of amphibians, reptiles, birds and mammals [14]. The virus is formed by a non-enveloped icosahedral capsid with circular double-stranded DNA [15-16]. The genome is small, comprising to 8.000 base pairs, but it is complex, composed of three distinct regions: early region (E), late region (L) and upstream regulatory region (URR) or long region control (LCR).

The E region contains from seven to eight genes (E1, E2, E3, E4, E5, E6, E7 and E8), of which E1 is related with viral replication, E2 with viral transcription and DNA replication, E4 with maturation and alteration of extracellular matrix cell and E5, E6 and E7 are involved in cellular transformation. The E3 and E8 genes have been recently described only in a few HPV types but their function is unknown [16-18].The L region containing two genes, L1 and L2, which encode structural proteins necessary for viral capsid formation in the final stages of replication. Both E and L are coding region therefore called open reading frames (ORF), however the region URR does not fit in this description because it is a non-coding region. The URR region is found between E and L region and contain promoter and enhancer DNA sequences critical to regulate viral replication and transcription by both viral and cellular genes [19].

Based on phylogenetic analysis, the HPV is classified into genera (alpha, beta, gamma, mu and nu), species and types [15]. The classification of HPV types is based mainly on analyses of the L1 gene, which is the most conserved gene in all known papillomaviruses. When the DNA sequence of the L1 ORF differs by more than 10% from the closest known virus type, a new papillomavirus is recognized. Differences between 2% and 10% homology define a subtype and less than 2% a variant. A viral variant can differ between 2% in coding regions and 5% in non-coding regions [13,15]. Currently, approximately 150 different types are recognized and 120 HPV types are fully sequenced [18]. Types classified as members of the same species with approximately 80-90% of similarities trend to share biological properties such as the tissue tropism, disease manifestation, and pathogenicity [14].

According to their tropism, the HPV also can be classified as cutaneous and mucosal type. The cutaneous type are associated with skin lesions, being HPVs 1, 2 and 4 the most prevalent in common and plantar warts, and the types 5, 8, 9, 12, 14, 15, 17, 19-25, 36, 46 and 47 the most frequent in epidermodysplasia verruciforme. HPV-5 and -8 are associated with skin carcinoma [20-21]. HPV with mucous tropism infects the anogenital tract, upper aero digestive tract, other head and neck mucosa and are generally subdivided into high-risk and low-risk type based on their oncogenical potential. The most relevant low-risk type are HPV-6 and 11, however the types 40, 42, 43, 44, 54, 61, 70, 72 can be observed in genital benign lesions. Among the high-risk types, the HPV 16 and 18 are most common; especially type 16, which can be found in various cancers such as cervical, oropharyngeal and penile carcinomas. Types 31, 33, 35, 52, 58 and 67 belong to a category of moderate to high-risk [20,22-24].

HPV life cycle is closely linked to the differentiation program of infected epithelial cells, more specifically the keratinocytes. Infection is initiated through microlesions in the epithelium, which allow virions come in contact with the basal cell layer by direct HPV receptor connection to surface host cell ligands. The receptors involved are not fully identified, but some data revealed a role for α6 integrin and heparin sulfate. Following infection, the virus probably maintains its genome as a low copy number episome in the basal cells of the epithelium, providing a reservoir of viral DNA for further use in cell divisions. When infected basal cells begin to divide, viral DNA is distributed among the daughter cells with a massive upregulation of expression of all early genes mainly the E6 and E7. After mitosis some daughter cells may persist in the basal layers, whereas other move toward the upper layers of the epithelium and begin to differentiate. During this differentiation process there is viral DNA replication that amplifies the amount of virus at least 1000 copies per cell, and finally expression of the coat proteins L1 and L2 followed by assembly of infectious virus [25-28].

The mechanism of viral-induced cell growth is analogous to other tumors viruses that deregulate the cell cycle. Cancer appearance in lesions with persistent HPV is related to the overexpression of E6 and E7 proteins. E6 interfere with the function of p53 whereas E7 with the function of Rb protein, leading to abnormal cells growth by promoting inhibition of apoptosis and dysregulation of cell cycle, respectively. [28]. Basically, HPV infection occurs through sexual contact, non-sexual contact and maternal contact. In healthy individuals most (around 80%) HPV infections clear spontaneously but in some cases, HPV infection persist, leading to cancer development [26,29]. A series of events allows the viral persistence: differentiation-specific organization of the virus life cycle, mechanisms to maintain genome copy-number in undifferentiated cells, angiogenesis promotion, and strategies to evade both innate and adaptive immune surveillance [28].

4. HPV and head and neck sites

Twenty-five percent of HNSCC are associated with HPV [30]. There is increasing evidences that sexual practices are the means by which HPV-Positive HNSCC patients are exposed to virus. Therefore, changes in sexual practices (young people with their first sexual experience at an earlier age, numbers of sexual partners and higher probability of engaging in oral sex compared to individuals from earlier decades) may be associated with HPV-infection prevalence [31].

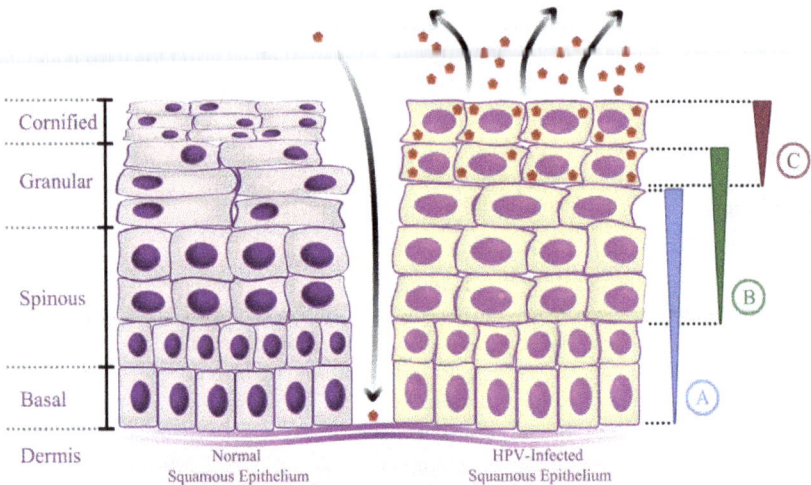

Figure 1. Human Papillomavirus Life Cycle: A: Early gene expression E1, E2, E6 and E7; B: Viral genome amplification; C: Virion assembly and release (Adapted from Moody & Laimins 2010).

Recently, a specific correlation between HPV-positive patients and sexual behavior has been established in HNSCC [32]. This study shown, in patients with HNSCC, that high-risk HPV-16 was correlated with vaginal/oral sex partners, casual sex habits and infrequent users of barriers during vaginal/oral sex. Heck et al. [31] presents association between HNSCC subtypes and sexual behavior. In Oropharynx Cancer the prevalence of HPV infection is close to 36% [30] and this entity was associated with the number of sexual partners and lifetime oral sex partners [31]. A similar result was described by D'Souza et al. [33], which presented an association between HPV-16 measurements and presence of oral HPV-infection. The authors has also found HPV-16–positive oropharyngeal cancer correlated with oral-sex or vaginal-sex partners, engagement in casual sex, early age at first intercourse, and infrequent use of condoms. In tonsillar cancers, Hemminki et al. [34] demonstrated that women with cervical lesions present an increased risk of tonsillar cancer. In addition, increased risk was also found among husbands of women with invasive cervical malignancies. Heck et al., [31] has also found correlation among tonsillar cancers, number of oral sex partners, and earlier age at sexual debut. At the same study, another subtype of HNSCC (Cancer of the Base of the Tongue) was associated with sexual behavior; it was related with oral sex among women, number of sexual partners, and among men presenting history of same-sex sexual contact.

The sexual behavior has been associated with oral HPV-infection. Univariate analysis showed that oral HPV-infection was significantly increased with the lifetime number of oral/vaginal sex partners. Multivariate analysis demonstrated that oral HPV-infection was significantly elevated among individuals who reported having either 10 oral or 25 vaginal sex partners during their life [35]. In addition, a curious fact was demonstrated: the open-mouthed kissing was associated with oral HPV-infections and could contribute to HPV-infection among individuals who might not otherwise be exposed. To summarize, all these findings suggests that HPV- infection sexually transmitted could play an important role in HNSCC carcinogenesis [35].

5. Oral premalignant lesions

The transformation of normal oral mucosa in OSCC entities can be linked to the emergence of Pre-Cancerous lesion [36]. This association with several oral mucosa disorders such as oral leukoplakia, oral erythroplakia, oral lichen planus, nicotine stomatitis, tobacco pouch keratosis and oral submucous fibrosis (Table1) could be seen. However, that kind of disorders presents a varied spectrum of malignant transformation potential [37]. Reviewing the clinical features of oral Pre-Cancerous lesions and OSCC, the literature emphatically agrees that the early detection is the most important strategy for diagnosis and prevention of OSCC [37]. Applying this diagnosis strategy the OSCC-patients reduces the treatment in advanced stages, thereby increasing the chances of cure [36]. One of the extensive efforts in the clinical management of patients diagnosed with Pre-Cancerous lesions is to delineate clinical outcome, since it is difficult to separate lesions that follow a benign transformation from the entities that are predisposed to malignant course [38]. However, can be observed only a subset of Pre-Cancerous lesions following the malignant course blowing in OSCC.

Disease Name	Malignant Potential
Proliferative Verrucous Leukoplakia (PVl)	6
Nicotine Palatinus in Reverse Smokers	5
Erythroplakia	5
Oral Submucous Fibrosis	5
Erythroleukoplakia	4
Granular Leukoplakia	4
Laryngeal Keratosis	3
Actinic Cheilosis	3
Smooth. Thick leukoplakia	2
Smooth. Red Tongue of Plummer-Vinson Syndrome	2
Smokeless Tobacco Keratosis	1
Lichen Planus (erosive forms)	1
Smooth Thin Leukoplakia	+/-

Table 1. Malignant transformation Potential of *Precancerous Lesions* (adapted from Neville et al. 2009).

The role of HPV in cancer has been exhausted discuss during the recent years. However, HPV in Pre-Cancerous lesions malignant transformation remains under study. Currently, some of the most studied Pre-Cancerous lesions in the literature are: Oral leukoplakia, Oral erythro-plakia, Oral lichen planus Oral submucous fibrosis and Smokeless tobacco keratosis. Aimed to understand the malignant potential of theses lesions some author have attempted to relate the disorder progression with HPV malignant mechanism. Even so, the complete knowledge of viral infection and malignant transformation still remains obscure and controversial.

5.1. Oral leukoplakia and HPV

Oral leukoplakia (OL) is considered an uncommon potentially malignant lesion of the oral mucosa. In 1978, Kramer and colleagues defined Oral leukoplakia as "a white patch or plaque that cannot be characterized clinically or histopathologically, as any other disease" [39]. Observing only oral Pre-Cancerous Lesions, OL is the most frequent potentially malignant lesion of this mucosa, represents 85% of oral Pre-Cancerous Lesions presenting a predilection to male gender [40-42]. However, additional reports found no differences among gender [43]. OL affects 3% of white adults [42] with age distribution in the developed countries between the fourth and seventh decades of life, whilst in the developing countries might occur up to 5-10 years earlier [41].

Clinically, OL can be separated in homogeneous and non-homogeneous leukoplakias entities. The first group (homogeneous) was classified into flat, corrugated, wrinkled and pumice-like, and the latter group of leukoplakias (non-homogeneous) was classified into verrucous, nodular, ulcerated and erythroleukoplakia. The authors has also describes that a non-homo-geneous leukoplakias presents an increased malignant potential when compared to homoge-neous entities [44]. OL can be microscopically characterized by a hyperkeratosis of squamous epithelium. This hyperkeratosis consists of hyperparakeratosis or hyperorthokeratosis; however, a combination between hyperparakeratosis and hyperorthokeratosis also can be seen. In spite of hyperkeratosis, the underlying epithelium layer can show atrophy or thinning. However, spinous layer can presents acanthosis process and the subjacent connective tissue can present a chronic inflammatory infiltrate, ranging from spread foci of inflammatory cells presented in smooth leukoplakia to the numerous foci observed on speckled leukoplakia [42].

Through the years, OL increases the tendency to malignant transformation [45]. The causes of OL remain unclear, in spite of that tobacco intake is considered the most common risk factor for oral leukoplakia development [41-42]. This relation seems to be universal; it appears both in the developing and developed world [41,46]. HPV-infection was well established as etiologic factor of almost 100% of cervical malignancies [6]. Through this establishment, several studies have addressed to find presence and prevalence of HPV-infection in different tumor sites. In the oral cavity, benign lesions have been associated with 24 types of HPV (1, 2, 3, 4, 6, 7, 10, 11, 13, 16, 18, 30, 31, 32, 33, 35, 45, 52, 55, 57, 59, 69, 72 and 73) and malignant entities have been associated with HPV types 2, 3, 6, 11, 13, 16, 18, 31, 33, 35, 52 and 57 [47-48].

Presence of HPV-DNA was more frequent in pre-cancerous lesions and OSCC when compared with control samples. However, only pre-cancerous lesions reach a statistical significance (P =0.0216) [49]. Comparing OSCC and control samples with pre-cancerous lesions pre-cancerous lesions the authors also found a significant prevalence of Low- risk HPV in pre-cancerous lesions. Significant prevalence of Low-risk HPV in pre-cancerous lesions has also observed by Miller & Johnstone [1] meta-analysis. They reported that low-risk HPV DNA was more prevalent in OL and; on the contrary, observed that high-risk HPVs was 2.8 times more frequent in OSCC.

The presence of HPV has been analyzed in potentially malignant lesions, and HPV DNA has been found in different proportions. Sugiyama et al. [50] detected HPV-16 and -18 in normal, dysplastic, and malignant oral epithelium and found statistical significance between the HPV-16 detection in epithelial dysplasia group and OSCC group. A study comparing normal oral mucosa, OL and OSCC was coordinated by Llamas-Martinez et al. [51], aiming to determinate the HPV genome as an independent clinicopathological factor and detect different HPV-genotypes. The data do not show relationship between HPV-genotypes and clinicopathological factors. However, the presence of HPV-16 was increased in OL and OSCC (14/35 cases 40%, 11/33 cases 33.3% (p=0,0005); respectively). These results suggest that HPV-16 is related with OL and OSCC pathogenesis. Campisi et al. [52] investigating the relation among High-Risk HPV infection, apoptosis (bcl-2 and survivin) and proliferation biomarkers (PCNA) observed HPV-DNA in 38.1% of samples. HPV infection was associated with survivin and PCNA suggesting the interference of HPV on epithelial maturation. A year before, Lo Muzio et al. [53] showed increased rates of HPV-positive OL related with a survivin expression and suggested an unfavorable clinical outcome to these lesions. This unfavorable behavior was induced by influence of survivin on apoptosis process.

In conclusion, the correlation between OL malignant transformation and HPV infection were not totally understood. However, these data suggests that HPV-infection could play an important role in oral carcinogenesis leading to OL malignant transformation.

5.2. Oral erythroplakia and HPV

The expression 'erythroplasia' initially was used to describe a reddish precancerous lesion that develops on the glans of penis [55]. Due to clinical and histopathological similarities with genital process, the reddish precancerous oral lesion has also named erythroplakia. The *Oral erythroplakia* (OE) is presented like an unknown-causes lesion. However, it is assumed the same association with OSCC [42]. The authors has also describes that OE presents an increased malignant potential when compared with others pre-cancerous entities [42,55], Older men are predominantly affected by OE with peak prevalence in the sixth decade of life (65 to 74 years). Floor of mouth, tongue, and soft palate are the most common sites of involvement [42].

Clinically, OE may be associated with leukoplakia (erythroleukoplakia) and OSCC [56]. Usually, the lesions do not present symptoms but, is not uncommon some patients reporting a burning sensation and / or sore. The altered mucosa can present a well-demarcated erythematous macule or plaque with a soft, velvety texture [55]. Microscopically, reddish color of erythroplakia can be explained by a combination of features. Red color is presented by underlying microvasculature, and additionally, this color can be due to low keratinization and epithelial thinness [42]. Generally, OE can be associated to severe epithelial dysplasia and, at the time of biopsy, may presents 'carcinoma in situ' or 'invasive carcinoma' [55].

Information about the role of HPV infection in OE is limited. Reichart & Philipsen (2004) discussed the role of hpv infection in OE together with p53 alterations [56]. Nielsen et al. [57] immunohistochemically detected hpv-infection (by situ hybridisation and PCR) in potentially malignant oral lesions. Fifty percent of OE studied cases were HPV-positive. The authors suggest that HPV may be an etiologic co-factor involved in development of oral cancer. However, we can not assume that HPV is the major etiologic factor involved in malignant transformation of OE

5.3. Oral lichen planus and HPV

In 1869, Dr. Erasmus Wilson provided the first medical report about the chronic derrnatologic disorder *lichen planus*. The British physician appointed the disorder *"lichen planus"* because the skin lesions appear to be quite similar to the symbiotic algae and fungi relationship (*lichen*) [42]. *Oral lichen planus* (OLP) is a chronic mucocutaneous disorder presenting a potentially prema-lignant behavior. However, less than 1% of OLP progress to malignancy state [58]. This injury is most common in middle-aged adults within preponderance for female gender (3:2 ratio) [42]. Mattila et al. [58] characterized the OLP in 6 variants: reticular, papular, plaque-type, atrophic, erosive and bullous. Clinically, Neville et al. [42] mentioned reticular and erosive forms as the most common variants presented in the oral mucosa. Although, not common as reticular and erosive, the bullous form was considered a rare oral disorder [59]. Three most common oral mucosa sites involved in OLP are: buccal mucosa, gingivae and lateral borders of the tongue. Additionally, its can be originated in any site of oral mucosa and frequently, is seen as bilateral lesions [59].

Microscopically, the OLP is presented like a non-specific lesion. Moreover, some oral disorders may also demonstrate a similar histopathologic pattern to the OLP-lesions. The injured epithelium may present orthokeratosis and parakeratosis. A spinous cells layer thickness can be observed in different degrees. The rete ridges may be presented as a classically "saw toothed" shape. Due to hydropic degeneration is evident a destruction of the epithelium basal cell layer and, subjacent to epithelium an intense T lymphocytes band-like infiltrate can be observed [42].

Some authors attempt to elucidate the correlation between HPV-infection and malignant transformation of OLP; however, results from pertinent literature are conflicting. The High-risk HPV-16 was described in 26.3% of OLP, with significant statistical difference between High-risk HPV-16 prevalence and OLP when compared to control samples [60]. A study performed by Sand et al. [61] demonstrated the High-Risk HPV-18 in approximately 27% of lichen planus cases but do not found statistical difference between HPV infection and oral lesions suggesting the unclear pathologic correlation between HPV and OLP. On the other hand, Campisi et al. [62] demonstrated the presence of HPV-DNA in 19.7% (n = 14/71) of patients with OLP, with significant statistical difference in comparison with controls cases (5/90; 5.6%) (P = 0.005). In the present study, the High-risk HPV-18 was the most frequent genotype found, it was present in 71.4% (10/14) of samples. In a second analysis, all of cases were pooled in 2 clinical groups: (1) atrophic-erosive (AE) (atrophic, erosive, bullous, and mixed AE variants); and (2) nonatrophic-erosive (non-AE) (reticular, plaque-like, popular, and mixed non-AE variants) to evaluate the association between OLP variants and HPV-infection. However, this analysis failed to find particular correlation between OLP variants and HPV-infection. Analyzing 82 patients diagnosed with atrophic OLP, Mattila et al. [58] found that HPV-infection was present in 15,9% of lesions and was related with High-risk HPV-16. In addition, the HPV-positive cases presented a higher proliferation index and overexpression of Topoisomerase IIa (protein responsible for removal of DNA positive supercoils) in supra-basal layers in comparison with HPV-negative cases.

Ostwald et al. [63] studying prevalence and influence of Low-risk Hpv 6/11 and high-risk Hpv16/18 in benign oral lesions and OSCC detected the HPV-infection in 15.4% of OLP cases. Low-risk HPV presented the higher prevalence in OLP, whereas the High-Risk HPV presented the higher prevalence in OSCC. These interesting results demonstrated that High-risk HPV infection was successively increased from low-level premalignant lesion to OSCC, suggesting a correlation between High-Risk HPV and malignant potential [64]. The conflicting results of studies involving HPV-infection and malignant transformation of OLP lesions may occur due to differences in sample size of patients, associated comorbidities, and other external factors.

5.4. Oral submucous fibrosis and HPV

The name *"Oral submucous fibrosis"* (OSF) was firstly presented by Joshi in 1953; however, Schwartz had described this condition in five cases originated from Kenya, a year before, as *'atropica idiopathica mucosae oris'* [65]. OSF is frequently found in South Asian and South-East Asian patients (India, Bangladesh, Sri Lanka, Pakistan, Taiwan, Southern China) aged of 20–40 years [63]. This potentially malignant disorder has been close related to chronic consumption of Betel quid and Paan [42].

Microscopically, OSF can be characterized by the submucosal deposition of connective tissue. This deposition is extremely dense and presents a reduced vascular tissue. In early-stage lesion, sub-epithelial vesicles can be observed. On the other hand, the older-stage lesion presents epithelial atrophy with hyperkeratosis. In conjunction with these epithelial changes, 10% to 15% of biopsied tissues present epithelial dysplasia [42].

Although, OSF presents a multifactorial etiology, Betel quid and Paan consumption are considered the major causative agents. In pertinent literature only four studies evaluating the HPV and OSF were found: two studies evaluating an Indian population; one study analyzing differences between HPV-infection prevalence in OCSS and pre-malignant lesion; one study comparing two different HPV detection methods). Study performed by Luo et al. [49] presented only two cases of OSF infected by HPV-virion. Although, the lesions had been positive for HPV-infection was not possible to perform other conclusions, because this study used a small number of cases. Chaudhary et al. [66], comparing two HPV-detection methods identified around of 27% (total of 208 cases) of OSF patients' positive for HPV-infection. These two reports do not allow us to establish any positive correlation between HPV-infection and malignant transformation. In addition, evaluation of a hundred thirteen cases of OSF, designed by Mehrotra et al. [67], to assess the relationship of human papilloma virus infection and OSF showed no significant correlation between these two entities. Although, the hpv-infection do not show association with OSF an Indian population study, investigating the prevalence of

HPV-16 in OSF and OSCC cases, found a 91% prevalence of HPV-DNA in OSF and speculated that epithelium lesions in OSF could be an important factor to integration of HPV in basal cells genome (Jaloull et al. [68]. In conclusion, these studies do not have strength to sustain the idea that HPV has an important role in the malignant transformation of OSF.

5.5. Smokeless tobacco keratosis and HPV

Several oral manifestations have been associated to use of *Smokeless Tobacco*. Oral manifestations occur at the site of Smokeless Tobacco placement including mucosal lesions (Smokeless Tobacco Keratosis "STK") and gingival-periodontal disorders such as gingival recession, gingival inflammation, changes in gingival blood flow and interproximal periodontal attachment loss [69]. The use of *Smokeless Tobacco* and the STK has been suggested to be involved in development of oral cancers [70].

Clinically, the site of Smokeless Tobacco placement presents a leukoplakic lesion referred as "snuff dippers" lesions [71] STK presents a non-specific histopathologic appearance [42]. Squamous epithelium is hyper keratinized [42,70] and acanthotic; in addition, the intra-cellular edema is not uncommon on superficial cells glycogen-rich. In some cases, subjacent connective tissue can present an amorphous eosinophilic material. An increased sub-epithelial vascularity and vessel engorgement also can be seen. [42]. In STK the epithelial dysplasia does not common. In a study conducted by Leopardi et al. [72] they not evidenced cases of epithelial dysplasia. However, when present, epithelial dysplasia is usually mild [42]. Studies on STK pointed to three clinical grades [73].

Studies on smokeless tobacco keratosis pointed to three clinical grades: 1) Grade I superficial lesions presenting modest wrinkling and no mucosal thickening. Grade I lesions tends to present similar color to the surrounding mucosa. 2) Grade II superficial whitish lesions with undulating areas displaying moderate wrinkling and no mucosal thickening. 3) Grade III white entities with normal mucosal color areas, STK Grade III shows mucosal thickening and wrinkling [71]. However, this lesion is reversible when the product is discontinued [42]. Related to HPV a work aimed to detect p16 (INK4a) protein expression in smokeless tobacco keratosis as reliable precancerous marker. The author detected HPV-DNA in 15 of 62 (24%) cases and an apparent relation between the three standard grades of STK lesions and HPV-infection was observed. [71]

6. Malignant oral lesions and HPV

In the oral cavity, 24 types of HPV (1, 2, 3, 4, 6, 7, 10, 11, 13, 16, 18, 30, 31, 32, 33, 35, 45, 52, 55, 57, 59, 69, 72 and 73) have been associated with benign lesions and 12 types (2, 3, 6, 11, 13, 16, 18, 31, 33, 35, 52 and 57) with malignant lesions [47-48]. Since the first report of the presence of HPV DNA in head and neck cancer, 65 high-risk types have been consistently detected at different sites; however, these types are specifically found in transcriptionally active tumor cells [74]. According to data from a review, 99% of HPV-infections in head and neck cancers are by high-risk types 16, 18, 31 and 33 [75]. Infection with HPV 33 accounts for up to 10% of positive head and neck cancers; however, the HPV 16 type is by far the most common subtype detected in head and neck cancer ([75-77], and also, oropharyngeal cancer (OPC) is more likely to have HPV 16 than other types at head and neck sites. Just to demonstrate the high levels of HPV-16 genotype in OPC, this genotype accounts for 78% to 100% of positive cases, while HPV-18 accounts for only 1% of cases [75]. An interesting prevalence profile of the HPV types has been observed in some investigations in the countryside of Sao Paulo state in Brazil, where a higher prevalence of HPV 18 than HPV 16 was found in oral and cervical carcinomas. Furthermore, the presence of HPV 18 was found to be associated with metastasis to the lymph nodes and shorter patient survival [78-80].

Several HNSCC have been analyzed for the presence of HPV, and HPV-DNA has been found in different proportions of tumors from different head and neck sites [75,81]. Some evidence has indicated that some subtypes of HPV are specifically linked to head and neck cancer, especially those arising from specific oropharyngeal subsites (e.g., tonsil and the base of the tongue) [82]. The HPV prevalence in HNSCC ranges from 3% to 40% and could vary more according to the specific site and HPV has been found in 4-80% of oral squamous cell carcinoma. Brazilian observations in the countryside of São Paulo state have found a low prevalence of HPV in tumors of the larynx [83] and an increase in the presence of HPV-DNA in oral cavity cancers during the past two decades [79-80,84]. The wide variation in HPV prevalence can be attributed to different detection techniques, small sample numbers, differences in the lesions and sampling techniques and epidemiological characteristics of the populations studied [85]. Among the many methods to detect HPV infections, both polymerase chain reaction (PCR) and in situ hybridization assays have been well validated, although not perfect.

In terms of incidence, it is now believed that HPV-infection could be responsible for approximately 20% of oral cancers and 60-80% of OPC. Recently, in 2011, International Agency of Research of Cancer (IARC) declared that there is sufficient evidence that HPV-16 is causally associated with oral cancer cases [86]. More important, these HPV-related oral cancers are now considered to be completely different entities, differing remarkably from HPV-negative tumors in their clinical response and overall survival [76,87].

Currently, the identification of distinct epidemiological profiles in HPV-positive and HPV-negative HNSCCs is possible. The main factors studied are heavy or no tobacco/marijuana exposure, heavy or mild alcohol consumption, poor or intact dentition, low or high oral sex exposure, age > 50 years or < 45 years, lower or higher socioeconomic status and deceasing or increasing incidence [82]. The epidemiological trend suggests that HPV-positive HNSCC occurs more often in younger patients (age < 50 years), which differs from the typical characteristics of head and neck cancer (which is more frequent in men above 40 years old). Tumors that show association with the presence of HPV usually appears strawberry-like and exophytic lesions on gross inspection and occur more frequently in the tonsil and the base of tongue with a basaloid aspect, poor differentiation and cystic changes within metastatic lymph nodes [82]. In addition, gene expression profiles are known to be different in HPV- positive OPCs compared with HPV-negative cases [88].

Molecular evidences have shown that HPV-associated oral tumors differ significantly from the classic "tobacco and alcohol"-associated oral tumors. First, HPV-positive HNSCCs harbor wild type p53, while classical HNSCC have usually a mutated form of the protein, in accordance with the expected better development of HPV-associated lesions. Indeed, among HPV-positive tumors, the worst outcome is related to smoking, showing evidence that tobacco-derived carcinogens could potentiate the transformation effect of HPV [89-90]. But p53 status in HPV-related tumors, especially those presenting HPV-16 infection led to a confusion involving HPV detection methods and even HPV-related carcinogenesis itself. Initially, it was expected that HPV-16 positive tumors to have a predominantly mutated p53 status, given that HPV-16 E6 inactivates p53, and therefore, mutations in TP53 would be, and indeed are rarely present in cervical carcinomas. But in HNSCC, TP53 is mutated in 60-80% of all cases, and it was expected that HPV-infected tumors would be among the 20-40% of wild-type TP53, although this is not what was found in HNSCC. These findings highlighted the importance of the detection method of HPV infections. For example, the HPV DNA PCR assay is too sensitive, since it detects only a few copies of viral DNA, and may detect more than oncogenic infections, but also productive infections, laboratory artefacts and virions [91]. The following additional techniques can also provide data regarding the presence of HPV: light and electron microscopy, ELISA, gene expression by DNA microarray, Dot blot, Southern blot, hybrid capture and ligase chain reaction for probe amplification. Due to the existence of numerous options for HPV detection in HNSCC, a standardization of procedures for routine application has yet to be developed [77,85]. Among other important pathways in HPV-induced HNSCC are: (1) p53 and pRb pathways, involved in cell cycling; (2) EGFR pathway, which are an important therapeutical target in other cancers (as breast and lung cancers); (3) TGFβ pathway; (4) PI3K-PTEN-AKT pathway and (5) angiogenesis and hypoxia pathways [91].

Aimed to investigate the HPV frequency in Brazilian patients diagnosed with OSCC we performed a study to establish the HPV clinicopathological profile and its possible influence on prognosis of disease [84]. HPV expression in primary tumors (PTs), and their matched samples (MSs) of recidives, lymph nodal metastasis (LNM) or necropsies were correlated with survival of patients. Through polymerase chain reaction using one general and two type-specific HPV primers, 87 PTs and their corresponding MSs were tested. As first step, HPV-DNA detection was performed, using a GP5+/GP6+ primer (Bioneer Inc.) to amplify a 150-bp fragment from L1 gene of general HPV types (GP5+, 5'-TTTGTT ACTGTGGT AGA T ACT AC-3'; GP6+, 5'- GAAAAATAAACTGTAAATCATATTC-3'). At second step, PCR reaction was performed on HPV-positive DNA samples to determine if contained the genotypes -16 and -18, using specific primers targeting ~100 bp in the E7 ORF: HPV-16E7.667 (5'- GAT-GAAATAGATGGTCCAGC-3'), HPV-16E7.774 (5'-GCTTTGTACGCACAACCGAAGC- 3'), HPV-18E7.696 (5'-AAGAAAACGATGAAATAGATGGA-3') and HPV-18E7.799 (5'-GGCTTCACACTTACAACACA-3') (Bioneer Inc.). All of 87 OSCC patients analyzed, 17 (19.5%) presented tumors HPV-DNA positive. Analyses of all paraffin-embedded samples (87 primary tumors plus 87 matched samples) revealed the presence of HPV-DNA in 18 of 174 samples (10.4%), 10 samples (11.5%) from PTs, and 8 samples (9.2%) from MSs. In addition, no virus infection was detected in 7 (8.1%) MSs samples, and only one patient has demonstrated HPV-DNA positivity in both samples. HPV genotypes -16 and -18 were detected in 4 (22.2%) and 3 (16.7%) of the positive samples, respectively. Infection with both genotypes was found in 6 (33.3%) investigated samples, and HPV genotype was not identified in 5 (27.8%)

samples. The most prevalent infected anatomical site was the tongue. The main result of the present study was the significant number of positive HPV samples among non-smoking patients and although, a possible influence of HPV infection on carcinogenesis cannot be ruled out, the low frequency of HPV-positive OSCC cases found in our analysis leads us to suggest that this virus has not the same etiological influence on patients, as tobacco consumption does. Although we cannot to exclude a possible transient role for HPV in the OSCC induction, we believe that occasional detection of HPV-infection in OSCC resulting from the incidental colonization of tumoral lesions might reflect the true correlation of HPV in most analysis. [84].

7. HPV — Prognosis and treatment

In last decades no significant improvement of overall survival has been observed in patients with HNSCCs. It is believed that loco-regional recurrences, distant metastases and a second primary tumor are factors for this phenomenon [91]. Several studies have now established that head and neck HPV-positive tumors have better prognoses [76,88] and treatment-response rates when compared with HPV-negative tumors [88]. In a study comparing tumors in the same stage Leemans et al., [91] observed favorable prognoses after treatment of HPV-infected HNSCCs as compared to HPV-negative tumors. Univariate analyses for 5-year survival rate have pointed that HPV-positive patients surviving longer than HPV-negative patients ($p <$ 0.05); the 5-year survival rate was 54% for HPV-positive versus 33% for HPV-negative tumors [92]. In addition, a study performed by Fakhry et al. [76] evaluating the correlation between HPV infection and survival rate suggested that HPV-positive HNSCC have a significantly better survival (5-year survival of approximately 70%) when compared with HPV-negative patients (5-year survival of approximately 35%). Dayyani et al. [87] published a Meta-analysis, analyzing the impact of human papillomavirus (HPV) on head and neck squamous cell carcinomas, described that patients HPV-positive presented increased risk for HNSCC (adjusted OR = 1.83; 95% CI = 1.04-2.62; $p < 0.0001$). However, survival rate was improved in HPV-positive patients when compared to HPV-negative patients (HR = 0.42; 95% CI = 0.27-0.56, $p < 0.0001$). In other example, evaluation of prognosis and response rates to chemotherapy of oropharyngeal or laryngeal carcinomas showed that HPV-positive tumors present a significantly better overall 2-year survival rate than HPV-negative patients (2-year survival rate of HPV-positive tumors 95% (95% CI = 87%-100%), and 2-year survival rate of HPV-negative tumors 62% (95% CI = 49%- 74%)). The same study found that HPV-positive oropharyngeal carcinomas present higher response rates to chemotherapy compared with HPV-negative (82% vs 55%, difference = 27%, 95% CI = 9.3% to 44.7%, P =.01). Additionally, Dayyani et al. [87] described that HPV-positive head and neck squamous cell carcinomas presented an improved response to radiotherapy (non-adjusted OR = 4.07; 95% CI = 1.48-11.18, p = 0.006) and had a better response to chemo-radiation (non- adjusted OR = 2.87; 95% CI = 1.29-6.41, p = 0.01) as compared to HPV-negative head and neck squamous cell carcinomas.

A meta-analysis performed by Ragin & Taioli [93] aimed to analyze the impact of tumor HPV status on survival outcomes showed that patients diagnosed with head and neck squamous cells carcinoma HPV-positive had a lower risk of dying in comparison with HPV-negative tumors (combined HR: 0.85, 95% CI: 0.7–1.0). At the same study, HPV-positive patients had lower risk of disease-failure (recurrence of tumor) as compared to HPV-negative patients (meta HR: 0.62, 95%CI, 0.5–0.8). The evidence for association of OSCC with HPV-infection and its possible role as an oncogenic agent remains controversial. Schwartz et al. (2001) evaluating the HPV-16 influence on survival rate in OSCC demonstrated that patient's HPV-16 positive presented significantly reduced disease-specific mortality in OSCC (HR = 0.17, 95% CI = 0.04, 0.76) when compared with HPV-16 negative patients. This result suggests the HPV-16 infection could be associated with a favorable prognosis in OSCC. However, the mechanism responsible for this improved prognosis conferred by HPV is still unclear [94].

Several hypotheses have been proposed to explain the improved prognosis in tumors HPV-positive. The benefit on survival rate has been attributed to an enhanced radiosensitivity of tumors HPV-positive [95-96], and an improvement of apoptotic secondary response to the presence of unmutated p53 in HPV-associated tumors [95,97]. The improvement of disease-specific survival rate could be associated with a reduction risk of second primary tumor, since these HPV-positive patients tend to have no prior history of tobacco and/or high alcohol consumption [95]. This finding reduces the field cancerization process (upper respiratory epithelium repeatedly exposed to carcinogens) [98].

8. HPV vaccines (Therapeutic and prophylactic)

Several epithelial lesions are originated by infection with human papillomaviruses (HPVs), mainly benign hyperplasia with low malignant potential like warts or papillomas. However, there is a subgroup of HPVs that are associated with precancerous lesions, which could become a cancer in a small fraction of people [99]. As example of those high-risk HPV subtypes, HPV 16 and 18 [100] are responsible for approximately 70% of cervical cancer cases and are present in more than 60% of HPV-infected penile cancer and HPV-16 is the genotype most frequently detected in head and neck carcinomas, found in up to 90% of HPV-positive cases [99]. Other high-risk HPV types account for virtually all of the remaining cases of cervical cancer, although in other primary sites they do not appear to have a similarly important role [101]. Therefore, cancer of the uterine cervix is most widely accepted malignancy as being associated with HPV infection. HPV high-risk subtypes are also associated with some others anogenital carcinomas, including penile, anal and vulvar cancers [102-103] and a subset of head-and-neck squamous cell carcinomas [104].

Taken together, these findings supports in several countries, vaccination against some HPV types on girls and young women with the goal of protecting them against HPV-induced cervical cancer [105-106]. Trials with vaccines against cervical cancer shown that cross-protection is possible, because this vaccines also have the potential to prevent other cancers that are caused by the same types of HPV, including some of head and neck cancers [107], and the most of anogenital cancers outside the cervix, including cancer of the vulva, vagina, penis, and anus [108-109]. In theory, these vaccines should target the same viruses at other anatomical sites, as head and neck. This approach could provide important information about the final proof of HPV etiology in these tumors [110].

Prophylactic vaccines work primarily by inactivating HPV before the virus infects the host cells, stimulating humoral immunity [111]. Nowadays, there are two types of prophylactic HPV vaccine available in United States: the quadrivalent vaccine (Gardasil®) and bivalent vaccine (Cervarix®). The quadrivalent vaccine was first licensed for use in females to prevent cervical, vaginal and vulvar cancers and are effective against infection with HPV types 6, 11, 16 and 18 [112]. In 2009 the licensure was expanded to include males demonstrating effectiveness to prevent genital warts in both genders [113]. Bivalent vaccine was licensed for use in the U.S. in 2009 providing cervical cancers protection against HPV types 16 and 18 [114]. The impact of HPV prophylactic vaccination will address not only the incidence of cervical and anogenital cancers in women and men but also the incidence of some head and neck tumors. Growing number of head and neck cancers HPV-positive highlights the importance of routine prophylactic vaccination against HPV and, associated with alcohol and tobacco control, may be crucial in head and neck cancer prevention [115].

Also, therapeutic vaccines against HPV have to request cell mediated immunity and can also help prevent the progression of low-grade disease and lead existing lesions to regress, avoiding the recurrence of cancer lesions after treatment [116,117]. However, recent studies demonstrated the reduced effectiveness of therapeutic HPV-vaccine in established tumors. This could be explained by the fact that they have especially been tested in patients with compromised immune systems due advanced stage cancer [118]. A vaccine that possesses both prophylactic and therapeutic properties could be most effective HPV-vaccine strategy, preventing new and clear established HPV-infections. Additionally, the vaccine could be administered in, sexually inexperienced young individuals or older individuals HPV-infected, beneficiating them [119].

9. Final considerations

In recent decades, controversial results were not being able to provide the real role of HPV infection in OSCC genesis. An interesting fact that supports the controversial role of HPV-infection in OSCC is the highly fluctuating HPV-prevalence in comparison with cervical cancer. It may be due to HPV-detection influenced by: a reduced number of viral-copies, a viral-infection in a particular cell population, biopsy samples and detection methods (numerous methods and protocols for detection). Several details elucidating the relationship between pre-cancerous lesions, OSCC with HPV-infection must to be understood. The genomic detection of HPV-DNA, primarily in Pre-Cancerous lesions, provides stronger support for a viral etiology of HNSCC and OSCC. However the correlation between malignant transformation of Pre-Cancerous lesions and HPV-infection were not completely elucidated. Recently, numerous studies have suggested that HPV-infection could play an important role in oral carcinogenesis through the Oral leukoplakia malignant transformation. Although some synergies between HPV oncogenes and other carcinogens have been hypothesized, some researchers have showed, specifically in oral mucosa, that positive HPV-infection in OSCC might not result from viral infection but rather from an incidental HPV colonization. In addition, targeted therapy for HNSCCs and OSCC currently request an increased number of predictive biomarkers, such as the HPV-infection status and mutation-status of crucial genes, to personalize the treatment for individual patients. However, for a better understanding about real therapeutic implications of HPV-status of tumors on OSCC clinical outcome, the next generation of clinical trials could be significantly improved and standardized in their design. According to exposed in the present issue, and defended by our research group and other authors [36-37], we believe that diagnosis strategy based in early detection in oral Pre-Cancerous lesions and OSCC reduces the treatment at the advanced stage, thereby increasing the cancer cure chances. Our group also believes that the increasing effects of HPV vaccination in several cancers could help to reduce the number of new HNSCC and OSCC cases. Although knowledge of the accurate effects of HPV vaccination on cancer incidence will probably continue for several years, monitoring the current effects of HPV vaccination is crucial, not only in cervical cancer, but also in HNSCC and OSCC.

Author details

Danilo Figueiredo Soave[1*], Mara Rubia Nunes Celes[2], João Paulo Oliveira-Costa[3], Giorgia Gobbi da Silveira[3], Bruna Riedo Zanetti[3], Lucinei Roberto Oliveira[4] and Alfredo Ribeiro-Silva[3]

*Address all correspondence to: dsoave@usp.br

1 Department of Pathology – Ribeirão Preto Medical School – University of Sao Paulo, Brazil

2 Institute of Tropical Pathology and Public Health, Federal University of Goias, Brazil

3 Department of Pathology – Ribeirão Preto Medical School – University of Sao Paulo, Brazil

4 Department of Pathology – Vale do Rio Verde University, Brazil

References

[1] Miller CS, Johnstone BM. Human papillomavirus as a risk factor for oral squamous cell carcinomas: a meta-analysis 1982–1997. Oral Surg Oral Med Oral Pathol Oral Radiol Endod 2001 91:622–635

[2] Onon TS. History of human papillomavirus, warts and cancer: what do we know to-day? Best Pract Res Clin Obstet Gynaecol. 2011 Oct;25(5):565-74. Epub 2011 Jun 25.

[3] McCaffery M. Autopsy of a mummy - warts and all. . Can Fam Physician. 1974 Sep; 20(9):89-91.

[4] zur Hausen H. Papillomaviruses in the causation of human cancers - a brief historical account. Virology. 2009 Feb 20;384(2):260-5. Epub 2009 Jan 8.

[5] zur Hausen H, Gissmann L, Steiner W, Dippold W, Dreger I. Human papilloma vi-
     ruses and cancer. Bibl Haematol. 1975 Oct;(43):569-71.

[6] Kumaraswamy, K. L. & Vidhya, M. (2011). Human papilloma virus and oral infec-
     tions: An update. Journal of Cancer Research and Therapeutics, 7, 2, pp. 120-127,
     DOI: 10.4103/0973-1482.82915.

[7] Chang F, Syrjänen S, Kellokoski J, Syrjänen K.Human papillomavirus (HPV) infec-
     tions and their associations with oral disease. J Oral Pathol Med. 1991 Aug;20(7):
     305-17.

[8] Syrjänen KJ, Syrjänen SM, Lamberg MA, Pyrhönen S. Human papillomavirus (HPV)
     involvement in squamous cell lesions of the oral cavity. Proc Finn Dent Soc.
     1983;79(1):1-8.

[9] Syrjänen KJ, Syrjänen SM, Lamberg MA, Happonen RP. Local immunological reac-
     tivity in oral squamous cell lesions of possible HPV (human papillomavirus) origin.
     Arch Geschwulstforsch. 1983;53(6):537-46.

[10] Syrjänen KJ, Pyrhönen S, Syrjänen SM, Lamberg MA. Immunohistochemical demon-
     stration of human papilloma virus (HPV) antigens in oral squamous cell lesions. Br J
     Oral Surg. 1983 Jun;21(2):147-53.

[11] Syrjänen K, Syrjänen S, Lamberg M, Pyrhönen S, Nuutinen J. Morphological and im-
     munohistochemical evidence suggesting human papillomavirus (HPV) involvement
     in oral squamous cell carcinogenesis. Int J Oral Surg. 1983 Dec;12(6):418-24.

[12] Cox MF, Scully C, Maitland N. Viruses in the aetiology of oral carcinoma? Examina-
     tion of the evidence. Br J Oral Maxillofac Surg. 1991 Dec;29(6):381-7.

[13] Lizano, M., Berumen, J., García-Carrancá, A. HPV-related carcinogenesis: basic con-
     cepts, viral types and variants. Archives of medical research, Arch Med Res. 2009
     Aug;40(6):428-34.

[14] Chow, L. T., Broker, T. R., Steinberg, B. M. The natural history of human papilloma-
     virus infections of the mucosal epithelia. APMIS: acta pathologica, microbiologica, et
     immunologica Scandinavica, 2010 Jun;118(6-7):422-49.

[15] de Villiers, E.-M., Fauquet, C., Broker, T. R., Bernard, H.-U., Zur Hausen, H. Classifi-
     cation of papillomaviruses.Virology 2004 Jun 20;324(1):17-27.

[16] Buck, C. B., Cheng, N., Thompson, C. D., Lowy, D. R., Steven, A. C., Schiller, J. T.,
     Trus, B. L. Arrangement of L2 within the papillomavirus capsid. Journal of virology,
     2008 Jun;82(11):5190-7. Epub 2008 Mar 26.

[17] Zur Hausen, H. Papillomaviruses and cancer: from basic studies to clinical applica-
     tion.Nat Rev Cancer, 2002 May;2(5):342-50.

[18] Rautava, J., Syrjänen, S. Biology of human papillomavirus infections in head and
     neck carcinogenesis.Head Neck Pathol. 2012 Jul;6 Suppl 1:3-15. Epub 2012 Jul 3..

[19] Stanley, M. Pathology and epidemiology of HPV infection in females. Gynecol Oncol. 2010 May;117(2 Suppl):S5-10.

[20] Cardoso, J. C., Calonje, E. Cutaneous manifestations of human papillomaviruses: A review. Acta Dermatovenerol Alp Panonica Adriat. 2011 Sep;20(3):145-54.

[21] Lazarczyk, M., Cassonnet, P., Pons, C., Jacob, Y., & Favre, M. The EVER proteins as a natural barrier against papillomaviruses: a new insight into the pathogenesis of human papillomavirus infections.Microbiol Mol Biol Rev. 2009 Jun;73(2):348-70.

[22] Stoler, M. H. Human papillomaviruses and cervical neoplasia: a model for carcinogenesis. International journal of gynecological pathology: official journal of the International Society of Int J Gynecol Pathol. 2000 Jan;19(1):16-28.

[23] Kreimer, A. R., Clifford, G. M., Boyle, P., & Franceschi, S. Human papillomavirus types in head and neck squamous cell carcinomas worldwide: a systematic review. Cancer epidemiology, biomarkers & prevention: a publication of the American Association for Cancer Research, cosponsored by the American Society of Preventive Oncology, 2005 Feb;14(2):467-75.

[24] Miralles-Guri, C., Bruni, L., Cubilla, A L., Castellsagué, X., Bosch, F. X., de Sanjosé, S. Human papillomavirus prevalence and type distribution in penile carcinoma. J Clin Pathol. 2009 Oct;62(10):870-8. Epub 2009 Aug 25.

[25] Doorbar, J. The papillomavirus life cycle. Journal of clinical virology: the official publication of the Pan American Society for Clinical Virology, 2005 Mar;32 Suppl 1:S7-15.

[26] Vidal, L., & Gillison, M. L. Human papillomavirus in HNSCC: recognition of a distinct disease type. Hematology/oncology clinics of North America, 2008 Dec;22(6): 1125-42, vii

[27] Moody CA, Laimins LA. Human papillomavirus oncoproteins: pathways to transformation. Nat Rev Cancer. 2010 Aug;10(8):550-60. Epub 2010 Jul 1.

[28] Bodily, J., Laimins, L. A. Persistence of human papillomavirus infection: keys to malignant progression. Trends in microbiology, 2011 Jan;19(1):33-9. Epub 2010 Nov 1.

[29] Lacour, D. E.,Trimble, C. Human papillomavirus in infants: transmission, prevalence, and persistence. Journal of pediatric and adolescent gynecology, 2012 Apr; 25(2):93-7. Epub 2011 May 20.

[30] Ragin, C.; Edwards, R.; Larkins-Pettigrew, M.; Taioli, E.; Eckstein, S.; Thurman, N.; Bloome, J. & Markovic, N. (2011). Oral HPV Infection and Sexuality: A Cross-Sectional Study in Women. International Journal of Molecular Science, 12, 6, pp. 3928-3940.

[31] Heck, J.E.; Berthiller, J.; Vaccarella, S.; Winn, D.M.; Smith, E.M.; Shan'gina, O.; Schwartz, S.M. et al. Sexual behaviours and the risk of head and neck cancers: a pooled analysis in the International Head and Neck Cancer Epidemiology (IN-

HANCE) consortium. International Journal of Epidemiology 2010. 39, 1, pp. 166–181, DOI:10.1093/ije/dyp350.

[32] Gillison, M.L.; D'Souza, G.; Westra, W.; Sugar, E.; Xiao, W.; Begum, S. & Viscidi, R. Distinct risk factor profiles for human papillomavirus type 16-positive and human papillomavirus type 16-negative head and neck cancers. Journal of the National Cancer Institute 2008.100, 6, pp. 407–420, DOI: 10.1093/jnci/djn025.

[33] D'Souza, G.; Kreimer, A.R.; Viscidi, R.; Pawlita, M.; Fakhry, C.; Koch, W.M. et al. (2007). Case-control study of human papillomavirus and oropharyngeal cancer. The New England journal of medicine, 356, 19, pp. 1944-1956.

[34] Hemminki K, Dong C, Frisch M. Tonsillar and other upper aerodigestive tract cancers among cervical cancer patients and their husbands. Eur J Cancer Prev 2000; 9:433–7.

[35] D'Souza G, Agrawal Y, Halpern J, Bodison S, Gillison ML. Oral sexual behaviors associated with prevalent oral human papillomavirus infection. J Infect Dis 2009;199:1263–9.

[36] Mishra R. Biomarkers of oral premalignant epithelial lesions for clinical application. Oral Oncol. 2012 Jul;48(7):578-84. Epub 2012 Feb 18.

[37] Neville BW, Day TA. Oral cancer and precancerous lesions. CA Cancer J Clin 2002;52(4):195–215.

[38] William WN Jr. Oral premalignant lesions: any progress with systemic therapies? Curr Opin Oncol. 2012 May;24(3):205-10.

[39] Kramer IRH, Lucas RB, Pindborg JJ, Sobin LH.Definition of leukoplakia and related lesions: an aid to studies on oral pre- cancer. Oral Surg Oral Med Oral Pathol 1978 Oct;46(4): 518-39.

[40] Baric JM, Alman JE, Feldman RS et al. Influence of cigarette, pipe, and cigar smoking, removable partial dentures, and age on oral leukoplakia. Oral Surg Oral Med Oral Pathol 1982 Oct;54(4):424-9.

[41] Napier SS, Speight PM. Natural history of potentially malignant oral lesions and conditions: an overview of the literature. J Oral Pathol Med 2008 Jan;37(1):1-10.

[42] Neville BW., Damm DD., Allen CM., Bouquot JE. Oral & Maxilofacial Pathology. Philadelphia-W.B. Saunders Company; 2009.

[43] Cowan CG, Gregg TA, Napier SS et al. Potentially malignant oral lesions in northern Ireland: a 20-year population- based perspective of malignant transformation. Oral Dis 2001 Jan;7(1):18-24.

[44] Pindborg JJ., Reichart PA., Smith CJ. Histological typing of cancer and precancer of the oral mucosa. Berlim-Springer; 1997

[45] Liu W, Shi LJ, Wu L, Feng JQ, Yang X, Li J, Zhou ZT, Zhang CP.Oral Cancer Development in Patients with Leukoplakia – Clinicopathological Factors Affecting Outcome PLoS One. 2012;7(4):e34773. Epub 2012 Apr 13.

[46] Lim K, Moles DR, Downer MC, Speight PM. Opportunistic screening for oral cancer and precancer in general dental practice: results of a demonstration study. Br Dent J 2003; 194: 497–502.

[47] Bouda, M.; Gorgoulis, V.G.; Kastrinakis, N.G.; Giannoudis, A.; Tsoli, E.; Danassi-Afentaki, D. et al. "High risk" HPV types are frequently detected in potentially malignant and malignant oral lesions, but not in normal oral mucosa. Modern Pathology, 2000 Jun;13(6):644-53.

[48] Kojima, A.; Maeda, H.; Sugita, Y.; Tanaka, S. & Kameyama, Y. (2002). Human papillomavirus type 38 infection in oral squamous cell carcinomas. Oral Oncology, 2002 Sep;38(6):591-6.

[49] Luo CW, Roan CH, Liu CJ. Human papillomaviruses in oral squamous cell carcinoma and pre-cancerous lesions detected by PCR-based gene-chip array. Int J Oral Maxillofac Surg. 2007 Feb;36(2):153-8. Epub 2006 Nov 15.

[50] Sugiyama M, Bhawal UK, Dohmen T, Ono S, Miyauchi M, Ishikawa T. Detection of human papillomavirus-16 and HPV-18 DNA in normal, dysplastic, and malignant oral epithelium. Oral Surg Oral Med Oral Pathol Oral Radiol Endod. 2003 May;95(5): 594-600.

[51] Llamas-Martínez S, Esparza-Gómez G, Campo-Trapero J, Cancela-Rodríguez P, Bascones-Martínez A, Moreno-López LA, García-Núñez JA, Cerero-Lapiedra R. Genotypic determination by PCR-RFLP of human papillomavirus in normal oral mucosa, oral leukoplakia and oral squamous cell carcinoma samples in Madrid (Spain). Anticancer Res. 2008 Nov-Dec;28(6A):3733-41.

[52] Campisi G, Di Fede O, Giovannelli L, Capra G, Greco I, Calvino F, Maria Florena A, Lo Muzio L. Use of fuzzy neural networks in modeling relationships of HPV infection with apoptotic and proliferation markers in potentially malignant oral lesions. Oral Oncol. 2005 Nov;41(10):994-1004. Epub 2005 Aug 29.

[53] Lo Muzio L, Campisi G, Giovannelli L, Ammatuna P, Greco I, Staibano S, Pannone G, De Rosa G, Di Liberto C, D'Angelo M. HPV DNA and survivin expression in epithelial oral carcinogenesis: a relationship? Oral Oncol.2004 Aug;40(7):736-41.

[54] Campisi G, Panzarella V, Giuliani M, Lajolo C, Di Fede O, Falaschini S, Di Liberto C, Scully C, Lo Muzio L. Human papillomavirus: its identity and controversial role in oral oncogenesis, premalignant and malignant lesions (review). Int J Oncol. 2007 Apr;30(4):813-23.

[55] Villa A, Villa C, Abati S. Oral cancer and oral erythroplakia: an update and implication for clinicians. Aust Dent J. 2011 Sep;56(3):253-6. doi: 10.1111/j. 1834-7819.2011.01337.x. Epub 2011 Jul 10.

[56] Reichart PA, Philipsen HP. Oral erythroplakia—a review. Oral Oncol. 2005 Jul;41(6): 551-61. Epub 2005 Apr 9.

[57] Nielsen H, Norrild B, Vedtofte P, Praetorius F, Reibel J, Holmstrup P. Human papillomavirus in oral premalignant lesions. Eur J Cancer B Oral Oncol. 1996 Jul;32B(4): 264-70.

[58] Mattila R, Rautava J, Syrjänen S. Human papillomavirus in oral atrophic lichen planus lesions. Oral Oncol. 2012 Jun 1. [Epub ahead of print]

[59] Epstein JB, Wan LS, Gorsky M, Zhang L. Oral lichen planus: Progress in understanding its malignant potential and the implications for clinical management. Oral Surg Oral Med Oral Pathol Oral Radiol Endod. 2003 Jul;96(1):32-7.

[60] O'Flatharta C, Flint SR, Toner M, Butler D, Mabruk MJ. Investigation into a possible association between oral lichen planus, the human herpesviruses and the human papillomaviruses. Mol Diagn 2003;7:73-83.

[61] Sand L, Jaiouli J, Larsson PA, Hirsch JM. Human papilloma viruses in oral lesions. Anticancer Res. 2000 Mar-Apr;20(2B):1183-8.

[62] Campisi G, Giovannelli L, Aricò P, Lama A, Di Liberto C, Ammatuna P, D'Angelo M. HPV DNA in clinically different variants of oral leukoplakia and lichen planus. Oral Surg Oral Med Oral Pathol Oral Radiol Endod. 2004 Dec;98(6):705-11.

[63] Ostwald C, Rutsatz K, Schweder J, Schmidt W, Gundlach K, Barten M. Human papillomavirus 6/11, 16 and 18 in oral carcinomas and benign oral lesions. Med Microbiol Immunol. 2003 Aug;192(3):145-8. Epub 2002 Nov 1.

[64] Szarka K, Tar I, Fehér E, Gáll T, Kis A, Tóth ED, Boda R, Márton I, Gergely L. Progressive increase of human papillomavirus carriage rates in potentially malignant and malignant oral disorders with increasing malignant potential. Oral Microbiol Immunol. 2009 Aug;24(4):314-8.

[65] More CB, Das S, Patel H, Adalja C, Kamatchi V, Venkatesh R. Proposed clinical classification for oral submucous fibrosis. Oral Oncol. 2012 Mar;48(3):200-2. Epub 2011 Nov 8. Review

[66] Chaudhary AK, Pandya S, Mehrotra R, Bharti AC, Singh M, Singh M. Comparative study between the Hybrid Capture II test and PCR based assay for the detection of human papillomavirus DNA in oral submucous fibrosis and oral squamous cell carcinoma. Virol J. 2010 Sep 23;7:253.

[67] Mehrotra R, Chaudhary AK, Pandya S, Debnath S, Singh M, Singh M. Correlation of addictive factors, human papilloma virus infection and histopathology of oral submucous fibrosis. J Oral Pathol Med. 2010 Jul;39(6):460-4. Epub 2010 Jan 8.

[68] Jalouli J, Ibrahim S, Mehrotra R, Jalouli MM, Sapkota D, Larsson P, Hirsch J. Prevalence of viral (hpv, ebv, hsv) infections in oral submucous fibrosis and oral cancer from India. Acta Otolaryngol. 2010 Nov;130(11):1306-11.

[69] Chu YH, Tatakis DN, Wee AG. Smokeless Tobacco Use and Periodontal Health in a Rural Male Population. J Periodontol. 2010 Jun;81(6):848-54.

[70] Accortt NA, Waterbor JW, Beall C, Howard G. Cancer incidence among a cohort of smokeless tobacco users. Can- cer Causes and Control 2005: 16: 1107– 1115.

[71] Greer RO Jr, Meyers A, Said SM, Shroyer KR. Is p16INK4a protein expression in oral ST lesions a reliable precancerous marker? Int J Oral Maxillofac Surg. 2008 Sep;37(9): 840-6. Epub 2008 Jul 7.

[72] Leopardi EA, Poulson TC, Nieger BL, Lindenmuth JE, Greer RO. Smokeless tobacco usage patterns and male athlete sequellae: A Report of two surveys and associated intervention strategies among Utah adolescents. J Cancer Ed 1989: 4: 125–134.

[73] Greer RO, Poulson TC. Oral changes associated with the use of smokeless tobacco by teenagers. Oral Surg Oral Med Oral Pathol Oral Radiol Endod 1983: 56: 275–284.

[74] Vidal, L. & Gillison, M.L. Human papillomavirus in HNSCC: recognition of a distinct disease type. Hematol Oncol Clin North Am. 2008 Dec;22(6):1125-42, vii. DOI: 10.1016/j.hoc.2008.08.006.

[75] Kreimer, A.R.; Clifford, G.M.; Boyle, P. & Franceschi, S. Human papillomavirus types in head and neck squamous cell carcinomas worldwide: a systematic review. Cancer Epidemiol Biomarkers Prev. 2005 Feb;14(2):467-75. Review. DOI: 10.1158/ 1055-9965.

[76] Fakhry C, Westra WH, Li S, et al. Improved survival of patients with human papillomavirus-positive head and neck squamous cell carcinoma in a prospective clinical trial. J Natl Cancer Inst. 2008;100:261–9.

[77] Snow, A.N. & Laudadio, J. Human Papillomavirus Detection in Head and Neck Squamous Cell Carcinomas. Adv Anat Pathol. 2010 Nov;17(6):394-403. Review. DOI: 10.1097/PAP.0b013e3181f895c1.

[78] Guimarães, M.C.; Soares, C.P.; Donadi, E.A.; Derchain, S.F.; Andrade, L.A.; Silva, T.G. et al. Low Expression of Human Histocompatibility Soluble Leukocyte Antigen-G (HLA-G5) in Invasive Cervical Cancer With and Without Metastasis, Associated With Papilloma Virus (HPV). J Histochem Cytochem. 2010 May;58(5):405-11. Epub 2009 Sep 28.DOI: 10.1369/jhc.2009.954131.

[79] Lira, R.C.; Miranda, F.A.; Guimarães, M.C.; Simões, R.T.; Donadi, E.A.; Soares, C.P. & Soares, E.G. BUBR1 expression in benign oral lesions and squamous cell carcinomas:

Correlation with human papillomavirus. Oncol Rep. 2010 Apr;23(4):1027-36. DOI: 10.3892/or_00000729.

[80] Mazon, R.C.; Gerbelli, T.R.; Neto, C.B.; de Oliveira, M.R.B.; Donadi, E.A.; Goncalves, M.A.G. et al. Abnormal cell-cycle expression of the proteins p27, mdm2 and cathepsin B in oral squamous-cell carcinoma infected with human papillomavirus. Acta Histochem. 2011 Feb;113(2):109-16. Epub 2009 Oct 6. DOI: 10.1016/j.acthis. 2009.08.008.

[81] Syrjänen, S. Human papillomavirus (HPV) in head and neck cancer. J Clin Virol. 2005 Mar;32 Suppl 1:S59-66.DOI: 10.1016/j.jcv.2004.11.017.

[82] Gillespie, M.B.; Rubinchik, S.; Hoel, B. & Sutkowski, N. Human Papillomavirus and Oropharyngeal Cancer: What You Need to Know in 2009. Curr Treat Options Oncol. 2009 Dec;10(5-6):296-307. Epub 2009 Sep 19. DOI: 10.1007/s11864-009-0113-5.

[83] Miranda, F.A.; Hassumi, M.K.; Guimarães, M.C.; Simões, R.T.; Silva, T.G.; Lira, R.C. et al. Galectin-3 Overexpression in Invasive Laryngeal Carcinoma, Assessed by Computer-assisted Analysis. J Histochem Cytochem. 2009 Jul;57(7):665-73. Epub 2009 Mar 30.DOI: 10.1369/jhc.2009.952960.

[84] Oliveira, L.R.; Silva, A.R.; Ramalho, L.N.Z.; Simões, A.L. & Zucoloto, S. HPV infection in Brazilian oral squamous cell carcinoma patients and its correlation with clinicopathological outcomes. Mol Med Report. 2008 Jan-Feb;1(1):123-9.

[85] Feller, L.; Wood, N.H.; Khammissa, R.A. & Lemmer, J. Human papillomavirus-mediated carcinogenesis and HPV-associated oral and oropharyngeal squamous cell carcinoma. Part 2: Human papillomavirus associated oral andoropharyngeal squamous cell carcinoma. Head Face Med. 2010 Jul 15;6:15. DOI: 10.1186/1746- 160X-6-15.

[86] IARC Monographs on the Evaluation of Carcinogenic Risks to Humans. Part B: biological agents LYON, France 2011, Volume 100B pp. 278–80

[87] Dayyani F, Etzel CJ, Liu M, et al. Meta-analysis of the impact of human papillomavirus (HPV) on cancer risk and overall survival in head and neck squamous cell carcinomas (HNSCC). Head Neck Oncol. 2010;2:15. Published online 2010 June 29.

[88] Lajer, C.B. & Von Buchwald, C. The role of human papillomavirus in head and neck cancer. APMIS. 2010 Jun;118(6-7):510-9. Review. DOI: 10.1111/j. 1600-0463.2010.02624.x.

[89] Ang, K.K.; Harris, J.; Wheeler, R.; Weber, R.; Rosenthal, D.I.; Nguyen-Tân, P.F. et al. Human Papillomavirus and Survival of Patients with Oropharyngeal Cancer. N Engl J Med. 2010 Jul 1;363(1):24-35. Epub 2010 Jun 7.DOI: 10.1056/NEJMoa0912217.

[90] Sinha, P.; Logan, H.L. & Mendenhall, W.M. (2011). Human papillomavirus, smoking, and head and neck cancer. Am J Otolaryngol. 2012 Jan-Feb;33(1):130-6. Epub 2011 May 5. Review. DOI: 10.1016/j.amjoto.2011.02.001.

[91] Leemans CR, Braakhuis BJ, Brakenhoff RH. The molecular biology of head and neck cancer. Nat Rev Cancer. 2011;11:9–22. Review

[92] Hannisdal, K.; Schjølberg, A.; De Angelis, P.M.; Boysen, M. & Clausen, O.P. Human papillomavirus (HPV)-positive tonsillar carcinomas are frequent and have a favourable prognosis in males in Norway. Acta Otolaryngol. 2010 Feb;130(2):293-9.

[93] Ragin CC, Taioli E. Survival of squamous cell carcinoma of the head and neck in relation to human papillomavirus infection: review and meta-analysis. Int J Cancer. 2007 Oct 15;121(8):1813-20.

[94] Hennessey, P.T.; Westra, W.H. & Califano, J.A. Human papillomavirus and head and neck squamous cell carcinoma: recent evidence and clinical implications. J Dent Res. 2009 Apr;88(4):300-6.

[95] Gillison ML, Koch WM, Capone RB, Spafford M, Westra WH, Wu L, et al. Evidence for a causal association between human papillomavirus and a subset of head and neck cancers. J Natl Cancer Inst. 2000 May 3;92(9):709-20.

[96] Lindel K, Beer KT, Laissue J, Greiner RH, Aebersold DM. Human papillomavirus positive squamous cell carcinoma of the oropharynx:a radiosensitive subgroup of head and neck carcinoma. Cancer. 2001 Aug 15;92(4):805-13.

[97] Butz K, Geisen C, Ullmann A, Spitkovsky D, Hoppe-Seyler F. Cellular responses of HPV-positive cancer cells to genotoxic anti-cancer agents: repression of E6/E7-oncogene expression and induction of apoptosis. Int J Cancer. 1996 Nov 15;68(4):506-13.

[98] Califano J, van der Riet P, Westra W, Nawroz H, Clayman G, Piantadosi S, et al. Genetic progression model for head and neck cancer: implications for field cancerization. Cancer Res 1996;56:2488–92

[99] Psyrri A, DiMaio D. Human papillomavirus in cervical and head-and-neck cancer. 24 Nat Clin Pract 5: 24-31.

[100] IARC Working Group on the Evaluation of Carcinogenic Risks to Humans (1995) Human papillomaviruses. IARC Monogr Eval Carcinog Risks Hum 64: 1–378.

[101] zur Hausen H. Papillomaviruses and cancer: from basic studies to clinical application. Nat Rev Cancer. 2002 May;2(5):342-50. Review.

[102] Crum CP, McLachlin CM, Tate JE, Mutter GL. Pathobiology of vulvar squamous neoplasia. Curr Opin Obstet Gynecol. 1997 Feb;9(1):63-9.

[103] Kayes O, Ahmed HU, Arya M, Minhas S. Molecular and genetic pathways in penile cancer. Lancet Oncol. 2007 May;8(5):420-9. Review.

[104] Gillison ML, Koch WM, Capone RB, Spafford M, Westra WH, Wu L, Zahurak ML, Daniel RW, Viglione M, Symer DE, Shah KV, Sidransky D. Evidence for a causal association between human papillomavirus and a subset of head and neck cancers. J Natl Cancer Inst. 2000 May 3;92(9):709-20.

[105] Villa, L.L.; Costa, R.L.; Petta, C.A.; Andrade, R.P.; Ault, K.A.; Giuliano, A.R. et al. Prophylactic quadrivalent human papillomavirus (types 6, 11, 16, and 18) L1 virus-like particle vaccine in young women: a randomized double-blind placebo- controlled multicentre phase II efficacy trial. Lancet Oncol. 2005 May;6(5):271-8. DOI: 10.1016/S1470-2045 (05)70101-7.

[106] Muñoz, N.; Kjaer, S.K.; Sigurdsson, K.; Iversen, O.E.; Hernandez-Avila, M.; Wheeler, C.M. et al. Impact of human papillomavirus (HPV)-6/11/16/18 vaccine on all HPV-associated genital diseases in young women. J Natl Cancer Inst. 2010 Mar 3;102(5): 325-39. Epub 2010 Feb 5.DOI: 10.1093/jnci/djp534.

[107] Herrero, R. Human papillomavirus and cancer of the upper aerodigestive tract. J Natl Cancer Inst Monogr. 2003;(31):47-51.

[108] Daling, J.R.; Madeleine, M.M.; Johnson, L.G.; Schwartz, S.M.; Shera, K.A.; Wurscher, M.A. et al. Penile cancer: importance of circumcision, human papillomavirus and smoking in situ and invasive disease. Int J Cancer 2005 Sep 10;116(4):606-16.

[109] Gross, G. & Pfister, H. Role of human papillomavirus in penile cancer, penile intrae-pithelial squamous cell neoplasias and in genital warts. Med Microbiol Immunol. 2004 Feb;193(1):35-44. Epub 2003 Jun 28.

[110] Syrjänen, S. The role of human papillomavirus infection in head and neck cancers. Ann Oncol. 2010 Oct;21 Suppl 7:vii243-5.

[111] Zinkernagel, R.M. On natural and artificial vaccinations. Annu Rev Immunol. 2003;21:515-46. Epub 2001 Dec 19.

[112] U.S. Food and Drug Administration, a. FDA Licenses Quadrivalent Human Papillo-mavirus (Types 6, 11, 16, 18) Recombinant Vaccine (Gardasil) for the Prevention of Cervical Cancer and Other Diseases in Females Caused by Human Papillomavirus [Online]. Available at: http://www.fda.gov/AboutFDA/CentersOffices/CDER/ ucm095647.htm. Accessed May 10, 2011.

[113] Centers for Disease Control and Prevention (CDC), 2010b. FDA licensure of quadri-valent human papillomavirus vaccine (HPV4, Gardasil) for use in males and guid-ance from the Advisory Committee on Immunization Practices (ACIP). MMWR Morb. Mortal. Wkly. Rep. 59, 630–632.

[114] U.S. Food and Drug Administration. FDA News Release: FDA approved new vac-cine for prevention of cervical cancer. [Online]. Available at: http://www.fda.gov/ NewsEvents/ Newsroom/PressAnnouncements/ucm187048.htm. Accessed Novem-ber 30, 2009.

[115] Klozar, J.; Tachezy, R.; Rotnáglová, E.; Koslabová, E.; Saláková, M. & Hamsíková, E. Human papillomavirus in head and neck tumors: epidemiological, molecular and clinical aspects. Wien Med Wochenschr. 2010 Jun;160(11-12):305-9. DOI: 10.1007/ s10354-010-0782-5.

[116] Chu, R.N. Therapeutic vaccination for the treatment of mucosotropic human papillo-
      mavirus-associated disease. Expert Opin Biol Ther. 2003 Jun;3(3):477-86.

[117] Stanley, M. Genital human papillomavirus infections—current and prospective
      therapies. J Natl Cancer Inst Monogr. 2003;(31):117-24. Review.

[118] Brinkman, J.A.; Caffrey, A.S.; Muderspach, L.I.; Roman, L.D. & Kast, W.M. The im-
      pact of anti-HPV vaccination on cervical cancer incidence and HPV-induced cervical
      lesions: consequences for clinical management. Eur J Gynaecol Oncol. 2005;26(2):
      129-42.

[119] Franceschi, S. The International Agency for Research on Cancer (IARC) commitment
      to cancer prevention: the example of papillomavirus and cervical cancer. Recent Re-
      sults Cancer Res. 2005;166:277-97.

Permissions

The contributors of this book come from diverse backgrounds, making this book a truly international effort. This book will bring forth new frontiers with its revolutionizing research information and detailed analysis of the nascent developments around the world.

We would like to thank Prof. Dr. Davy Vanden Broeck, MSc, PhD., for lending his expertise to make the book truly unique. He has played a crucial role in the development of this book. Without his invaluable contribution this book wouldn't have been possible. He has made vital efforts to compile up to date information on the varied aspects of this subject to make this book a valuable addition to the collection of many professionals and students.

This book was conceptualized with the vision of imparting up-to-date information and advanced data in this field. To ensure the same, a matchless editorial board was set up. Every individual on the board went through rigorous rounds of assessment to prove their worth. After which they invested a large part of their time researching and compiling the most relevant data for our readers. Conferences and sessions were held from time to time between the editorial board and the contributing authors to present the data in the most comprehensible form. The editorial team has worked tirelessly to provide valuable and valid information to help people across the globe.

Every chapter published in this book has been scrutinized by our experts. Their significance has been extensively debated. The topics covered herein carry significant findings which will fuel the growth of the discipline. They may even be implemented as practical applications or may be referred to as a beginning point for another development. Chapters in this book were first published by InTech; hereby published with permission under the Creative Commons Attribution License or equivalent.

The editorial board has been involved in producing this book since its inception. They have spent rigorous hours researching and exploring the diverse topics which have resulted in the successful publishing of this book. They have passed on their knowledge of decades through this book. To expedite this challenging task, the publisher supported the team at every step. A small team of assistant editors was also appointed to further simplify the editing procedure and attain best results for the readers.

Our editorial team has been hand-picked from every corner of the world. Their multi-ethnicity adds dynamic inputs to the discussions which result in innovative outcomes. These outcomes are then further discussed with the researchers and contributors who give their valuable feedback and opinion regarding the same. The feedback is then collaborated with the researches and they are edited in a comprehensive manner to aid the understanding of the subject.

Apart from the editorial board, the designing team has also invested a significant amount of their time in understanding the subject and creating the most relevant covers. They scrutinized every image to scout for the most suitable representation of the subject and create an appropriate cover for the book.

The publishing team has been involved in this book since its early stages. They were actively engaged in every process, be it collecting the data, connecting with the contributors or procuring relevant information. The team has been an ardent support to the editorial, designing and production team. Their endless efforts to recruit the best for this project, has resulted in the accomplishment of this book. They are a veteran in the field of academics and their pool of knowledge is as vast as their experience in printing. Their expertise and guidance has proved useful at every step. Their uncompromising quality standards have made this book an exceptional effort. Their encouragement from time to time has been an inspiration for everyone.

The publisher and the editorial board hope that this book will prove to be a valuable piece of knowledge for researchers, students, practitioners and scholars across the globe.

List of Contributors

Angela Adamski da Silva Reis
Federal University of Goiás - Biological Sciences Institute - Department of Biochemistry and Molecular Biology, Brazil

Daniela de Melo e Silva
Federal University of Goiás - Biological Sciences Institute - Department of General Biology, Brazil

Cláudio Carlos da Silva and Aparecido Divino da Cruz
Pontifical Catholic University of Goiás - Department of Medicine and Biology, Brazil

Santiago Melón, Marta Alvarez-Argüelles and María de Oña
Virology Unit (Microbiology Service), Hospital Universitario Central de Asturias (HUCA), Oviedo, Asturias, Spain

Fátima Galán-Sánchez and Manuel Rodríguez-Iglesias
Department of Microbiology, School of Medicine and Clinical Microbiology Laboratory, Puerta del Mar Univ. Hosp. University of Cádiz, Spain

Evanthia Kostopoulou and George Koukoulis
Pathology Department, Faculty of Medicine, University of Thessaly, Greece

Ralf Hilfrich
Cytoimmun Diagnostics GmbH Pirmasens, Germany

Lis Ribeiro-Müller, Hanna Seitz and Martin Müller
German Cancer Research Center (DKFZ), Program Infections and Cancer, Heidelberg, Germany

Miguel Ángel Arrabal-Polo, Jacinto Orgaz-Molina, Sergio Merino-Salas, Fernando Lopez-Carmona Pintado and Miguel Arrabal-Martin
San Cecilio University Hospital, Spain

María Sierra Girón-Prieto
Granada District, Spain

Salvador Arias-Santiago
Baza Hospital, Granada School of Medicine, Spain

Fernando Augusto Soares
AC Camargo Cancer Hospital - Antonio Prudente Cancer Care Center, Brazil

Giórgia Gobbi da Silveira, Danilo Figueiredo Soave, Andrielle de Castilho Fernandes and Alfredo Ribeiro-Silva
Ribeirão Preto Medical School, University of São Paulo, Brazil

Lucinei Roberto Oliveira
Vale do Rio Verde University, Brazil

João Paulo Oliveira-Costa
AC Camargo Cancer Hospital - Antonio Prudente Cancer Care Center, Brazil
Ribeirão Preto Medical School, University of São Paulo, Brazil

Claudie Laprise and Helen Trottier
Department of Social and Preventive Medicine, University of Montreal, Montreal, Sainte-Justine Hospital Research Center, Montreal, Canada

Maria Filippova and Penelope Duerksen-Hughes
Department of Basic Science, Loma Linda University School of Medicine, Loma Linda, CA, USA

Ron Swensen
Department of Gynecology and Obstetrics, Loma Linda University School of Medicine, Loma Linda, CA, USA

Whitney Evans
Department of Basic Science, Loma Linda University School of Medicine, Loma Linda, CA, USA
Center for Health Disparities and Molecular Medicine, Loma Linda University School of Medicine, Loma Linda, CA, USA

Danilo Figueiredo Soave
Department of Pathology – Ribeirão Preto Medical School – University of Sao Paulo, Brazil

Mara Rubia Nunes Celes
Institute of Tropical Pathology and Public Health, Federal University of Goias, Brazil

João Paulo Oliveira-Costa, Giorgia Gobbi da Silveira, Bruna Riedo Zanetti and Alfredo Ribeiro-Silva
Department of Pathology – Ribeirão Preto Medical School – University of Sao Paulo, Brazil

Lucinei Roberto Oliveira
Department of Pathology – Vale do Rio Verde University, Brazil